Manual of Singing Voice Rehabilitation

A Practical Approach to Vocal Health and Wellness

Manual of Singing Voice Rehabilitation

A Practical Approach to Vocal Health and Wellness

Leda Scearce, MM, MS, CCC-SLP

Plural Publishing Inc.

PLURAL PUBLISHING INC.

5521 Ruffin Road
San Diego, CA 92123

e-mail: info@pluralpublishing.com
Website: http://www.pluralpublishing.com

Typeset in 10½/13 Palatino by Flanagan's Publishing Services, Inc.
Printed in the United States of America by McNaughton & Gunn, Inc.

Library of Congress Cataloging-in-Publication Data

Names: Scearce, Leda, author.
Title: Manual of singing voice rehabilitation : a practical approach to vocal health and wellness / Leda Scearce.
Description: San Diego : Plural, [2016] | Includes bibliographical references and index.
Identifiers: LCCN 2015042419 | ISBN 9781597565684 (alk. paper) | ISBN 1597565687 (alk. paper)
Subjects: | MESH: Voice Disorders--rehabilitation. | Singing—physiology.
Classification: LCC RF540 | NLM WV 500 | DDC 616.85/56—dc23
LC record available at http://lccn.loc.gov/2015042419

Contents

Foreword

As we live into the 21st century, our world is a place in constant motion, all time and matter seeming to move faster by the minute. Every aspect of our culture is affected by an exponential rate of change and in no place is that demonstrated more than the field of Western medicine. Extraordinary leaps in scientific research and knowledge coupled with technological developments have paved the way for meaningful, applied advances in the understanding, diagnosis, and treatment of human disease. It is an exciting and challenging time to be involved in any aspect of the medical field.

Voice medicine is one of a growing number of subspecialties that has benefited from this evolutionary process. The past 50 years have seen improvements in care of the voice and treatment of voice disorders that previous generations could not have imagined. Many of these advances can be attributed to meaningful collaborations among the many disciplines involved in voice, including laryngology, speech pathology, voice science, singing, and acting pedagogy in addition to contributions from singers and actors and many others. We have learned that a "team approach" to medical diagnosis and treatment can positively impact treatment outcomes. This has given rise to the role of the singing voice rehabilitation specialist in the field of voice medicine. This area of expertise was originally defined as a singing teacher with specific training to work with injured voices and was commonly referred to as a singing voice specialist.

As more people have become interested in pursuing this path and as demand in medical settings for this particular expertise has grown, it has become imperative that appropriate, standardized, and authorized training protocols be established. This pathway to certification is now being vigorously discussed and pursued. In the meantime, any training program for singing voice rehabilitation is going to require educational materials. Naturally included will be knowledgeable textbooks written by individuals in the field whose unquestionable credentials, vast experience, and peer recognition have solidified their reputations as expert in singing voice rehabilitation. Leda Scearce is just such a person.

Leda is the ideal individual to have written what I believe is the most comprehensive examination, explanation, and overall directive on singing voice rehabilitation to date. As a highly trained and accomplished professional singer, speech therapist, and singing voice rehabilitation clinician, she is in the unique position to understand every element necessary to the development of those wishing to enter this field. In her very thorough book, she has left no stone unturned. Using the most accessible prose, she leads us from a basic history of this nascent profession through chapters covering everything from voice disorders to vocal hygiene and from building a multidisciplinary voice team to the nitty gritty of documentation and session planning. Her extensive passages on vocal pacing were a welcome reminder to me about the need to establish clear guidelines and goals for the patient and to make sure that the patient at all times understands the plan for his or her return to vocal health. The inclusion of chapters by other experts in the field of voice, such as the chapters on vocal apps and sound equipment, provides very current information while also representing the kind of collaborative approach that is needed in all areas of medicine.

This book is written with the understanding that a voice disorder in a singer has enormous emotional-psychological implications for the patient and that to successfully treat the voice of the injured singer, you must treat the whole person. This is a construct that had sadly fallen out of fashion in modern Western medicine and is only now being readdressed in our medical universities. The importance of the book's consistent reference to the compassion we need to show the injured singer cannot be overstated. And yet, Leda balances this point of view with the objectivity necessary to clearly assess a patient's needs and establish an effective treatment plan.

While the target audience for this book may be those who already possess extensive background knowledge in voice anatomy, physiology and neuroanatomy, voice science and acoustics, singing pedagogy, voice disorders, and other areas of voice, this book can be valuable to many others. For individuals with some basic background in voice, it can provide important insight into the knowledge base and skill sets needed to work with injured voices.

As an experienced singing voice specialist, Leda's book has provided me not only with new insights about how to approach common problems I encounter daily in the clinic but also validation for long-held treatment paradigms shared by many of us in voice care.

Manual of Singing Voice Rehabilitation: A Practical Approach to Vocal Health and Wellness is a comprehensive, systematic, and current text for those wishing to better practice the science and art of singing voice rehabilitation. It was written by one of our best clinicians whose singular combination of intellectual integrity, rigorous scholarship, and generous heart and spirit is evident in the message of holistic healing that resounds through this entire work. I can honestly say that this book has inspired me to raise the bar in my daily work and has enabled me to clarify my thinking about many of the questions I face as a voice clinician. Thank you, Leda for your amazing work. We are in your debt for this important contribution to the field.

—Margaret Baroody
Singing Voice Specialist
Philadelphia Ear, Nose and Throat Associates

Acknowledgments

I count myself extremely fortunate to have many teachers, mentors, colleagues, collaborators, students, allies, and friends who, over the years, have shared gifts of knowledge, wisdom, guidance, insight, support, kindness, encouragement, opportunity, and camaraderie. I am thankful for all of them, especially Maya McNeilly, Angus Reuben, Cesare DeLac, Peggy Baroody, Kate McGarry, Don Wilder, Karyn Friedman, Gary Poster, Laurina Uribe, Brenda Smith, Glenn Bunting, Elizabeth Gavett, Mary Klimek, Debra Albrecht, Judith Coffey, Wafaa Carter, Art Jolin, Benee and Lee King, Chris Hvezda, Nancy McMillan, Kathleen Evans, David Witsell, Tara Nixon, Emily Scheuring, Melissa Stark, Karen Stark, Seth Cohen, Gina Vess, Caroline Banka, Hilary Bartholomew, Eileen Raynor, and Ray Esclamado. I am grateful for the gracious contributions of Matthew Edwards, Mirabelle Sajisevi, Alissa Collins, Chad Whited, and Jarrod Keeler and for the special assistance of Erika Juhlin and Gerrit Heinrich.

This book would not be possible without you.

About the Editor

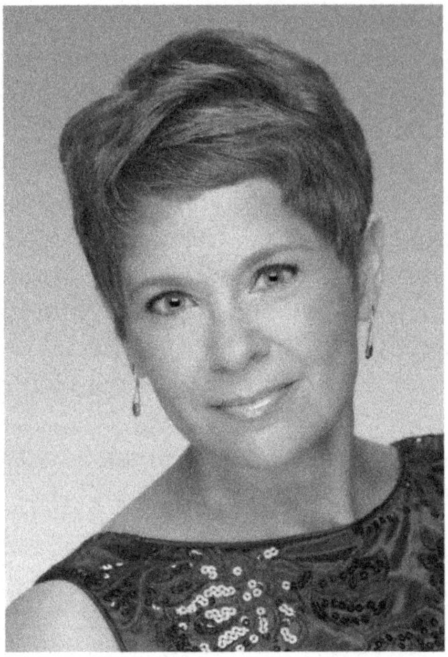

Soprano Leda Scearce has been featured in leading roles with the National Opera Company, Hawaii Opera Theatre, Long Leaf Opera Festival, Triangle Opera, the Ohio Light Opera Company, and Whitewater Opera Company, and has appeared as a concert soloist with orchestras including the North Carolina, Toledo, and Honolulu Symphonies. An active proponent of new music, Ms. Scearce has given world premiere performances of works written for her with the Berkeley Contemporary Chamber Players, Nashville Chamber Orchestra, Orchestra Nashville, Mallarme Chamber Players, the American Chamber Music Festival, and Chamber Music Hawaii. A winner of the Birmingham Opera Vocal Competition, Ms. Scearce has also been a regional finalist in the Metropolitan Opera National Council Auditions. Ms. Scearce is a graduate of Indiana University with both bachelor's and master's degrees in vocal performance. A voice teacher for more than 25 years, Ms. Scearce has served on the artist faculties of Bowling Green State University, Meredith College, Brigham Young University of Hawaii, and the University of Southern Maine.

Ms. Scearce obtained a master of science degree in speech-language pathology from Boston University, where she completed an internship in voice disorders and voice rehabilitation for the performing voice at the Massachusetts Eye and Ear Infirmary. She is currently singing voice specialist, clinical associate faculty, and director of performing voice programs and development at the Duke Voice Care Center, where she provides rehabilitation therapy to singers, actors, and other vocal performers with voice injuries. Ms. Scearce is a frequent speaker on the topic of the singing voice at national and international voice conferences, including the American Academy of Otolaryngology-Head and Neck Surgery, the Voice Foundation, National Association of Teachers of Singing, the International Conference on the Physiology and Acoustics of Singing, The National Center for Voice and Speech, the McIver Lecture in Vocal Pedagogy, and the North Carolina Regional Chapter of the Acoustical Society of America. She is a member of the American Speech-Language-Hearing Association, the Voice Foundation, National Association of Teachers of Singing, the American Academy of Otolaryngology-Head and Neck Surgery, and is a founding member of the Pan-American Vocology Association. Ms. Scearce maintains an active performance career.

Contributors

Caroline Warren Banka, MS, CCC-SLP
Senior Clinical Specialist
Duke Voice Care Center
Durham, North Carolina
Chapter 19

Seth M. Cohen, MD, MPH
Associate Professor
Division of Head and Neck Surgery & Communication Sciences
Duke University Medical Center
Durham, North Carolina
Chapters 3 and 17

Alissa Collins, MD
Duke University Medical Center
Durham, North Carolina
Chapter 3

Matthew Edwards, DMA
Associate Professor of Voice and Voice Pedagogy
Shenandoah Conservatory
Associate Director
CCM Voice Pedagogy Institute
EdwardsVoice.com
Winchester, Virginia
Chapter 18

Jarrod Keeler, MD
Department of Otolaryngology-Head and Neck Surgery
Division of Facial Plastic Surgery
Stanford University
Stanford, California
Chapter 17

Mirabelle B. Sajisevi, MD
Duke University Medical Center
Durham, North Carolina
Chapter 4

Leda Scearce, MM, MS, CCC-SLP
Clinical Singing Voice Specialist
Director of Performing Voice Programs and Development
Duke Voice Care Center
Clinical Associate Faculty
Duke University School of Medicine
Raleigh/Durham, North Carolina

Chad W. Whited, MD
Austin Voice and Swallow Center
Clinical Lecturer
University of Texas at Austin
Austin, Texas
Chapter 17

David L. Witsell, MD, MHS
Professor
Duke University Medical Center
Director
Duke Voice Care Center
Division of Head and Neck Surgery & Communication Sciences
Durham, North Carolina
Chapter 4

To the brave singers who inspire me every day.
In bocca al lupo.

PART I

Setting the Stage

CHAPTER 1

Singing Voice Rehabilitation: A Hybrid Profession

If you have picked up this book, you have already demonstrated your interest in helping singers recover from voice problems. Although many pathways intersect with the act of singing (including performance, voice pedagogy, conducting, music education, music therapy, speech-language pathology, and otolaryngology, to name just a few), singing voice rehabilitation is a hybrid profession that represents a very specific *amalgam* of voice pedagogy, voice pathology and voice science. Becoming a singing voice rehabilitation specialist requires in-depth training and thorough preparation across these fields. Before you become a practitioner, you must lay the groundwork for this fusion of faculties.

UNDERSTANDING THE HYBRID NATURE OF SINGING VOICE REHABILITATION

The Road Hereto

For many decades, helping singers recover from a voice injury has presented a conundrum: Who is the best person to provide singing voice rehabilitation: the singing teacher or the speech-language pathologist (SLP)? Experienced singing teachers are typically better prepared to train singers, having the appropriate knowledge and skill set to build technique in healthy voices. However, speech-language pathologists have the clinical and scientific background necessary for voice assessment, they understand the differential impact of voice disorders on vocal function, and they are conversant in therapeutic paradigms.

Additional questions spring from this supposed dichotomy: Must one have dual training in both fields to provide singing voice rehabilitation? What training and experience should singers seek in the person who provides their rehabilitation? How is singing voice rehabilitation different from speaking voice rehabilitation and from voice lessons?

Let's take a look at how some of these questions have been and are being addressed.

Clinical Singing Voice Rehabilitation Specialists

For those who wish to practice *clinical* singing voice rehabilitation (or singing voice *therapy*), the training "package" must include at least a master's degree in speech-language pathology due to requirements for obtaining licensure and billing insurance. In the United States, these practitioners are typically certified by the American Speech-Language-Hearing Association (ASHA) and licensed by the state to provide rehabilitation services in a medical setting or private practice (requirements in other countries vary: International readers must of course become familiar with the competency standards for the country in which they practice).

Training in voice performance/pedagogy is also a necessity for those seeking a clinical career in singing voice rehabilitation, as speech-language pathology education does not adequately prepare clinicians to address the specialized needs of the performing voice patient, even if the clinician has obtained advanced training in clinical *speaking voice* rehabilitation as part of their graduate training, professional internship experiences, and continuing education. Ideally, speech-language pathologists who provide singing voice rehabilitation should also be experienced teachers of singing (ASHA, 2005; National Center for Voice and Speech [NCVS], 2013). This makes intuitive sense if you consider that one must be proficient at building technique in healthy instruments before embarking on the more complex endeavor of rehabilitation for singers with injured instruments. Speech-language pathologists should consider the ethical implications of engaging in singing voice rehabilitation if they do not possess a significant performing and teaching background.

Historically, people who have pursued this career have assembled the necessary expertise through self-designed pathways (NCVS, 2013). Some are dual-degreed, having obtained at least a master's degree in both speech-language pathology and voice pedagogy/performance. There are variations on this theme, with some first pursuing the performance and teaching part of their training and later obtaining the clinical portion. Others have taken the clinical pathway first (although usually with at least a modicum of singing training and performing experience in their backgrounds), augmenting their training later with deeper study and additional degrees in vocal performance and/or pedagogy. According to Dr. Robert T. Sataloff and other experts, this type of dual training is the optimal background for the practice of singing voice rehabilitation (Emerich, Baroody, Carroll, & Sataloff, 2006; NCVS, 2013; Sataloff, 2006). We might refer to such practitioners as *clinical singing voice rehabilitation specialists, singing voice therapists,* or *clinical vocologists.*

The Singing Teacher and Singing Voice Rehabilitation

A number of notable singing voice rehabilitation specialists—indeed, many of the pioneers of this profession—do not have degrees in speech-language pathology. In fact, some voice centers employ singing teachers who have a thorough background and knowledge of voice disorders to provide singing voice rehabilitation even if they are not speech-language pathologists (in such cases, speaking voice therapy is usually provided separately by an SLP). In this situation, there are complexities as to how payment is made for the singing portion of the rehabilitation (since singing teachers are not able to bill insurance) as well as potential liability issues. Nonetheless, in many cases, this arrangement works effectively and well with the singing teacher acting as part of the team with the medical and speech-language pathology providers.

Still another scenario is the voice teacher working solo in an academic or private studio setting who includes singers who have voice disorders as a part of his or her practice, often with excellent results. In some cases, singers are referred to these practitioners by a clinical voice care team and the voice teacher works in collaboration with the medical providers, albeit at a separate location.

Whether in the clinic or the studio, having a singing teacher who is not an SLP deliver rehabilitation services may present potential financial, time, and convenience disadvantages for the singer, as he or she will not be able to take advantage of insurance benefits and will have to seek voice therapy for speaking voice with a separate provider (NCVS, 2013). However, if a clinical singing voice rehabilitation specialist is not readily available, the investment of time and money may be well worth it to the singer.

Singing voice teachers who do not have clinical training and certification must be cognizant of the legal ramifications of characterizing the services they provide as "therapy." Doing so may render them liable for damages if a singer decides to take legal action against them. Singing teachers who work with singers who have vocal injuries may wish to consider obtaining liability insurance.

An ASHA (2005) position statement asserts that "the preparation of the teachers of singing needs to be augmented . . . to include training in anatomy and physiology, behavioral management of voice problems, development of the speaking voice, and the singing teacher's role in working with the speech-language pathologist and the physician in the medical management of voice disorders." However, in the United States, no clearly defined criteria have been established as yet for voice teachers (whether they work within a medical practice or not) as to what education and training is needed to work with singers who have voice injuries. A number of programs have sought to provide this background information for singers and teachers of singing, including the Summer Vocology Institute at NCVS, the PhD in Voice Pedagogy at the University of Kansas, the Singing Health Specialization cognate offering at the Ohio State University (all reported in NCVS, 2013), and a program in Singing Voice Rehabilitation developed by Karen Wicklund (Wicklund, 2010). It is important to point out that although many of these are excellent programs for *augmenting* the knowledge typically gained in academic music or speech-language pathology programs, none are recognized by ASHA or state licensing organizations, and thus these programs do not prepare or qualify the voice teacher to provide voice *therapy*.

The Way Forward

Although there is currently much debate about what form and direction the future of singing voice rehabilitation will take, one thing is very clear: There is a tremendous need for providers who can help singers recover from voice problems in a manner that is first and foremost effective but also scientifically and evidence based.

In April 2013, a symposium was held at the National Center for Voice and Speech to explore the topic of singing voice health, titled "Proposed Specialty Training in Vocal Health: Why, Who, What and How?" This symposium—which led directly to the formation of the Pan American Vocology Association (PAVA) in 2014 —featured much discussion relative to the topic of singing voice rehabilitation: Who is best qualified to provide it, what training should be obtained, and what critical skills must be demonstrated by those who practice it?

Although there are currently no credentialing processes or training programs that specifically prepare one for singing voice rehabilitation, the establishment of organizations like the Pan American Vocology Association (PAVA) and of academic degrees in clinical singing voice rehabilitation currently under way (Scearce, Scheuring, Nixon, Wells, & Lundgren, 2014) make it likely that the coming decades will see increasing educational opportunities for those who seek this specialized training, as well as clarification and specification of professional standards. It is indeed an exciting time to be part of this emerging profession.

What's in a Name? Clarifying the Terminology

- As the language surrounding singing voice rehabilitation has historically been inexact, inconsistent, and unclear, an attempt was made at the NCVS symposium in 2013 to clarify terminology used to refer to the practice of working with singers who have voice disorders as detailed in the Summary Statement of the symposium. This included defining the difference between voice habilitation and voice rehabilitation:

  > The major demarcation drawn was between voice *habilitation* and voice *rehabilitation* for the performance voice. It was generally agreed that voice habilitation describes maintenance, building and enhancing vocal skills and knowledge in a healthy performer, and that voice rehabilitation describes restoration of lost vocal function for a performer who has suffered a voice disorder or voice injury. It was pointed out multiple times that there can be considerable overlap of these functions, but there was general agreement that the distinction was valid and deserving of differentiating terminology. (NCVS, 2013, p. 5)

- People who provide singing voice rehabilitation are sometimes referred to as "singing voice specialists" (or SVSs). However, it is important to realize that to date, no formal process has been established by any relevant organization or institution for determining the criteria for this designation, there is currently no oversight as to the use of this title, and it has been applied to those with widely varying backgrounds and experience, from speech-language pathologists with advanced degrees in voice pedagogy to voice teachers who work in a clinical context to voice teachers who have undergone training in supplementary vocal health programs to people who simply self-designate the title.
- The NCVS summary statement (2013) acknowledges the importance of establishing clear terminology relative to providers of singing voice rehabilitation:

(1) to ensure that titles/nomenclature surrounding vocal health reflect the provider's qualifications so that the public will be able to identify the appropriate provider to address their needs (i.e., voice training vs. voice rehabilitation; acting voice vs. singing voice, etc.), and (2) to improve the specificity of the language we use to describe the roles and responsibilities of singing voice health providers so that the public is adequately informed of the provider's level of education, training, experience, depth of scientific and clinical knowledge, and scope of practice. (NCVS, 2013, p. 5)

In the Meantime

It may appear that I am presenting conflicting views as to who should provide singing voice rehabilitation, endorsing dual training in speech-language pathology and voice pedagogy while commending the trailblazing work of many singing voice teachers who have augmented their training to prepare themselves to work with singers who have voice disorders. My purpose is not to confuse matters but to acknowledge the reality that this is a dynamic and emerging profession in which historical and contemporary approaches are both currently in play. A more clearly delineated pathway will likely arise in the not-too-distant future, but at present issues of "who should do what" have not yet been fully resolved. In the meantime, my intention in this book is to provide practical resources to illuminate and enhance the necessary skills and competencies for conducting singing voice rehabilitation. Throughout this text, we will continually explore the integration of these critical skills and their application in creating targeted, personalized intervention programs for the singers you will work with, as well as recommendations for recognizing where and how scopes of practice converge and diverge for providers with differing backgrounds and experience.

WHAT YOU WILL NEED TO KNOW

To get the most out of this book, you will need to have a deep and broad knowledge of voice science, voice disorders, and voice pedagogy. Details of the critical skills the singing voice rehabilitation specialist must possess are enumerated below. This book assumes that you have already acquired such knowledge and that you are ready to put it into practice. For this reason, you will not find much in these pages on "the basics" relative to these topics.

Critical Skills for Singing Voice Rehabilitation

If singing voice rehabilitation is a hybrid profession, then the singing voice rehabilitation specialist—whether on the clinical or pedagogical track—must demonstrate a level of competency in all component disciplines of voice science, voice disorders, vocal performance, voice pedagogy, voice assessment, and intervention. The wealth of knowledge that the singing voice rehabilitation specialist endeavors to acquire must then be integrated into assessing voice and developing and executing appropriate intervention plans. What elements of each facet are most critical in the training and acquisition of skills?

Anatomy, Physiology, and Acoustics of Voice and Singing

Obviously, the singing voice rehabilitation specialist must possess a thorough and in-depth understanding of voice anatomy and physiology, including neuroanatomy and physiology related to voice. This must comprise not only the ability to label anatomical structures and understand their function but to understand the interconnection between body systems and their impact on voice. For example, body alignment and posture have a tremendous influence on vocal function, as do respiratory mechanics and the interaction between air and tissue movement.

Anatomy and physiology also form the foundation for understanding principles of motor learning and how they may be applied in the context of rehabilitation in general and of singing voice in particular. This knowledge is necessary for effectively shaping voice and for the development of appropriate exercise and practice regimens in the rehabilitation process.

The singing voice rehabilitation specialist must thoroughly grasp principles of the physics of sound, particularly as they relate to acoustics of voice. The critical skill lies in using this knowledge to fathom the complexity of how acoustics and physiology interact.

Knowledge of voice science must form the basis for understanding different kinds of singing, realizing that acoustics and physiology play an enormous role in the distinguishing sound characteristics we associate with various singing styles. This has a direct impact on developing appropriate therapy exercises relative to the singer's chosen vocal style.

Voice Pathology

The singing voice rehabilitation specialist's knowledge of voice disorders must be vast, systematic, and comprehensive. A cursory perusal of common voice problems and ability to recognize images of different types of voice injuries will not suffice, as different types of voice injuries impact not only vocal output but the mechanics of the entire phonatory system. The ability to acutely understand this is crucial in decision making relative to the recovery process for any individual singer. The medical diagnosis of voice disorders is made by a physician, but the singing voice rehabilitation specialist must be able to differentially identify voice anomalies, accurately assess the underlying cause, and realize how the disorder will impact respiratory mechanics, tissue dynamics, muscular engagement, resonance (natural sound reinforcement), articulatory movement, acoustic output, sound quality, pitch range, dynamic range, and stamina. All of this information will factor into accurate diagnosis, the prognosis for improvement and recovery with intervention (medical, surgical, and/or behavioral), and development of an individualized rehabilitation protocol.

Performance and Pedagogy

The singing voice rehabilitation specialist's training must span both science and art. It is assumed that the person who provides singing voice rehabilitation will be a well-trained and accomplished performer, preferably with professional performing experience. This not only affords an important basis for shaping voice but endows awareness of the language that singers use, insight into what singers go through when they have a voice disorder, and credibility in interacting with singers and the performing voice community. Given the wide range of singing styles, it is not necessarily expected that the singing voice rehabilitation specialist will have professional experience in performing all types of singing but should have adequate familiarity with and proficiency in demonstrating various styles of singing so that he or she can model them as needed in rehabilitation sessions. The singing voice rehabilitation specialist should be familiar with repertoire associated with a wide variety of singing styles and genres and should be especially mindful of staying abreast of current trends in contemporary singing.

The singing voice rehabilitation specialist must also have a high level of demonstrated expertise in teaching singing. This should begin with training singers who do not have a voice injury. Once excellence in building technique in healthy instruments has been achieved, training may be undertaken for the more complex task of rehabilitation. Knowledge and experience relative to voice pedagogy must encompass both classical and contemporary singing techniques, as well as historical knowledge and familiarity with a wide span of pedagogical theories and approaches.

Voice Assessment

All of this training and experience will be utilized in developing proficiency in assessing voice. In addition to the components of clinical assessment typically included in voice evaluation—laryngeal imaging, acoustic assessment, perceptual assessment, and administration of standardized evaluation tools—the clinical singing voice rehabilitation specialist must be adept at assessing singing voice. This will encompass assessment of parameters of singing technique such as body alignment, respiration, registration, resonance, vocal quality, balance of muscle activation, presence of maladaptive muscle tension, pitch range and accuracy, loudness range, vocal stability, use of vibrato, and stylistic appropriateness of technique. Assessment should also evaluate vocal hygiene, vocal pacing (how much, how intensely, and in what situations the voice is being used), whether the singer has an adequate vocal warm-up routine, whether typical repertoire is suited to the singer, use of amplification, and duration and intensity of performances. The professional and emotional ramifications of a voice injury for the singer should also be explored as part of the evaluation. Details of singing voice evaluation are covered in the next chapter.

Shaping Voice

Science and art are conjoined in what is possibly the most critical skill for the singing voice rehabilitation specialist: consummate expertise in shaping voice. This aptitude has perceptual (or receptive) and communicative (or expressive) components, both of which must be perfected. The singing voice rehabilitation specialist must possess a keen ear for hearing minute changes in vocal quality. Although there is a certain degree of innate ability to this skill, dedicated training will enhance both the accuracy and specificity of perceptual voice assessment. This perception must then be interpreted, translated, and communicated in a manner that is relevant and meaningful to the singer—through verbal and/or auditory feedback, visual demonstration, modeling, or instruction—in a fashion that incrementally moves the singer toward a method of vocal production and sound quality that is safe, healthy, and appropriate for his or her style of singing. This is shaping voice.

It is vital that the clinical singing voice rehabilitation specialist understands principles of shaping voice relative to speaking *and* singing voice. Training of the speaking voice is typically not a part of voice pedagogy curricula, where misperceptions of what constitutes healthy speaking voice often abound (Michael, 2012). The clinical singing voice rehabilitation specialist must address the entire vocal instrument and thus cannot afford to be misinformed regarding training of the speaking voice. For those without a clinical background, appropriate referrals should be made for speaking voice therapy.

Auxiliary Skills

Additional areas for expertise that may be incorporated into training include keyboard skills, music theory, music notation, use of recording equipment, electronic amplification and sound engineering for live performance, venue acoustics, and solo versus ensemble voice production (NCVS, 2013). Comprehension of the demands of various singing voice professions (such as music educators, worship leaders, music directors, choral conductors, music therapists, etc.) will also ensure that the singing voice rehabilitation specialist is well prepared to address the particular needs of these populations.

The Journey Ahead

There are numerous resources through which you may acquire this knowledge; however, I caution you to avoid limiting yourself to "self-teaching" or book learning. Your training may of course include this but should also incorporate course work from accredited academic programs, hands-on instruction in singing, observation of experienced professionals, and supervised experience in voice pedagogy and voice rehabilitation. Ideally, you will have acquired appropriate relevant academic degrees in speech-language pathology and vocal performance and pedagogy.

If you have gained this knowledge and experience, you are prepared to enter a new phase of your training, transitioning from the acquisition and integration of information to practical application of that information, from "knowing" in the abstract to the concrete action of "doing." I invite you to embark on this journey in which you will put your knowledge into practice, moving from the conceptual to the experiential as you learn to work directly with singers to guide them on their journey back to vocal health and the joy of singing.

HOW TO USE THIS BOOK

This book should not be considered a "how-to" instructional guide in the abstract. The information you will find here is intended to provide you with tools that you will use to lay the foundation of your practice or to augment your existing practice. As in any skill-based endeavor, a book is no substitute for gaining experience under the tutelage of a master teacher. My expectation is that your exploration of the content of this book will occur in tandem with the guidance and supervision of an experienced singing voice rehabilitation specialist.

Each chapter will expose you to important concepts of singing voice rehabilitation and factors that will need to be addressed in the singing voice rehabilitation process. This includes exploration of the special needs of singers and how you can optimize your singing voice rehabilitation sessions to create an environment of safety and trust. Although this book is not intended to provide in-depth exploration of the vocal impact of medical problems and medications, you will find information and resources here that will aid you in ensuring these critical factors are adequately addressed for the singers you work with. The book contains a wealth of information for developing exercises and technical interventions to target specific vocal problems and—importantly—guidance in customizing the exercises based on injury, singing style, skill level, professional level, and the particular vocal demands of each singer. In addition, we will plumb the depths of vocal hygiene and vocal pacing so that you can tailor your education on these topics to each singer's unique lifestyle. The chapters will include clinical case studies to illustrate real-life examples and practical application.

Your singing voice rehabilitation sessions will involve educating singers about principles of vocal health and giving them the tools they will need to regain optimal vocal condition. To aid in this educational component, the book includes supplements that may be downloaded from the companion website in handout format for you to distribute as you see fit. Much of this information is also useful in prevention of voice injuries and will be valuable to all singers you work with, whether they have a voice injury or not.

When you complete this book, you should have a clear idea of how to interact with singers in an effective and supportive way, what factors to address, how to structure your singing voice rehabilitation sessions, how to ensure that singers are getting adequate exercise while allowing their injuries to heal, how to customize vocal exercise regimens to each singer on an individual basis, and what resources and materials to provide to singers to optimize the outcome of their rehabilitation.

Although the intended audience for this book is speech-language pathologists and teachers of singing who are accomplished performers, experienced pedagogues, and clinically and scientifically well informed, there is information herein that may also be of value to all singers, to physicians interested in learning more about the behavioral side of singing voice rehabilitation, to nonsinging speech-language pathologists, or to anyone seeking knowledge about singing health, including music educators, music therapists, conductors, vocal coaches, worship leaders, and music directors.

REFERENCES

American Speech-Language-Hearing Association. (2005). *The role of the speech language pathologist, the teacher of singing, and the speaking voice trainer in voice habilitation* (Technical report). Rockville, MD: American Speech and Hearing Association Ad Hoc Joint Committee with the National Association of Teachers of Singing and the Voice and Speech Trainers Association. Retrieved from http://www.asha.org/members/deskref-journals/deskref/default

Emerich, K., Baroody, M., Carroll, L., & Sataloff, R. T. (2006). The singing voice specialist. In R. T. Sataloff (Ed.), *Vocal health and pedagogy, Volume II: Advanced assessment and treatment* (2nd ed.). San Diego, CA: Plural.

Michael, D. (2012). Dispelling vocal myths. Part IV: "Talk higher!" *Journal of Singing, 69,* 167–172.

National Center for Voice and Speech (NCVS). (2013). *NCVS Symposium on Specialty Training in Vocal Health Summary Report; April 25–26, 2013, Salt Lake City, UT.* Retrieved from http://www.ncvs.org/STVH_Summary_Report_2013.pdf

Sataloff, R.T. (2006) *Vocal health and pedagogy, Volume I: Science and assessment* (2nd ed.). San Diego, CA: Plural.

Scearce, L., Scheuring, E., Nixon, T., Wells, R., & Lundgren, K. (2014, May). *Toward a training paradigm for clinical singing voice rehabilitation.* Paper presented at The Voice Foundation 43rd Annual Symposium, Philadelphia, PA.

Wicklund, K. (2010). *Singing voice rehabilitation: A guide for the voice teacher and speech-language pathologist.* Clifton Park, NY: Delmar.

CHAPTER 2

It Takes a Team: Multidisciplinary Voice Care for the Singer

THE MULTIFACTORIAL NATURE OF VOICE PROBLEMS

Voice problems are almost always multifactorial. Depending on the diagnosis and severity of the voice problem, the treatment plan may include surgical management, medications, lifestyle adjustments (e.g., changes in diet and sleep habits), optimizing vocal hygiene, improving vocal pacing (how much and how intensely one uses the voice and in what situations), and training to improve the efficiency of the speaking voice. For singers, the treatment plan becomes even more complex, as their rehabilitation will likely also include therapy that directly addresses the singing voice, including targeted rehabilitation exercises, counseling, and guidance in applying principles of optimal vocal coordination into real-life performance situations. No single provider will have the education, training, experience, and qualifications to address all of these factors thoroughly, effectively, and efficiently. It takes a team to manage a singer's voice problem.

The focus of this book will be on rehabilitation. For the chapters that follow, the assumption will be that the singer has already been evaluated by appropriate voice care providers, a diagnosis has been made, and a course of singing voice rehabilitation has been recommended as part of the overall treatment plan. There are numerous resources available through which you may learn about clinical voice assessment. I am assuming that you have already acquired this knowledge through coursework, clinical internships or observation experiences, and your reading and research. If this is not the case, now is the time to do so. Whether you work as a clinical singing voice therapist or as a nonclinical member of the voice care team, you must have a thorough understanding of all of the clinical aspects of voice care. Our discussion here will be limited to a review of the clinical components of voice evaluation and treatment, the members of the voice care team, and their roles and responsibilities.

WHAT A VOICE PROBLEM MEANS TO A SINGER

For all people, the voice is intricately bound to personal identity, self-esteem, and self-image. The voice is our primary means of communication and expression, and it can be central to occupation, creativity, worship, and spirituality. This phenomenon becomes magnified for singers, for whom voice is the source of artistic and creative expression and may also represent livelihood and income. The voice is the singer's instrument, and unlike other instruments, it can never be replaced if irreparable damage occurs. A voice problem represents a crisis for the singer. Furthermore, the athleticism of singing and the demands of the singing career put vocal performers at high risk for developing a voice injury. When a voice injury occurs, it is essential that singers receive comprehensive care that addresses all elements of their vocal health and that ensures efficient and effective outcomes so that they can return to performing at their optimal level as quickly as possible.

THE VOICE CARE TEAM

The most important individual on the voice care team is the singer. The singer must know his or her own voice, must value his or her voice enough to seek care, must be dedicated enough to make the lifestyle changes necessary for recovery, and must commit to voice rehabilitation by attending rehabilitation sessions and completing home practice regularly. Other key players on the singer's voice care team include the laryngologist, the speech-language pathologist, and the singing voice rehabilitation specialist. If the singer is currently taking voice lessons, the singing teacher is a critical member of the team as well. Depending on the nature of the voice disorder, referrals may be made to other physicians (such as neurologists, endocrinologists, gastroenterologists, pulmonologists, etc.) and/or to other health care providers such as physical therapists, dentists, or massage therapists. The team may also include nurses, nurse practitioners, physician assistants, and voice scientists (Sataloff, 2006a, 2006b; Sataloff, Heman-Ackah, & Hawkshaw, 2006).

Credentials and Qualifications of the Voice Care Team

The Laryngologist

A laryngologist is an otolaryngologist who has specialized training in caring for voice problems. The laryngologist should be board certified in otolaryngology-head and neck surgery and fellowship trained in laryngology. Having said this, it is important to keep in mind that the laryngology fellowship was only established by the American Academy of Otolaryngology-Head and Neck Surgery in 1990. Physicians who completed their residency prior to this date may not be fellowship trained but may have achieved specialization in laryngology through other training paradigms (Sataloff, Heman-Ackah, & Hawkshaw, 2006).

The Speech-Language Pathologist

In the United States, the speech-language pathologist who works with voice disorders should have his or her Certificate of Clinical Competence (CCC-SLP) from the American Speech-Language-Hearing Association and should be licensed by the state in which he or she practices (American Speech-Language-Hearing Association, 2007, pp. 4–5). As noted in the last chapter, this text is primarily oriented to practice in the United States, although international readers are very welcome. If you practice outside the United States, you should familiarize yourself with the competency requirements of the country in which you work, if you haven't already done so.

Speech-language pathology is a very broad field, and training in evaluation and treatment of voice disorders is typically a very small part of the academic program. In most graduate speech-language pathology programs in the United States, students have a single course in voice disorders (sometimes only a half-semester course) and practical clinical experience may be limited to a single case. Some students complete their graduate program with no hands-on clinical experience in voice at all. Therefore, it is essential that the speech-language pathologist on the voice care team achieve specialization in voice beyond the minimum requirements. This can be accomplished by seeking clinical internship experiences at a voice care center as part of their graduate training and through professional internship experiences and continuing education. Training should include in-depth study of the complete gamut of voice disorders and their diagnosis and treatment paradigms; anatomy, physiology, and acoustics of voice; interpretation of laryngeal imaging, including stroboscopy and high-speed video; execution and interpretation of instrumental voice measures, including acoustic and aerodynamic measures of voice and electroglottography (EGG); perceptual evaluation of voice; administration and interpretation of self-assessment measures; and development and implementation of treatment plans.

As we discussed in Chapter 1, even if a speech-language pathologist is well prepared for rehabilitation of the speaking voice, singing voice rehabilitation is outside the realm of clinical practice for general speech-language pathologists. Therefore, if the speech-language pathologist (SLP) does not have the appropriate background in singing voice, it will be necessary for the SLP to collaborate with a suitable singing voice rehabilitation provider.

The Singing Voice Rehabilitation Specialist

The appropriate training, qualifications, and background for the singing voice rehabilitation provider have been thoroughly discussed in Chapter 1, and you should refer to that chapter for details.

Collaboration of the Voice Care Team

For optimal treatment results, the voice care providers should work as a team. This leads to a clearer diagnosis of the problem, a more comprehensive and integrated treatment plan, better monitoring of progress or identification of new problems, and better communication. This model also makes it easier for the singing patient to schedule care.

There are multiple paradigms for how such collaborative team management may be achieved. In some clinics, the laryngologist and speech-language pathologist and/or clinical singing voice rehabilitation specialist perform the evaluation in tandem, collaborating to make recommendations for medical, surgical, and behavioral components of the treatment plan all in the same visit. In other practices, the process occurs in a sequential or serial fashion, with the singing patient first seeing the laryngologist for medical evaluation and diagnosis. The laryngologist then refers the singer as needed to the speech-language pathologist and/or singing voice rehabilitation specialist.

These other providers may work in the same practice with the laryngologist or may work in a separate practice.

In many cases, the singing patient is currently receiving voice lessons at the time of the evaluation. When this is the case, the singer's current voice teacher is also a member of the voice care team, even if the direct singing voice rehabilitation will be provided by a clinical or nonclinical singing voice rehabilitation specialist. Thus, the voice teacher may function in a more auxiliary—*but no less essential*—role. Because the teacher is intimately acquainted with the singer's voice, voice history, and vocal habits, he or she can identify when subtle changes occur. In this way, singing teachers often represent the front line for identifying a voice problem and are in the best position to recommend evaluation. The current voice teacher's role may also include conferencing and consulting with the rehabilitation team to incorporate recommendations and rehabilitation exercises into ongoing voice lessons, or even attending singing voice therapy sessions so that he or she may ensure that strategies, techniques, and exercises are integrated into voice lessons and academic/professional singing activities while the singer is undergoing voice rehabilitation and after discharge.

THE VOICE EVALUATION

To be truly comprehensive, the clinical voice evaluation must encompass a number of key elements (Roy et al., 2013). These include a complete medical history and review of medications, complete head and neck examination, laryngeal imaging (videolaryngostroboscopy), acoustic and aerodynamic testing, and perceptual evaluation of speaking and singing voice, preferably including a standardized clinician administered assessment tool, such as the Consensus Auditory-Perceptual Evaluation of Voice (CAPE-V) or Grade, Roughness, Breathiness, Asthenia, Strain (GRBAS). Vocal history should include onset of the voice problem and any associated precipitating factors, voice training history, review of current vocal demands (speaking and singing), and assessment of vocal hygiene. The evaluation may also include use of a patient self-assessment tool to determine the impact of the voice complaint on quality of life, such as the Voice Related Quality of Life (V-RQOL), Voice Handicap Index (VHI), Singer's Voice Handicap Index (SVHI), or Singer's Voice Handicap Index-10 (SVHI-10). Some clinics are utilizing high-speed videography and videokymography in addition to videostroboscopy for laryngeal imaging, and some include electroglottography as part of the assessment.

Following completion of the voice evaluation, the voice care team will make medical and communication diagnoses and recommendations for the treatment plan, which may include surgical, medical, and/or behavioral interventions (Benninger & Murry, 2006; Hillman, 2013; Hirano & Bless, 1993; Roy et al., 2013).

ROLES AND RESPONSIBILITIES OF THE VOICE CARE TEAM

All members of the vocal health team should provide vocal hygiene education (including recommendations for hydration, smoking cessation and avoidance, illness resistance, and minimizing infection risk) as well as vocal pacing. Team members must also be acutely aware that the singer may present in a heightened emotional state, and they must interact with the singer with compassion and understanding. Everyone on the vocal health team needs to recognize that the singer may feel that he or she is in a crisis, as professional or academic success, self-esteem and self-worth, livelihood, reputation, and future performing opportunities may all be jeopardized by a voice problem. It is essential that the voice care team avoid use of the term "vocal abuse" as a concept and label. Voice injury is an occupational hazard and may reflect lack of education but is not "abuse." Use of such pejorative language may instill self-blame in the singer and may compromise the absolute trust that must be established between the singer and the voice care team. We will go into the ways in which such labeling can be harmful as well as other considerations for supporting the singer's emotional needs in greater depth in Chapter 8.

You will note in the discussion below the convergence, divergence, and overlapping of the roles of the speech-language pathologist who is not trained to work with singers, the speech-language pathologist who is trained to work with singers (clinical singing voice rehabilitation specialist), and the nonclinical singing voice rehabilitation specialist (voice teacher who is not an SLP). Again, this reflects the diversity and complexity of current treatment paradigms for the singing voice. The roles and responsibilities of these professionals will likely become more distinct and streamlined as progress is made toward certification and credentialing for the relevant professions.

The Laryngologist's Role and Responsibilities

The laryngologist takes the patient's medical and voice history and conducts a full head and neck examination. This includes laryngeal imaging as a means to diagnose laryngeal pathology via stroboscopy and, in some cases, high-speed video (in many practices, the laryngeal imaging procedure is executed by the speech-language pathologist). Based on the laryngeal imaging results, the laryngologist makes a medical diagnosis of the voice problem (e.g., vocal fold lesions, paralysis or paresis, laryngitis, etc.). The laryngologist assesses and treats medical factors that may include seasonal or chronic allergies, laryngopharyngeal reflux, acute laryngitis, upper respiratory tract infection, or sinus infection. The laryngologist provides surgical management of the voice problem when indicated and directs voice care with speech-language pathologists and singing voice rehabilitation specialists. Reevaluation with the laryngologist may be conducted at an interval appropriate to the diagnosis (Benninger & Murry, 2006; Sataloff, 2006a).

Steroids may be used as a diagnostic tool to get a clearer picture of underlying injury by temporarily resolving general edema. Steroids may also be necessary acutely to enable the singer to complete an important performance. It is important to avoid patient reliance on steroids, and stroboscopy should be conducted before prescribing steroids to ensure there is no contraindication and after treatment to ensure the injury has not been exacerbated (Alessi & Crummey, 2006; Sataloff & Hawkshaw, 2006).

Allergy management may be provided by the laryngologist or through consultation with an allergy specialist. Singers should avoid systemically drying medications if at all possible (decongestants/antihistamines). The laryngologist may instead prescribe nasal treatment for allergies such as nasal steroid or antihistamine sprays. Having said this, it is important to realize that some singers may in fact need oral antihistamines in addition to nasal medications to achieve optimal control of allergies, or when their allergy symptoms are more systemic (for example, when the singer has eye or skin reactions). Sinus irrigation may be recommended as well as education regarding optimal control of the patient's physical environment (bedding, floor covering, air filters, pets, etc.). Immunotherapy (allergy shots or sublingual immunotherapy) may also be part of the allergy regimen.

The laryngologist may prescribe medication for laryngopharyngeal reflux (LPR) and provide information about lifestyle changes (such as changing diet and timing of meals) that can help to control LPR. If reflux is determined to be inadequately managed through these interventions, the laryngologist may refer to a gastroenterologist for further assessment and recommendations.

The voice has a complex and intricate relationship with the rest of the body,

The Best of All Possible Worlds Is Not Always Possible

The standard of care for singing voice includes having a fellowship-trained laryngologist on the voice care team. The importance of having a medical voice expert on your voice care team cannot be overstated. However, the reality is that in relatively smaller communities, there may not be a laryngologist in the area. If this is the case, you have an obligation to exert yourself to find an otolaryngologist (ENT) who has an interest in working with singers, who has videostroboscopy equipment and is knowledgeable in interpreting stroboscopy, and who is amenable to a team-based approach to treatment. This will require considerable legwork on your part, researching the training and experience of the physician, initiating communication, seeking observation experiences in his or her practice, and sharing your knowledge regarding vocal health and rehabilitation through in-services, community education programs, literature, and any other means at your disposal. It will also be helpful to identify and develop a relationship with an experienced laryngologist—even on a long-distance basis—whom you can consult and ask questions of when you have concerns about medical management in a particular case. In some situations (and always if stroboscopy is not locally available), you will need to encourage the singer to be willing to travel to get the best care. Be prepared to back up your recommendation by citing the qualifications of the expert. This link provides a listing of voice centers in the United States: http://www.gbmc.org/nationalreferraldatabase

The American Speech-Language-Hearing Association Special Interest Group 3 (ASHA SIG 3) also provides a discussion forum on voice topics, which is sponsored by the University of Iowa Department of Otolaryngology-Head and Neck Surgery. This listserv is an excellent resource through which you may query a vast population of voice experts on a variety of voice topics, including locating appropriate voice professionals (laryngologists, singing voice rehabilitation specialists, speech-language pathologists, voice teachers, acting voice trainers, etc.). Any voice professional may join the listserv. Information on how to join is provided in Appendix 2–A.

and there are numerous medical problems that may contribute to dysphonia. Any such factors, if present, will need to be addressed to achieve resolution of the voice problem. The laryngologist will make appropriate referrals to other physicians and practitioners as indicated. For example, the laryngologist may refer to a neurologist for sleep disorders, dystonia, or neck pain. A pulmonologist may be consulted for asthma, a rheumatologist for autoimmune dysfunction, or an endocrinologist for hormonal imbalance (including thyroid disease). A dentist, oral surgeon, or physical therapist may be helpful in managing temporomandibular joint dysfunction (TMD). In some cases, referral to a psychiatrist or psychologist may be indicated (Sataloff, Heman-Ackah, et al., 2006).

The Speech-Language Pathologist's Role and Responsibilities

If the voice practice includes a clinical singing voice rehabilitation specialist, he or she will fulfill all of the protocols outlined below in addition to those listed for the singing voice in the next section. Otherwise, a clinical or nonclinical singing voice rehabilitation specialist may be consulted to assess and treat the singing voice.

At the evaluation, the speech-language pathologist takes a detailed voice history. This should include onset and duration of the voice problem and any associated precipitating factors. Typical vocal demands should be reviewed both for singing and speaking, including any phonotraumatic behaviors such as yelling or chronic throat clearing as well as vocal hygiene habits (such as hydration, caffeine, and alcohol intake) and smoking history. While interviewing the patient, the speech-language pathologist will perceptually assess speaking voice quality, coordination of phonation, evident muscle tension, resonance, pitch, loudness, and vocal characteristics such as vocal fry, diplophonia, or pitch/phonation breaks.

In some clinics, the speech-language pathologist conducts the videostroboscopy and/or high-speed video examination. This may include use of flexible (distal chip) and/or rigid endoscopes. Stroboscopy and high-speed video allow detailed examination of the laryngeal structures, glottic closure, and vibratory patterns at various pitches and provide information on vocal fold cover viscosity, vibration, and degree of closure (Hirano & Bless, 1993; Sataloff, 2006a).

The speech-language pathologist administers and interprets acoustic and aerodynamic testing. Acoustic testing should include average fundamental frequency and pitch range. Measures of perturbation, noise-harmonic ratio, tremor, subharmonic noise, and soft phonation index have historically been included in acoustic testing and are based on sustained vowel phonation. However, the results of some of these measures have not provided good correlation to perceptual ratings. New assessment programs have recently been developed that allow for acoustic assessment in continuous speech. The Analysis of Dysphonia in Speech and Voice (ADSV) from PentaxMedical performs cepstral-based measures. ADSV has shown promising outcomes related to dysphonia severity and voice analysis measurement. This type of program is already being utilized at a number of clinics and is becoming part of standard acoustic evaluation (Peterson, Roy, Awan, Merrill, & Tanner, 2013). Aerodynamic assessment typically includes measures of subglottic pressure, phonation threshold pressure, vital capacity, and characteristics of airflow and resistance.

The speech-language pathologist does not make a medical diagnosis but describes changes to laryngeal structures and appearance, vocal fold mobility, and mucosal parameters of vocal fold vibration based on laryngeal imaging. He or she also interprets results of perceptual and acoustic assessment, evaluates vocal hygiene and voice use habits, and assesses the impact of the injury on the patient's communication and quality of life. Once the medical diagnosis has been made by the laryngologist, the speech-language pathologist makes recommendations for voice therapy related to speaking voice, develops a treatment plan with measurable goals, and provides speaking voice therapy. Voice therapy includes developing exercises and intervention strategies to optimize coordination of phonation subsystems through a systematic, hierarchical training program. Speaking voice therapy will be explored in greater depth in Chapter 13. The voice therapy regimen will likely also include ongoing counseling regarding vocal hygiene, as well as regular review of voice use to optimize vocal pacing. If the SLP is also a clinical singing voice rehabilitation specialist, his or her treatment plan will include rehabilitation of the singing voice.

The Singing Voice Rehabilitation Specialist's Role and Responsibilities

As noted above, in some practices, the singing voice rehabilitation specialist is also a licensed, certified speech-language pathologist. If this is the case, clinical voice evaluation and behavioral therapy encompassing both speaking and singing can be conducted by the same person. This is an optimal arrangement, as it means fewer visits for the patient and allows for a more holistic approach to the behavioral intervention, addressing the patient's speaking and singing voice simultaneously. If he or she is not an SLP, the singing voice rehabilitation specialist will work collaboratively with the voice care team under the supervision of the clinical providers. In this scenario, speaking voice therapy and singing voice rehabilitation are typically conducted separately. Although this paradigm potentially increases the financial and time outlay of the singer, when implemented by expert professionals, it has the advantage of double reinforcement, with the patient getting the same core message from two different providers.

The singing voice rehabilitation specialist will obtain additional details regarding the history of the problem relative to singing, including the specific singing symptoms, the style(s) the singer typically sings in, voice type, professional status, training background, typical performance activities, and any impending performances. He or she will also review the singer's typical singing schedule, including individual practice time, rehearsals, performance, and recreational singing. If the singing voice rehabilitation specialist is conducting the evaluation with the laryngologist, this information may be collected simultaneously with the medical history of the voice problem, resulting in a thorough and efficient voice history.

The singing voice rehabilitation specialist will conduct further perceptual assessment focusing on the singing voice. This may be accomplished by having the singer perform a series of vocalises and/or repertoire. As this can be a time-consuming process, the singing voice evaluation may be conducted at a separate appointment. The assessment should include pitch and dynamic range, voice quality, breath support, resonance, projection, pitch accuracy, ease of phonation, register negotiation, vibrato characteristics, whether declared voice part is appropriate, posture, and body alignment. The singing voice rehabilitation specialist will also assess whether the singer's technique is effective and safe, and how well it aligns with his or her chosen singing style(s). Review of video and/or audio recordings of the singer (if available) can be very helpful. This allows clearer assessment of the singer's function in real-world situations. Recordings that predate the injury can be used as part of the evaluation process to determine the patient's baseline and current loss of function.

Based on results of evaluation, the singing voice rehabilitation specialist develops a rehabilitation plan to optimize vocal coordination and conditioning for singing and to unload maladaptive and nonproductive vocal behaviors. The exercises should be designed to promote healing and avoid further injury. This may include teaching basic vocal skills to untrained singers or optimizing vocal function and technique in trained singers. Vocal pacing and vocal hygiene will also be components of singing voice rehabilitation.

COLLABORATIVE INTERACTION AND DECISION MAKING

Clearly, voice care for singers is complex and multifactorial in nature. There are numerous elements of voice evaluation and management that cannot be addressed or decided on by only one member of the team. Regular communication and collaboration are required to achieve optimal results.

Obtaining a clear history of the voice problem can sometimes be hampered by communication breakdown, particularly if the singer uses technical singing language or abstract, imagery-based language to describe vocal activities and symptoms. Even the best-trained laryngologist may not be familiar with all the "singerese" that may arise in the discussion. A collaborative history taking between the laryngologist and the clinical or nonclinical singing voice rehabilitation specialist can be very beneficial in such a case, as the singing voice provider can function as an interpreter.

The speech-language pathologist and/or singing voice provider can also play an important role in follow-up education and ensuring the patient's adherence to medical recommendations, since they will likely see the patient on a regular basis for rehabilitation sessions. The patient may experience difficulty with a medication, may not have a clear understanding of the results of the evaluation or rationale for treatment recommendations, or may wish to explore options he or she had not previously wished to consider (such as surgery). In such cases, the voice pathologist and/or singing voice rehabilitation specialist can facilitate communication with the laryngologist and reinforce recommendations to ensure that all contributing factors are being addressed in an efficient and thorough manner.

Balancing Voice Rest and Vocal Exercise

Determining how much the singer should sing and whether to recommend voice

The Singing Voice Rehabilitation Specialist as Communication Facilitator

As a singing voice rehabilitation specialist, your encounters with the singer will occur much more frequently than the physician's. This regular interaction provides you with an excellent opportunity to continually review the status of any medical problem(s). If the singer has a contributing medical problem, you should make a point of asking him or her at each session about the symptoms, whether medications are being taken as directed, and whether the singer feels the problem is well managed with the current treatment. If the problem does not seem to be controlled or is not resolving, you can play an important role in expediting an update in treatment by communicating with the physician or urging the singer to do so. If you are working in a clinical setting on a voice care team with physicians, this is quite a simple process, as you are likely in regular contact with the treating doctor. If not, the process can be a little more complicated, particularly if you do not know the doctor well. If the physician is not used to treating singers or working with other members of a voice care team, her or she may not appreciate your involvement and may even perceive your questions as presumptuous or intrusive. In such cases, you will have to work hard to be a diplomatic but staunch advocate for the singers you work with. This obligation of advocacy extends to questions of surgical intervention. If your training, experience, and research suggest that surgery may be indicated—especially if the singer is not progressing despite adherence to the rehabilitation regimen—you should be prepared to discuss this option with the singer and surgeon. Conversely, if surgery has been recommended and you have questions about the level of experience of the surgeon or advisability of the procedure, you will need to take a role in the discussion. This is where your scientific and evidence-based knowledge will be critical. If you can back up your questions about treatment by pointing to relevant research, you will have much greater credibility. You must be prepared to provide specific citations from respected sources.

rest is often a team decision and depends largely on the professional status of the singer, style of singing, and degree of injury. Complete vocal rest is rarely indicated, as muscles need regular exercise and deconditioning may result from prolonged voice rest. If maladaptive behavior is contributing to the voice injury, voice rest is merely a "Band-Aid" that does not address the underlying functional problem. In addition, long-term voice rest can promote discouragement and fear of singing. Instead of blanket recommendations for voice rest, the voice care team must collaborate to determine a plan of action that will optimize recovery.

Should the Singer Continue Performing During Rehabilitation?

At the initial evaluation, a number of different scenarios may present relative to the singer's current performance status.

Some singers may have experienced a fairly recent change in voice, while others may have been struggling with a voice problem for a period of months or even years. If the voice problem has been prolonged, some may have soldiered on, pushing through performances in spite of lost range, quality, and stamina. Others may have drastically reduced their performance activities or ceased altogether. Some may depend on singing for their income, in which case any reduction in performing has financial consequences. For others, a reduction in performing may not necessarily affect livelihood but may significantly impact their quality of life, spiritual activity, or sense of purpose.

There are a number of factors to consider in determining whether a change in performance activities is advisable, such as severity of injury, risk of further injury, professional status, financial dependence on singing, impact on academic success, ability to fulfill community or spiritual commitments, risk of harming the singer's reputation as a performer, and the degree to which it would be frustrating to the singer to perform below personal standards. All of these elements must be assessed and carefully weighed. If the patient is currently working with a singing teacher, the clinical singing voice rehabilitation therapist and laryngologist may also consult him or her to determine the importance of any upcoming performances or other vocal activities. This type of collaboration is particularly critical when deciding whether a singer should proceed with a performance in an injured state, as we will explore below.

Depending on the severity of the singer's injury, he or she may be able to tolerate continued performing while undergoing singing voice rehabilitation by adjusting the current schedule, optimizing vocal pacing strategies, and beginning an appropriate vocal exercise regimen. For others, it will be better to briefly cease performing. In such cases, the voice care team must determine when the singer is ready to "get back on the horse" and return to regular performing. We will examine this process in Chapter 15. Conducting serial stroboscopy can be very beneficial in assessing progress and adjusting voice use recommendations.

Discharge and Follow-Up

Duration and intricacy of intervention will differ from case to case, depending on the severity of injury, whether surgery was necessary, the nature and complexity of the contributing factors, and the degree of support that is likely needed to ensure that the patient can safely engage in singing activities. In some cases, medical management may be all that is needed. In others, behavioral factors may be able to be addressed in only a few rehabilitation sessions. Still other singers may require rehabilitation over a period of months and may need intermittent "brush-up" sessions after discharge. The voice care team collaborates in determining the timing of discharge and developing an appropriate follow-up plan. The patient may be discharged by one member of the team while continuing to work with another.

The most important consideration in determining when to discharge the patient is level of function. Through medical or surgical management and improvement of vocal pacing, vocal hygiene, and vocal efficiency, the singer may be able to return to a level of performance that meets his or her professional or avocational needs, even if some degree of physical injury or impairment is still evident in laryngeal imaging results. Determining when to discharge from singing intervention can be a challenging decision. As singing voice rehabilitation inevitably and inherently addresses vocal technique, in many cases, the singer will continue to improve and make progress. The line between "singing rehabilitation" and "singing lessons" can be quite blurry. The singing voice rehabilitation specialist must keep in mind that the goal of singing rehabilitation is restoration of function that has been lost, whereas that of singing lessons is building technique in a healthy instrument. If the latter begins to be the case, it is likely time to discharge the patient. Discharge criteria and decision making will be covered in greater depth in Chapter 6.

Risk of reinjury is high if behaviors are not permanently changed and if necessary ongoing medical management is not continued. Periodic reexamination by all or part of the team may be recommended to monitor the singer's status and adjust the maintenance plan.

An excellent way to ensure continued improvement and help the singer stay on the path of vocal health is to encourage ongoing study with the current singing teacher or refer to a competent singing teacher in the community.

The Show Must Go On: Acute Laryngitis and the Singer

It is not unusual for singers to present with an acute change in voice, requiring immediate evaluation and rapid decision making. When this happens, you will not have the luxury of the steady course of events outlined thus far. In the face of an impending performance, acute laryngitis represents a vocal emergency, and in such cases, the collaborative process of the voice care team must be expedited.

Causes and treatments for acute laryngitis will be discussed in Chapters 3 and 4. Ideally, singing should be avoided or at least minimized when the singer is suffering from acute laryngitis. However, there are situations where cancellation of a scheduled performance presents adverse consequences and in which—with the proper medical support and behavioral modifications—the singer may safely get through the performance.

Only the physician can make the diagnosis and the recommendation of whether or not to go ahead with the performance but may collaborate with singing health providers in making decisions. If the determination is made that the singer may proceed, he or she will need additional guidance and strategies on how to safely weather the performance under the supervision of medical voice professionals, including a laryngologist and singing voice rehabilitation specialist, to be discussed further below.

Diagnosis and Medical Treatment of Acute Laryngitis

The diagnosis of acute laryngitis is outside the scope of practice for a singing voice rehabilitation specialist, regardless of whether or not that person is a speech-language pathologist. In many states, the SLP can perform videolaryngostroboscopy, but ultimately the examination must be reviewed by a physician, preferably a laryngologist. If acute laryngitis is suspected, is it of critical importance for the larynx to be examined (ideally with stroboscopy but at least with laryngoscopy) to determine whether it is safe to proceed with a given performance.

Steroids may be a part of the treatment plan for the acute problem, but other medical management may be recommended as well. Depending on the diagnosis, the physician may prescribe antibiotics and/or cough medications, mucolytics, allergy medications, or reflux treatment.

Use of Steroids for Acute Laryngitis. Many times, out of a sense of urgency regarding a pending performance, singers with laryngitis will consult a primary care physician or urgent care clinic and oral or injectable steroids will be provided without instrumental examination of the larynx. This route is inadvisable and you should routinely caution the singers you work with to avoid it. Without accurate diagnosis of the underlying pathology, the singer is at risk for exacerbation of injury or permanent damage to the vocal folds (Sataloff, 2006b; Sataloff & Hawkshaw, 2006). For some conditions (such as vocal fold hemorrhage and fungal laryngitis), steroid treatment is contraindicated. Furthermore, steroid treatment can mask the underlying injury so that the singer does not perceive the effects of "pushing through" a performance until it is too late. Acute hoarseness or other alteration of phonation can be considered to be the body's way of warning the singer that something is wrong, and this warning should be heeded. Oral or injectable steroids can be helpful in getting a singer through a critical performance, but ultimately this treatment is a "Band-Aid." Contributing factors must be addressed in the long term. If the singer has taken steroids to get through performances frequently in the past, it will be important to ascertain whether the singer is overusing this type of medication and whether behavioral intervention is needed to uncover factors that may be contributing to recurrent problems surrounding performance, such as insufficient vocal pacing, inadequate vocal coordination and conditioning, or poor vocal hygiene.

Considerations for Canceling a Performance

Temporary cessation of singing (including canceling a performance) should be recommended for acute vocal fold hemorrhage, vocal fold ulceration or mucosal tear, or any case in which there is a danger of increasing the degree of injury by singing (Sataloff, Cline, Lyons, & Rubin, 2006). This includes situations in which the singing voice rehabilitation specialist determines the singer does not have a sufficient level of vocal skill to compensate for the injury.

The recommendation for cancelling a performance cannot be taken lightly. Depending on the professional status of the singer and the importance of the performance, cancellation may result in significant financial repercussions that extend beyond the singer, as well as damage to the singer's reputation (Sataloff, Cline, et al., 2006). Although the singing voice rehabilitation specialist can and should weigh in on the decision, there are potential legal and liability risks associated with prognosticating the outcome of a medical condition. Thus, the recommendation should ideally be made by the physician. Cancelling a performance is usually a distressing prospect for a singer. When this recommendation is made, it will be vital to ensure that the singer fully understands that it is made in the interest of supporting his or her long-term vocal health and future performances.

Strategies to Support the Singer

The decision to proceed with a performance under suboptimal vocal conditions is equally weighty. The singer's reputation may be damaged by a performance that is not up to his or her standards (jeopardizing future engagements), or the singer may risk serious or even permanent injury. The singing voice rehabilitation specialist may assist in this decision-making process by assessing whether the singer has sufficient technical skill to compensate effectively; by providing information on vocal exercises to reduce vocal fold edema and optimize coordination of respiratory, phonatory, and resonance subsystems; by probing the details and importance of the performance; and by ascertaining whether performance adaptations can be made to support the singer. If the physician deems it medically safe for the singer to proceed with the performance, there are a number of strategies that may be implemented in addition to any medical management that has been provided to help the singer get through the acute phase.

Vocal Exercise. Depending on the circumstances, you may or may not have an opportunity to schedule a rehabilitation session with the singer prior to performance. If not, you can at least provide education regarding semi-occluded vocal tract (SOVT) exercises and encourage the singer to complete simple exercises (sustained single pitches, gentle pitch glides) using SOVT sounds (straw phonation, lip/tongue/ligual-labial trills, voiced fricatives, humming, etc.). For detailed discussion of the benefits of SOVT exercises, see Chapter 11. Recent research postulates that this type of vocal exercise may be more effective than voice rest in attenuating acute vocal fold inflammation (Verdolini Abbott et al., 2012). I typically recommend that the singer complete these exercises for 3 to 6 minutes several times per day and anytime he or she feels vocally fatigued.

Vocal Hygiene. If the singer does not already practice good vocal hygiene, review relevant recommendations (see Chapter 5 for details and materials). Improving hydration, minimizing alcohol consumption, and avoiding coughing and throat clearing are all steps the singer may take immediately to help support vocal health.

Vocal Pacing. When undertaking a performance with acute laryngitis, the singer should unload as much voice use outside the performance as possible. This may include minimizing rehearsing, eliminating unnecessary singing, and keeping time spent on the sound check to the bare minimum. The singer should reduce speaking voice use as much as possible, including audience interactions, "meet-and-greet" sessions, working a merchandise table, interviews, and social voice use (especially speaking in noisy environments). The singer may be tempted to "check" the voice frequently by singing exercises or phrases or may engage in a prolonged warm-up routine if the voice does not feel normal. Advise the singer to judiciously allocate warm-up time, "saving" the voice for the performance.

Adapting the Program. Review the program with the singer to see if any adaptations may be made. This can be difficult in theatrical productions (musical theater or opera) and in classical concerts, where the content is fairly fixed. However, it is worth exploring whether there is the potential for any numbers to be cut. Contemporary singers may have more options for altering the content of the program, cutting a few songs to shorten set-length, trading out songs that are particularly strenuous with those that are less demanding, adding instrumental breaks or solos, or delegating songs to other bandmates. They may also consider transposing songs into a range that is less challenging.

Advocate for the Singer. You may need to advocate for the singer with other important people involved in the performance. This may include the tour manager, director, conductor, producer, or artist's manager. Any of these people may at first be resistant to making a change in the program, rehearsal schedule, or associated events but typically will come around once they recognize that the singer may not be able to complete the performance unless permitted to follow the voice care team's recommendations for modifying vocal activities during and surrounding performances. Some singers feel that it can be helpful to arrange for a pre-performance announcement letting the audience know that the he or she is indisposed but has decided to perform anyway. This makes the singer a bit of a hero to the audience and may take off some of the performance pressure.

Importance of Follow-Up. Depending on the diagnosis and the situation, you may see the singer only for the evaluation, or for ongoing singing voice rehabilitation. In either case, follow-up is critical. If the singer has multiple performances, medical treatment and supportive strategies may need to be continued or revised. If the singer is not local to you and will be continuing a performance tour or going on to another performance, you can help ensure follow-up by providing contacts for voice care at the next stop on the road. In such cases, I always contact the singer after the performance to see how he or she did. If there are indications that chronic voice problems may persist past the acute stage, singing voice rehabilitation is indicated and should be initiated as soon as possible after the singer has recovered from the acute injury.

REFERENCES

Alessi, D. M., & Crummey, A. (2006). Medications: The positive and the negative impact on voice. In M. S. Benninger & T. Murry (Eds.), *The performer's voice* (pp. 153–164). San Diego, CA: Plural.

American Speech-Language Hearing Association. (2007). *Scope of practice in speech language pathology*. Retrieved from http://www.asha.org/policy/SP2007-00283/

Benninger, M., & Murry, T. (Eds.). (2006). *The performer's voice*. San Diego, CA: Plural.

Hillman, R. (2013, May). *The way forward in clinical voice assessment*. Paper presented at The Voice Foundation 42nd Annual Symposium Care of the Professional Voice, Philadelphia, PA.

Hirano, M., & Bless, D. (1993). *Videostroboscopic examination of the larynx*. San Diego, CA: Singular.

Peterson, E., Roy, N., Awan, S., Merrill, R., & Tanner, K. (2013, May). *Performance of the Cepstral/Spectral Index of Dysphonia (CSID) as an objective treatment outcomes tool*. Paper presented at The Voice Foundation 42nd Annual Symposium Care of the Professional Voice, Philadelphia, PA.

Roy, N., Barkmeier-Kraemer, J., Eadie, T., Sivasankar, M. P., Mehta, D., Paul, D., & Hillman, R. (2013). Evidence-based clinical voice assessment: A systematic review. *American Journal of Speech-Language Pathology, 22*(2), 212–226.

Sataloff, R. T. (2006a). *Vocal health and pedagogy, Volume I: Science and assessment* (2nd ed.). San Diego, CA: Plural.

Sataloff, R. T. (2006b). *Vocal health and pedagogy, Volume II: Advanced assessment and treatment* (2nd ed.). San Diego, CA: Plural.

Sataloff, R. T., Cline, S. E., Lyons, K. M., & Rubin, A. D. (2006). Voice rest. In R.T. Sataloff (Ed.), *Vocal health and pedagogy, Volume II: Advanced assessment and treatment* (2nd ed., pp. 253–257). San Diego, CA: Plural.

Sataloff, R. T., & Hawkshaw, M. J. (2006). Medications for traveling perfomers. In R. T. Sataloff (Ed.), *Vocal health and pedagogy, Volume II: Advanced assessment and treatment* (2nd ed., pp. 213–217). San Diego, CA: Plural.

Sataloff, R. T., Heman-Ackah, Y. D., & Hawkshaw, M. J. (2006). Voice care professionals: A guide to voice care providers. In R. T. Sataloff (Ed.), *Vocal health and pedagogy, Volume I: Science and assessment* (2nd ed., pp.121–126). San Diego, CA: Plural.

Verdolini Abbott, K., Li, N. Y., Branski, R. C., Rosen, C. A., Grillo, E., Steinhauer, K., & Hebda, P. A. (2012). Vocal exercise may attenuate acute vocal fold inflammation. *Journal of Voice, 26*(6), 814.e1–814.e13.

APPENDIX 2–A

How to Join ASHA SIG 3 Listserv

This discussion forum is sponsored by the University of Iowa Department of Otolaryngology-Head and Neck Surgery. Its purpose is to promote discussion among health care professionals, scientists, and professional voice users regarding clinical and scientific issues relating to the normal and disordered human voice.

Access the e-mail list website at http://list.healthcare.uiowa.edu/read/?forum=VOICESERVE to subscribe, unsubscribe, view archives, temporarily stop receiving messages, or otherwise manage your subscription.

1. A screen with the message, "You must log in to enter that forum" will appear for a moment, followed by another screen asking for your e-mail address. Type in your e-mail address in the line provided and select the "OK" button in the right-hand corner. The system will tell you if you are not already subscribed. If you are subscribed, you will be prompted for a password. See the "**Important**" note below about passwords. Enter your password if you created one when you subscribed. If you have not created a password for your subscription, leave the password field blank and select "OK."
2. If you are not subscribed, select the "**Search**" button on the left. A list of names will then appear in alphabetical order. Locate the blue slider control on the right side of the window. Drag the slider control all the way to the bottom to view the very end of the list. Locate "voiceserve" near the bottom and select the "**Subscribe**" link in the right-hand column.
3. Lyris, the e-mail list program, will automatically and immediately send an e-mail to the e-mail address you entered in Step 1 (above) advising that, "You have been subscribed to voiceserve." You may want to save this message. It includes instructions about how to unsubscribe.
4. You will be returned to the All Forums list. Now select **VOICESERVE** in the left-hand column of the list. You should now be granted access to the e-mail list. A list of submitted messages will appear for your review. Select a message to read its content. To create a new message to share with the group, select "create new message" in the upper right-hand corner.

Now that you are subscribed, please take a moment to explore this powerful e-mail list tool.

IMPORTANT—The Lyris program automatically establishes subscriptions without passwords. Passwords are optional. If you want to create a password for your subscription, select the "My Account" item in the left-hand list and then select the "Advanced" tab at the top of the next display. Follow directions from there.

Select "Logout" in the upper right-hand corner of the window when you want to leave Lyris. Log in to Lyris any time you want to manage your listserv account.

New Voiceserve messages will be sent to your e-mail inbox. You may respond to them directly from there.

All messages to the e-mail list should be addressed as follows: voiceserve@list.healthcare.uiowa.edu

If you have any problems, contact michael-karnell@uiowa.edu

(B. Petty, personal communication, September 9, 2012)

CHAPTER 3

Voice Disorders

Alissa Collins and Seth M. Cohen

As discussed in Chapter 1, a thorough and in-depth knowledge of voice disorders is considered to be part of the foundation for embarking on singing voice rehabilitation. It is assumed that the reader has already meticulously studied this topic. The information herein is intended to provide a framework of reference in the form of a brief review with special considerations for the performing voice.

STRUCTURAL PATHOLOGIES

Vocal Fold Nodules

Vocal fold nodules (Figure 3–1) are benign lesions of the vocal fold epithelium that are caused by phonotrauma, vocal overuse, and repetitive stress leading to inflammation of the vocal folds.

Phonotrauma and vocal overuse refer to phonation that is either too loud/forceful or of excessive duration, respectively. Chronic cough and habitual throat clearing are additional sources of phonotrauma. The true prevalence of vocal fold nodules in the general population is unknown but children, talkative individuals, and professionals with significant vocal demands are those most often afflicted with vocal fold nodules (Akif Kiliç, Okur, Yildirim, & Güzelsoy, 2004; Lira Luce, 2014; Pereira, Tavares, & Martins, 2015). Vocal nodules in singers may result from voice overuse or excessive vocal demands, inadequate vocal pacing, or from singing too loudly, outside the singer's range or with inadequate vocal technique.

With initial voice overuse, phonatory trauma occurs to the mucosal membrane of the vocal fold, leading initially to edema within the submucosa and with more chronic phonotrauma to the hyalinization or scarring of Reinke's space (Flint

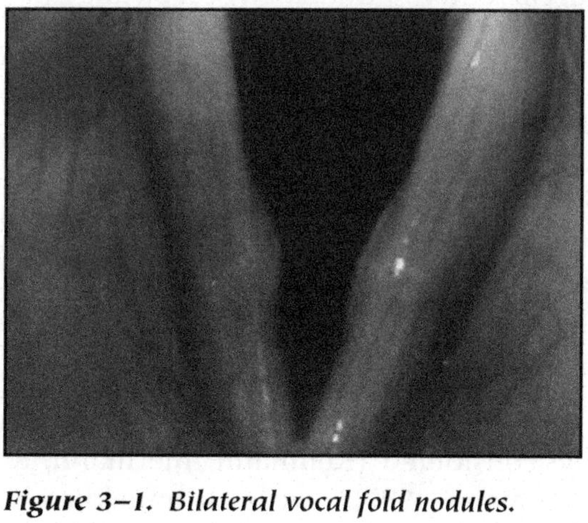

Figure 3–1. *Bilateral vocal fold nodules.*

et al., 2010, p. 865). Diagnosis is made with stroboscopic laryngeal examination. The nodules are bilateral sessile protrusions and typically form at opposing locations on the medial surfaces of the anterior two thirds of the vocal folds as this is the site of maximal collision force of the vocal folds during adduction. The nodules create an irregularity on the normally straight vocal fold edge, resulting in incomplete vocal fold closure during phonation. Vocal fold nodules are typically broad based, white, and bilateral. They can be distinguished from polyps, which tend to be unilateral (or asymmetrically bilateral) and are sometimes larger.

Speaking voice limitations are minimal until the nodules are of moderate size, at which point complaints often include hoarseness, breathiness, strain, decreased pitch, and vocal fatigue. However, the singing voice may be compromised with small nodules or even prenodular swelling. Singers will often complain of rough or harsh voice; vocal fatigue; difficulty with high, soft singing; unreliable voice; and the need for increased effort in singing (Flint et al., 2010, p. 865).

Treatment includes improved vocal hygiene (increased water intake, moderating caffeine intake, control of gastroesophageal reflux, optimizing vocal pacing) and voice therapy (Holmberg, Hillman, Hammarberg, Södersten, & Doyle, 2001; Ongkasuwan & Friedman, 2013; Pedersen & McGlashan, 2012). Nodules and prenodular swelling are usually very responsive to behavioral voice therapy and often do not require surgery. However, if the symptoms persist after an adequate trial of conservative management or if the singer reaches a plateau of improvement that is still below baseline, surgical excision can be considered (Keilmann, Biermann, & Hörmann, 1997). Voice rest immediately following surgery with graduated voice use is often recommended, followed by behavioral voice therapy.

It is important to note that although nodules are among the most benign of traumatic lesions and most responsive to nonsurgical management, the diagnosis of nodules is often the one most dreaded by singers. This has to do in large part with misguided perceptions in the singing and voice pedagogy communities that nodules portend the end of a career. When presenting this diagnosis to a singer, the vocal health provider should be prepared for an emotional reaction. This same perception of nodules as the worst diagnosis may lead the singer to be relieved if the diagnosis is a vocal fold polyp or cyst. Education on the nature of traumatic lesions and perspective on prognosis is often an important part of presenting the diagnosis.

Vocal Fold Polyp

Like nodules, polyps are benign vocal fold lesions caused by phonotrauma or overuse. Polyps are believed to result from shearing forces from vocal exertion, leading to rupture of capillaries and accumulation of blood in the superficial lamina propria. Infiltration of the area with inflammatory cells leads to deposition of extracellular matrix.

Polyps (Figure 3–2) can vary in their appearance. They can be sessile or pedunculated, edematous or hemorrhagic, gelatinous or hyalinized (containing myxoid-appearing fluid). Polyps are often unilateral and while usually in the mid-portion of the vocal fold, they can occur at any location on the vocal fold edge. There may be a reactive lesion (discussed later) on the opposite vocal fold.

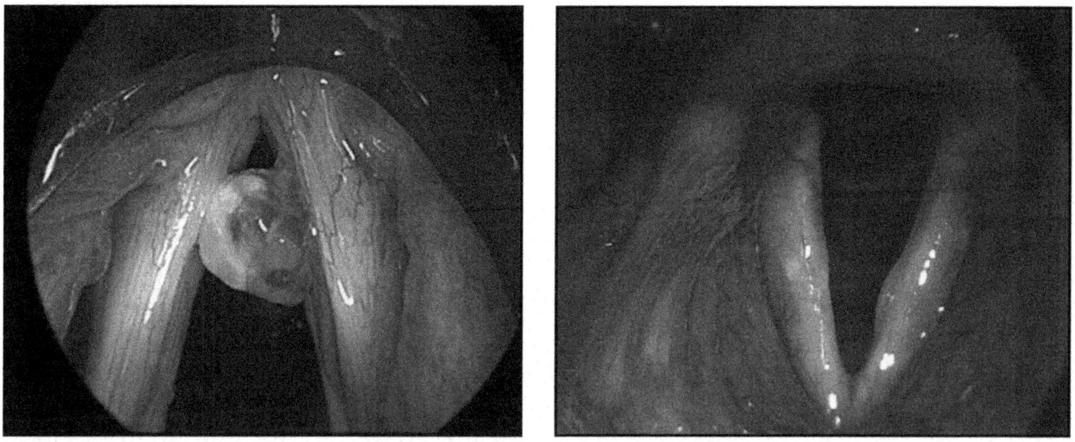

A B

Figure 3–2. A. Right hemorrhagic vocal fold polyp. B. Left vocal fold broad-based polyp.

Vocal fold polyps can interfere with glottic closure if they are located on the medial surface of the vocal fold. They can also interfere with vocal fold vibration. The presence of a unilateral polyp can lead to diplophonia if the vibrating frequencies of the vocal folds differ. A very large polyp may even cause dyspnea if the polyp ball-valves with inspiration. Patients with vocal fold polyps often complain of hoarseness, breathiness, and decrease in vocal range and loudness (Dursun et al., 2010). Diagnosis of vocal fold polyp is based on the history and stroboscopic laryngeal examination.

Treatment includes voice therapy and/or surgery. In 2007, Cohen and Garrett reported symptom resolution in 50% of patients with vocal fold polyps after a trial of improved vocal hygiene and voice therapy. Disappearance of the polyps was not necessary for symptom resolution. Garrett and Francis (2014) found polyps respond well to improved vocal hygiene and voice therapy and recommend surgical intervention for patients with larger polyps or those who prefer immediate resolution of symptoms. Inadequate symptom resolution with voice therapy alone, especially if symptoms continue to impair the singer's ability to perform, is also an indication for surgical intervention.

Vocal Fold Cyst

Cysts are self-contained sacs of fluid or semisolid substance within the vocal fold. There are two types of vocal fold cysts: mucous retention cysts and epithelial cysts.

Mucous Retention Cysts

The vocal folds contain mucous glands. When a duct of a mucous gland becomes plugged, the mucus is trapped and a mucous retention cyst results. Mucous retention cysts have been attributed to voice overuse, reflux, and upper respiratory infection. Mucous retention cysts often arise from the medial surface of the vocal fold just below the free edge and can be confused with vocal fold nodules. Singers' complaints may be similar to those with vocal fold nodules—rough or harsh voice; vocal fatigue; difficulty with high, soft singing; unreliable voice; and the need for increased effort in singing (Flint et al., 2010, p. 869; Martins, Santana, & Tavares, 2011). Definitive treatment for mucous retention cysts is surgery.

Epithelial Cysts

Epithelial cysts are collections of keratin debris within the vocal fold (Figure 3–3). There are two theories on the origin of epithelial cysts: They are believed to arise either from epithelial cells buried beneath the epithelial layer of the vocal fold prior to birth or following mucosal injury from the burying of epithelial cells that occurs with healing. The cysts can rupture spontaneously and the defect left behind is referred to as a glottic sulcus. Singers with epithelial cyst can experience diplophonia or a sudden transition to poor vocal quality in a specific frequency range. Treatment for epithelial cysts includes surgical excision with postoperative voice rehabilitation (Flint et al., 2010, p. 869; Martins et al., 2011).

Fibrous Mass

A fibrous mass (Figure 3–4) is a collection of amorphous fibrous material within the subepithelial or ligamentous part of the vocal fold.

Diagnosis is suspected based on stroboscopic evaluation when there is a pale, gray lesion within the vocal fold that causes significant reduction in the mucosal wave. Fibrous masses often do not respond to voice therapy and must be surgically excised for resolution. Intraoperatively, the fibrous masses are often found to have indistinct margins with extensions anteriorly and posteriorly within the vocal fold (Rosen et al., 2012).

Reactive Vocal Fold Lesion

A reactive vocal fold lesion arises on the vocal fold in a position directly opposite a unilateral vocal fold lesion (polyp, cyst, or fibrous mass). The shearing forces and mucosal irritation from the unilateral lesion lead to a reactive "callous" formation on the contralateral vocal fold. The paired primary and reactive vocal fold

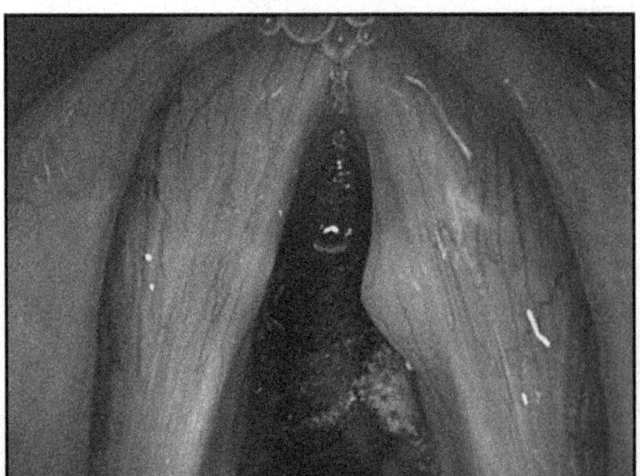

Figure 3–3. *Epithelial cyst in right vocal fold.*

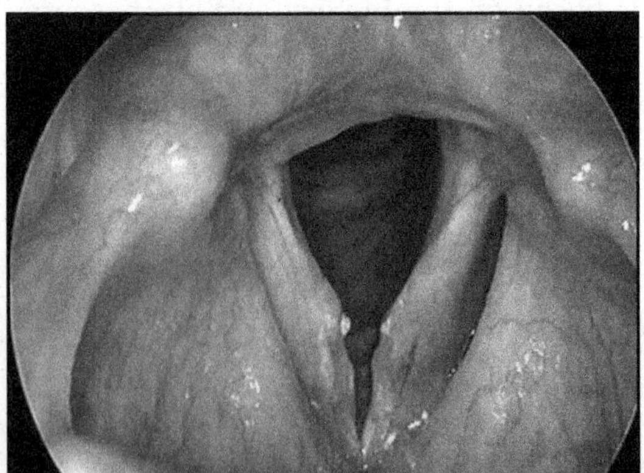

Figure 3–4. *Bilateral fibrous masses with varices.*

lesions can be confused with nodules, which are also bilateral. Vocal fold nodules will appear as mirror images of each other and result in hourglass closure. Stroboscopic exam for reactive vocal fold lesions may be notable for a unilateral lesion with a secondary reactive lesion where the primary lesion protrudes from the vocal fold surface and a slight indentation is made in the reactive lesion, giving it a "cup and saucer" or "lock and key" appearance. There is often incomplete closure of the vocal folds. Vibration of the vocal fold with the primary lesion is notably abnormal while the vibratory properties of the vocal fold with the reactive lesion are sometimes relatively spared (Rosen et al., 2012).

The patient may complain of hoarseness, rough voice, breathy voice, and/or vocal fatigue. Treatment should focus on management of the primary lesion. With conservative management of the primary lesion, the reactive lesion often will resolve.

Vocal Fold Sulcus

Vocal fold sulcus (Figure 3–5) is a depression, groove, or furrow in the vocal fold that can be congenital or forms as a consequence of repetitive stress to the vocal folds.

Vocal fold sulcus is caused by loss of the superficial lamina propria. In addition to other traumatic etiologies, a sulcus may result from a ruptured epidermoid cyst as described above. During phonation, the epithelium and superficial lamina propria glide freely over the deeper structures. In the case of vocal fold sulcus, the superficial structures are tethered to the deeper structures, thus limiting their free movement during phonation (Dailey & Ford, 2006). Vocal fold stiffness, and spindle-shaped glottic closure with compensatory hyperfunction may be noted on stroboscopic laryngeal examination (Selleck, Moore, Rutt, Hu, & Sataloff, 2015).

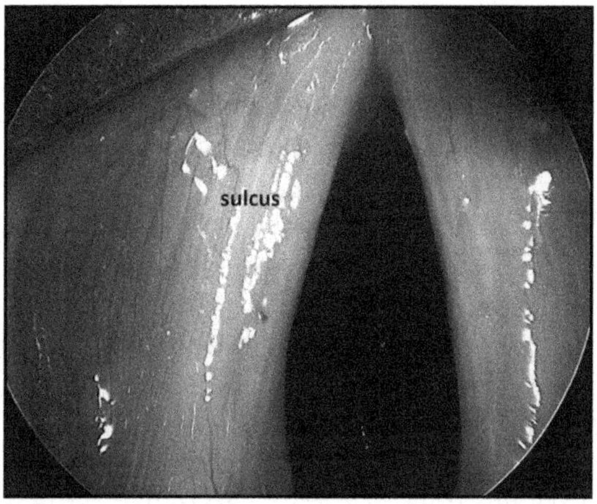

Figure 3–5. Sulcus vocalis in left vocal fold.

Although some individuals may have limited impairment with a sulcus, this type of lesion can be associated with significant impairments, as seen with deep sulci, which tether the epithelium to the vocal ligament (Ferrand, 2012, p. 221). Selleck's study identified hoarseness, vocal fatigue, and loss of range as the top three vocal complaints in patients with symptomatic sulcus (Selleck et al., 2015). Other symptoms include breathiness, loss of volume, vocal breaks, increased effort with phonation, diplophonia, and aphonia (Ferrand, 2012; Flint et al., 2010, pp. 221–222).

Treatment includes preoperative voice rehabilitation, as these patients tend to have significant compensatory vocal hyperfunction. Although voice therapy alone will not improve or resolve the lesion, in some cases it may adequately relieve symptoms so that surgery can be avoided. Definitive surgical treatment requires release of the tethered segment with or without injection of filler to augment the deficient vocal fold (Dailey et al., 2006).

Vocal Fold Scar

Vocal fold scar is the end result of wound healing following damage from infection, external trauma (e.g., intubation), phonotrauma, surgery, or neoplasm. The wound-healing process begins with blood clot formation at the site of injury. Macrophages (a type of white blood cell) arrive to remove damaged tissue. Cytokines (immune system mediators) signal epithelial cells and fibroblasts to the injured area. Fibroblasts are not capable of replacing the native structure of the vocal fold and instead fill the defect with collagen. Initially, the scar is thick and firm but over time it becomes thinner and softer. The collagen of the scar does not have the same vibratory properties as the normal vocal fold tissue. Contraction of the scar results in decreased pliability of the mucosa at the site of the prior vocal fold injury (Dailey & Ford, 2006; Ferrand, 2012, p. 218). Severity of the scar and its impact on vocal functioning are determined by the depth of the injury. Deeper injuries lead to worse scars and often worse vocal outcomes.

Vocal fold scar is related to vocal fold sulcus (discussed above) and their presentation is similar. Treatment for vocal fold scar is as above for vocal fold sulcus.

Varix

A vocal fold varix or capillary ectasia (Figure 3–6) is a tortuous, dilated vessel within the vocal fold. Most varices are located on the superior or medial edge of the phonating surface of the vocal fold and are usually oriented in the long axis of the vocal fold (Hochman, Sataloff, Hillman, & Zeitels, 1999).

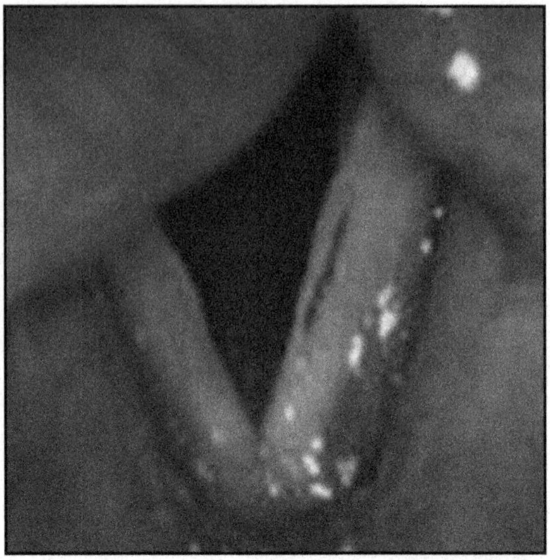

Figure 3–6. *Left vocal fold varix.*

They occur most frequently in female singers but are also seen following acute vocal trauma such as yelling, crying, or coughing (Gökcan & Dursun, 2009). Voice trauma and hormones are thought to be contributing factors, although the true etiology is unknown. It has been suggested that repetitive stress (such as that occurring with singing) leads to angiogenesis, formation of new blood vessels from preexisting vessels. Varices are also believed to contribute to mucosal edema following heavy voice use, although the mechanism is unclear (Flint et al., 2010, p. 866).

In the singer with varices, the speaking voice may be normal in the absence of mucosal edema. Singers with symptomatic varices may complain of relatively rapid onset of vocal fatigue or symptoms more characteristic of nodules. These symptoms could be related to edema as the varix may have a mass effect resulting in incomplete closure of the vocal folds. Stroboscopy often reveals a vascular lesion of the vocal fold with associated vocal fold stiffness and loss of the mucosal wave (Ferrand, 2012, p. 291). If there is an acute change in the vocal quality with significant dysphonia, a vocal fold hemorrhage (which will be discussed in the next section) may be the cause; therefore, sudden onset of severe dysphonia in the patient with known varix should trigger an immediate laryngeal examination.

Treatment for varices includes improved vocal hygiene and voice therapy. If medically appropriate, pharmacologic agents with known antiplatelet (aspirin, clopidogrel, nonsteroidal anti-inflammatory drugs) or anticoagulant (warfarin, heparin) activity should be stopped (Neely & Rosen, 2000). Asymptomatic varices can be approached conservatively with interval observation. Recurrent hemorrhagic varices can be detrimental to a singing career and often require surgical vaporization with a laser (Gökcan & Dursun, 2009).

Hemorrhage

Rupture of a capillary on the surface or just below the surface of the vocal fold due to aggressive or extensive voice use, coughing, or sneezing can lead to vocal fold hemorrhage (Figure 3–7).

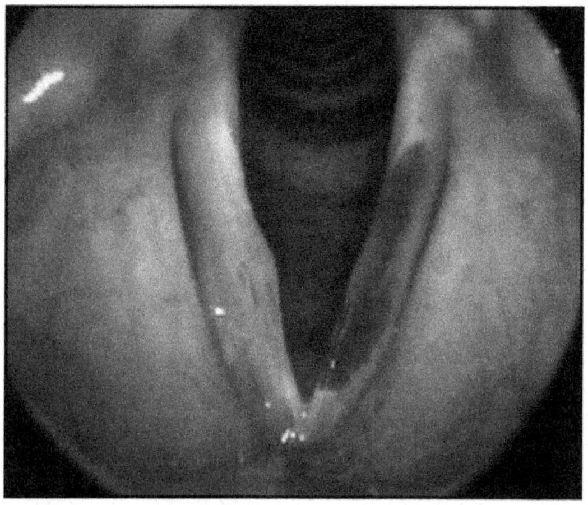

Figure 3–7. *Left vocal fold hemorrhage with right vocal fold fibrous mass.*

During extreme voice use, shearing forces acting on the mucosal surface of the vocal fold may lead to rupture of a superficial vocal fold capillary, resulting in a blush or bruise on the vocal fold surface without alteration in the contour of the medial edge. In contrast, rupture of a deeper capillary with extravasation of blood into the vocal fold leads to stiffness of the vocal fold and potentially an altered contour to the medial surface, called a hemorrhagic polyp. In the early stages, the hemorrhage will appear as a bright red lesion on the surface of the vocal fold and appears similar to a blood blister. As the hemorrhage resolves, the lesion may be in any stage of bruise resolution, and color may gradually fade to orange or yellow (Flint et al., 2010, p. 868).

The presentation of vocal fold hemorrhage varies but is often associated with phonotrauma. Some patients may have a normal speaking voice with only alterations in the extremes of their singing range while others may have sudden onset of severe dysphonia in both the speaking and singing voice. Treatment usually consists of strict voice rest for 1 week to minimize the risk of rebleeding and further damage to the vocal fold and repeat stroboscopy to confirm resolution (Gökcan & Dursun, 2009). If medically appropriate, antiplatelet and anticoagulant medications should be stopped (Neely & Rosen, 2000). Supplements with garlic, ginko, ginseng, ginger, or fish oil can affect coagulation and should be stopped. Most hemorrhages without hemorrhagic polyp will self-resolve within weeks and do not need surgical intervention. Approximately 50% of hemorrhagic polyps will require surgical excision to restore normal function of the vocal fold (Flint et al., 2010, p. 868; Klein, Lehmann, Hapner, & Johns, 2009).

Polypoid Corditis

Polypoid corditis (also called Reinke's edema or bilateral diffuse polyposis) (Figure 3–8) is characterized by diffuse edema and venous congestion that leads to polypoid changes of the vocal folds. Specifically, there is deposition of thick fluid within the superficial layer of the lamina propria, giving it a gelatinous appearance. The vocal folds appear pale with significant edema of the superior and medial surfaces. On rapid inspiration, the edematous tissue is drawn from the superior surface of the vocal fold into the glottis. The vocal fold is noted to have a convex contour.

Poplypoid corditis occurs more frequently in female smokers who use their voices extensively. Laryngopharyngeal reflux has been linked to poplypoid corditis as well. Virilization of the voice (most notable in women) is the most common complaint and there may also be respiratory difficulty and airway obstruction due to the diffuse polyposis (Zeitels et al., 2002).

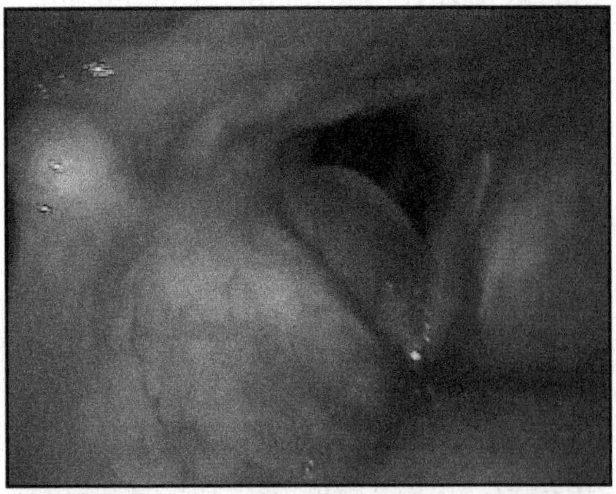

***Figure 3–8.** Right vocal fold poplypoid corditis (Reinke's edema).*

The condition is not naturally reversible. Smoking cessation and control of laryngopharyngeal reflux are encouraged to prevent progression of the condition. Voice rehabilitation can be helpful to optimize vocal behavior (Ferrand, 2012, p. 286; Zeitels et al., 2002). Office-based laser procedures or surgery to reduce the polypoid tissue are treatment options, but the polypoid edema may recur if the inciting behavior is not eliminated (Koszewski, Hoffman, Young, Lai, & Dailey, 2015). Poplypoid corditis edema can result in significant limitations to the singer relative to pitch and dynamic range, vocal quality, and vocal control, which may not be resolved with surgical intervention, as the loss of superficial lamina propria is often considerable. However, for some singers, the raspy or husky quality associated with poplypoid corditis is part of the "vocal signature." Treatment and prognosis will depend on the singer's goals and expectations of vocal function and quality.

Vocal Fold Granuloma

Vocal fold granulomas (Figure 3–9) are benign growths on the vocal fold that occur as part of the wound-healing response following injury.

The posterior glottis consists mostly of cartilage covered by a thin layer of perichondrium and mucosa. Injury leads to an exaggerated healing response, which results in formation of a granuloma. Granulomas often occur following endo-

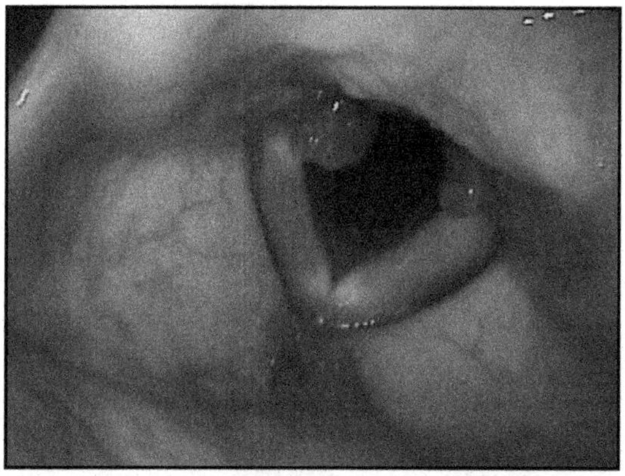

Figure 3–9. *Bilateral vocal process granulomas.*

tracheal intubation where the endotracheal tube rubs on the posterior aspect of the vocal fold (Flint et al., 2010, p. 875). Other sources include phonotrauma, chronic cough, and throat clearing (Zeitels et al., 2002). In the absence of recent endotracheal intubation, some authors assert untreated chronic laryngopharyngeal reflux may be the cause of vocal fold granulomas (Karkos, Thorley, Kaptanis, & Issing, 2011).

On stroboscopic or endoscopic laryngeal evaluation, vocal fold granulomas appear as spherical flesh-colored soft tissue growths arising from the posterior one third of the vocal fold at the vocal process. There may be incomplete glottic closure with large granulomas and significant hyperfunction. Large pedunculated granulomas may be seen flipping above and below the glottic plane with inspiration and expiration (Flint et al., 2010, p. 875). Patients may complain of discomfort or pain over the thyroid cartilage with occasional referred pain to the ipsilateral ear. They may have frequent throat clearing or coughing, and large granulomas may result in significant dysphonia (Zeitels et al., 2002).

Treatment is often conservative with a watchful waiting approach. Aggressive reflux management is undertaken even in patients with no reflux symptoms. Improved vocal hygiene and voice therapy are frequently used in cases where phonotrauma and chronic throat clearing are implicated in the etiology (Ferrand, 2012, p. 290; Zeitels et al., 2002). In most cases, the vocal fold granuloma is pedunculated (on a stalk). With maturation of the granuloma, the stalk becomes thinner and thinner and the granuloma eventually falls off (Flint et al., 2010, p. 875). Steroids may be useful adjuncts in the medical management of vocal fold granulomas (Hillel et al., 2010). Surgery is reserved for cases where the granuloma does not resolve despite months of adequate medical management, when there is impending airway compromise or for cases where the diagnosis is questionable. Recurrence of granulomas is not uncommon (Zeitels et al., 2002).

Leukoplakia

Leukoplakia (Figure 3–10) refers to a white, hyperkeratotic lesion on an epithelial surface.

The vocal folds are covered with nonkeratinizing epithelium so the presence of keratin is abnormal. The annual incidence of vocal fold leukoplakia in the United States is 2 to 10 lesions per 100,000 persons. Histopathologic evaluation of leukoplakia biopsy specimens includes evaluation for dysplasia (early changes in the epithelium that could progress to malignancy). Approximately 50% of the specimens in the study by Isenberg showed no dysplasia (Isenberg, Crozier, & Dailey, 2008).

Fiber-optic laryngoscopy and stroboscopy are useful tools for identifying

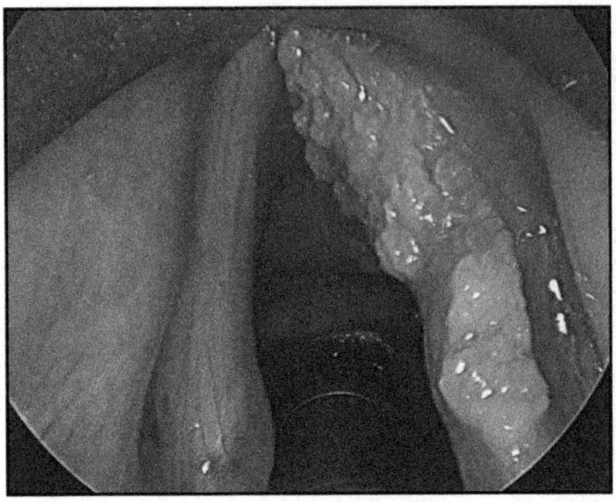

***Figure 3–10.** Right vocal fold leukoplakia with left vocal fold atrophy.*

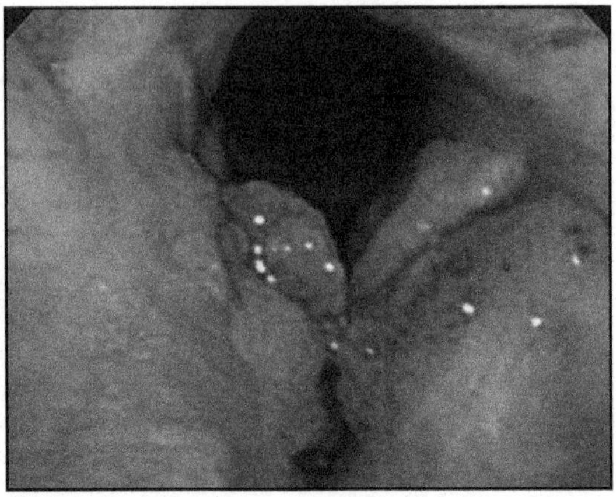

***Figure 3–11.** Bilateral papilloma involving the true and false vocal folds.*

leukoplakia, but they are unreliable in their ability to distinguish benign lesions from those with dysplasia or malignancy. Patients may seek medical evaluation for voice changes, but leukoplakia is often asymptomatic. Initial management is typically conservative with improved vocal hygiene, medical management of laryngopharyngeal reflux, and cessation of tobacco and alcohol use. Close follow-up and biopsy are imperative for high-risk lesions (such as those that progress over time) or in patients with tobacco and alcohol abuse history, history of radiation therapy, or prior head and neck squamous cell carcinoma (cancer) (Zeitels et al., 2002).

Papilloma

Recurrent respiratory papillomatosis (RRP) (Figure 3–11) is a benign condition in which wartlike tumors (papillomas) grow on the epithelial surfaces of the airway. These growths are caused by the human papillomavirus (HPV), with subtypes 6 and 11 being the most common. The vocal folds are the most common site for tumors, but they may also be found in the supraglottis or trachea.

Manifestations of the disease may begin in childhood or adulthood (Zeitels et al., 2002). Onset in childhood is associated with more aggressive and recurrent disease. The papillomas grow on the surface of the vocal folds, typically with a "clusters of grapes" type appearance. Children with RRP present with hoarseness and stridor. The child's airway is relatively narrow, and if RRP is not followed and treated aggressively, the airway can become obstructed. Adult-onset RRP is often less diffuse than childhood onset RRP, and the appearance is a "carpet variant" with a more smooth appearance and projections from the surface. It most often manifests with a rough vocal quality, vocal fatigue, and strain (Flint et al., 2010, pp. 878–879).

Treatment for RRP requires surgical excision in the operating room or office laryngeal laser procedures, but the growths will return, hence the name *recur-*

rent respiratory papillomatosis. Children often require reexcision more frequently, sometimes every few weeks. In adults, excision can range from monthly to once every 2 years. Patients should be followed regularly because in rare cases, RRP can progress to cancer (Flint et al., 2010, p. 878). Adjunctive therapies include intralesional injection with bevacizumab or oral supplements like indole-3-carbinol and cimetidine (Flint et al., 2010, pp. 879–880; Harcourt, Worly, & Leighton, 1999; Rosen & Bryson, 2004; Sidell, Nassar, Cotton, Zeitels, & de Alarcon, 2014; Zeitels et al., 2002). Patients may also benefit from improved vocal hygiene and voice therapy (Ferrand, 2012, p. 274).

Malignant Lesions

Cancer of the larynx (Figure 3–12) is the second most common malignancy of the upper aerodigestive tract, with over 13,000 new diagnoses predicted in the United States in 2015 ("Cancer of the larynx," 2015). There are three laryngeal subsites for laryngeal cancer: supraglottis, glottis, and subglottis. A variety of malignancies may occur in the larynx, but by far squamous cell carcinoma (SCC) is the most common. Fifty to 60% of laryngeal SCC are glottic, 35% to 40% supraglottic, and 5% subglottic ("What are the key statistics," 2015).

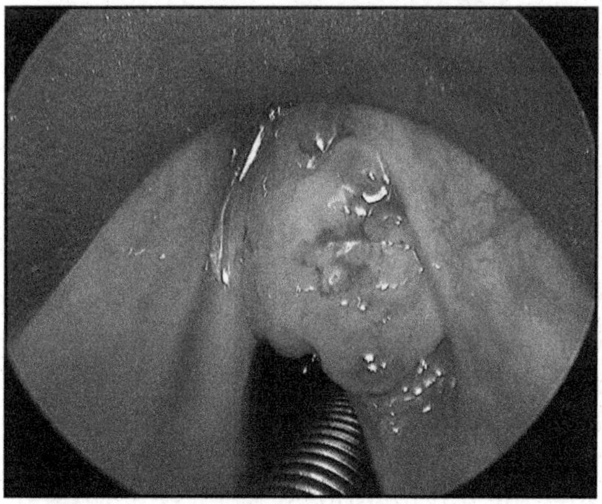

Figure 3–12. ***Squamous cell carcinoma involving the right vocal fold.***

Men are more than three times as likely as women to be diagnosed with laryngeal cancer ("What are the key statistics," 2015). Known risk factors for laryngeal cancer include tobacco and alcohol abuse. Other risk factors such as gastroesophageal reflux and infection with human papillomavirus have been suggested but limited data preclude definitive conclusions at this time (Coca-Pelaz et al., 2013; Torrente et al., 2011). Symptoms of laryngeal cancer depend upon the location of the cancer. Glottic cancers can cause hoarseness, breathiness, reduced volume, increased effort, and pain with phonation. Glottic cancers often present in the early stages owing to their impact on the patient's ability to phonate even with a small tumor. Supraglottic cancers can cause alterations in resonance, dysphagia, dyspnea, stridor, and hemoptysis. Subglottic cancers often present in advanced stages with stridor and dyspnea. Other symptoms for laryngeal cancers include weight loss, otalgia, globus sensation, throat clearing, and neck mass (indicates spread to the regional lymph nodes) (Flint et al., 2010, p. 1493).

Diagnosis of laryngeal cancer is based on the history, physical examination, and biopsy of suspicious lesions. Risk factors for laryngeal cancer, including tobacco and alcohol use, should be elicited. Examination of the upper aerodigestive tract with indirect laryngoscopy via mirror examination or flexible fiberoptic endoscope is of critical importance.

Identification of a suspicious laryngeal lesion necessitates evaluation in the operating room with direct laryngoscopy and esophagoscopy with biopsy for tissue diagnosis. Further evaluation of the extent of the disease is often performed with computed tomography (CT) or positron emission tomography (PET) scans.

Staging of laryngeal cancer is based on the TNM classification by the American Joint Commission on Cancer. T stands for tumor and defines the extent of the tumor. N stands for nodes and defines the involvement of the lymph nodes. M stands for metastasis and defines whether there is distant spread of disease. Higher T or N or presence of metastasis implies a higher stage of disease and often a worse prognosis.

Treatment for laryngeal cancer often utilizes a multidisciplinary team approach, which includes the surgeon, radiation oncologist, medical oncologist, pathologist, radiologist, dentist, speech language-pathologist, social worker, and dietitian. There are a variety of treatments available for laryngeal cancers that include surgery and radiation therapy with or without chemotherapy. The treatment is chosen based on the location and extent of disease, side effects, and outcomes with regard to speech and swallowing as well as the patient's goals of care. The details of the surgical treatment are beyond the scope of this book but may range from simple cordectomy with removal of the membranous vocal fold along with the vocalis muscle to total laryngectomy.

The voice outcomes following treatment of laryngeal cancer are largely dependent upon the size of the tumor, extent of invasion, and the type of treatment rendered. Outcomes for early superficial glottic cancers treated with surgery or radiation alone are comparable and usually good (Greulich, Parker, Lee, Merati, & Misono, 2015). Advanced laryngeal cancers treated with organ preservation (radiation with or without chemotherapy) have been shown to have better voice outcomes than with laryngectomy (Fung et al., 2005; Hillman, Walsh, Wolf, Fisher, & Hong, 1998). Voice complaints following treatment for advanced laryngeal cancer include reduction in loudness, lower pitch, vocal roughness, breathiness, and hoarseness (Stoicheff, 1975). These changes may be attributed to muscle atrophy, dryness of the laryngeal mucosa, and edema. Voice outcomes following laryngectomy depend on the patient's ability to successfully use an artificial electrolarynx or tracheoesophageal speech.

The survival rate for laryngeal cancer depends on the site of the tumor and how early the disease is detected and treated. The prognosis for cancers of the glottis is often good (>90% 5-year survival for Stage I cancers) as they are often detected early due to the presence of hoarseness, triggering patients to seek medical evaluation. Additionally, there are few lymph drainage pathways from the glottis, which limits the spread of the disease. Supraglottic and subglottic tumors are often detected later as they do not present with hoarseness in their early stages. They will also often involve the regional lymph nodes in the neck in later stages, portending a worse prognosis. The 5-year survival is approximately 75% for Stage I supraglottic cancers, and the survival rate decreases for the more advanced stages (Sessions, Lenox, & Spector, 2005). Vermund et al. (1990) report subglottic tumors of all stages have worse prognoses.

Obviously, malignant lesions involving the phonation system can present dire consequences relative to the singing voice. Even when the speaking voice is preserved to a level that is functional, singing may be extremely limited or in some cases, impossible. For some singers, surviving a life-threatening cancer may lead them to readjust their perspective on the importance of singing, but for others, the loss or reduction of singing activities may be devastating. Whenever possible, rehabilitation therapy should be considered as soon as feasible to maximize vocal function and optimize compensation for altered anatomy.

Subglottic Stenosis

Subglottic stenosis (Figure 3–13) refers to the narrowing of the airway between the glottis and the first tracheal ring. This area is naturally the narrowest and least expandable part of the airway.

Subglottic stenosis can be congenital or acquired (Ferrand, 2012, pp. 250–251; Flint et al., 2010, p. 2870). The degree of stenosis is graded using the Myer-Cotton system, which characterizes the stenosis according to the percent obstruction of the subglottic lumen (Myer, O'Connor, & Cotton, 1994).

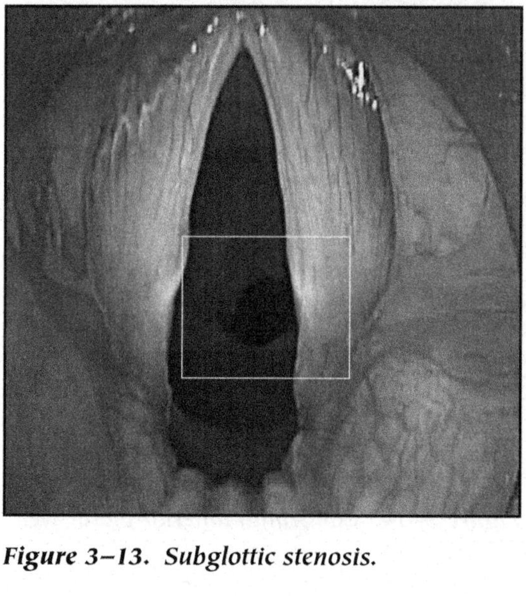

Figure 3–13. Subglottic stenosis.

Congenital subglottic stenosis (CSS) is defined as a subglottic diameter less than 4 mm in a full-term infant or 3.0 to 3.5 mm in a premature infant. The infant should not have a history of intubation or other acquired cause of subglottic stenosis when diagnosing CSS. CSS can be membranous or cartilaginous. In membranous CSS, the epithelial lining of the subglottic area is thickened, whereas in cartilaginous CSS, the cricoid is thickened. Symptoms and timing of presentation can vary depending on the severity of the stenosis. In cases of mild stenosis, symptoms may only be present when the patient experiences an upper respiratory tract infection, leading to edema of the airways. With more severe stenosis, symptoms may be persistent. Dyspnea, tachypnea, cyanosis, biphasic stridor, a hoarse weak cry, and failure to thrive are symptoms of CSS. Treatment of CSS depends on the severity of symptoms. Relatively asymptomatic infants can be observed as most children outgrow the problem. For more severe cases, surgical intervention is the mainstay of treatment (Flint et al., 2010, pp. 2913–2914). The details of surgical treatment are beyond the scope of this chapter.

Acquired subglottic stenosis (ASS) can occur in children and adults and can be caused by infection, laryngopharyngeal reflux, trauma, inflammatory conditions, radiation, or endotracheal intubation. By far, the most common cause of ASS is endotracheal intubation (Garnett, 2014). As mentioned previously, the subglottic area is the narrowest part of the airway and is not very compliant due to the complete cricoid ring. Pressure from the endotracheal tube causes edema and inflammation of the mucosa and cricoid cartilage. Inflammation of the cricoid causes it to weaken. As the subglottic area heals, it scars and the weakened cartilage and thickened scarred mucosa narrow the airway (Flint et al., 2010, pp. 2914–2915). With advances in the care of premature infants, more and more children are being diagnosed with ASS following prolonged periods of intubation for respiratory failure in the postnatal period (Johnson, Rutter, Cotton, Vijayasekeran, & White, 2008).

Diagnosis of CSS and ASS is made via flexible laryngoscopy, direct laryngoscopy with tracheoscopy in the operating room, or CT scan of the neck. The degree of stenosis is characterized by the percent narrowing of the lumen as well as the length of the narrowed segment. Pulmonary function tests may also be helpful to quantify the impact of the stenosis on inspiratory and expiratory function.

Other causes of ASS include uncontrolled reflux, granulomatosis polyangitis (formerly Wegener granulomatosis), sarcoidosis, and amyloidosis. Idiopathic subglottic stenosis is the cause in 5% of cases and is most commonly seen in women in the third to fifth decades in whom CSS and other causes of ASS have been eliminated (Damrose, 2008). Patients will often report progressive dyspnea and have likely been treated for asthma without improvement in symptoms. Other symptoms include stridor and noisy breathing. Endoscopic evaluation reveals a short segment (<2 cm) of circumferential narrowing of the subglottis (Liberman & Mathisen, 2009).

Treatment of subglottic stenosis includes medical management of reflux as this may incite ongoing edema and inflammation in the already narrowed subglottic tissues. Subglottic stenosis in an asymptomatic patient does not require surgery. Surgical treatments vary depending on the severity of stenosis and can range from balloon dilation of the stenotic segment to laryngotracheal reconstruction (Hseu, Benninger, Haffey, & Lorenz, 2014; Yamamoto, Monnier, Holtz, & Jaquet, 2014).

Anterior Glottic Web

Anterior glottic webs can be congenital (Figure 3–14) or acquired. Congenital anterior glottic webs are rare and compromise approximately 5% of all congenital laryngeal abnormalities. They are caused by failed resorption of the epithelial membrane covering the developing laryngotracheal lumen during embryogenesis.

Acquired anterior glottic webs are more common than congenital glottic webs and result from surgery, trauma, or intubation injury to the anterior com-

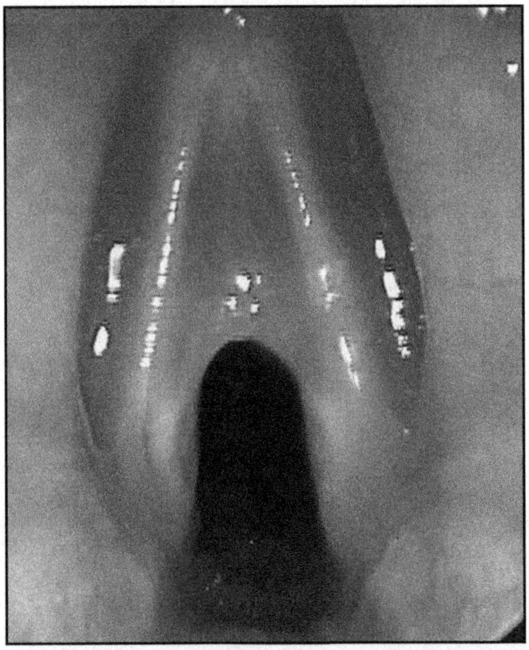

Figure 3–14. Congenital anterior glottic web.

missure. Anterior glottic webs can cause varying degrees of dysphonia and airway obstruction depending on their thickness and the length of vocal fold involved (Flint et al., 2010, pp. 2869–2870).

Treatment for anterior glottic webs is surgical. Thin anterior glottic webs with limited vocal fold involvement causing minimal dysphonia and no respiratory compromise can be observed. As anterior glottic webs effectively decrease the length of the vocal folds, pitch may be overall increased as a result, and ability to lower pitch may be compromised. Anterior glottic webs with involvement along the full length of the vocal folds will often cause severe dysphonia and respiratory compromise and a tracheostomy may be required (Flint et al., 2010, pp. 2869–2870; Rosen & Simpson, 2008, pp. 159–164).

INFLAMMATORY CONDITIONS AFFECTING VOICE

Acute Laryngitis

Acute laryngitis is an infection or inflammation of the larynx caused by viral, bacterial, or fungal pathogens. Viral laryngitis is often attributed to infection with the common cold viruses, rhinovirus and coronavirus. Direct inflammation of the pharynx and laryngeal mucosa from the viral infection as well as irritation due to postnasal drainage leads to symptoms. Examination reveals a pink or red color of the pharyngeal and laryngeal mucosa. Infection may cause throat discomfort and transient loss of voice. The infection is usually self-limited and treatment includes supportive care, hydration, and voice rest (Flint et al., 2010, p. 884). In severe cases, oral steroids can be helpful to hasten recovery but should be used with caution in patients with dilated varices due to risk of hemorrhage from voice use in an inflamed state.

One exception is viral croup or laryngotracheobronchitis, a viral illness caused by infection with respiratory viruses such as parainfluenza virus, respiratory syncytial virus, and rhinovirus. Children with croup can have varying presentations. Those with a barky cough, hoarseness, and fever may be managed conservatively while those with stridor, intercostal retractions, and increased work of breathing need urgent evaluation and stabilization of their airway (Petrocheilou et al., 2014).

Epiglottitis, a bacterial infection of the epiglottis, is a serious upper respiratory infection characterized by acute onset of fever, "hot potato voice," odynophagia, drooling, stridor, and increased work of breathing. In severe cases, the disease can be fatal if the airway is not protected. Widespread vaccination in children against *Haemophilus influenzae* type b has significantly reduced the number of cases of epiglottitis but it has not been eliminated (Guardiani, Bliss, & Harley, 2010).

The most frequent cause of acute fungal laryngitis is *Candida albicans*, an organism normally found in the upper aerodigestive tract. *Candida* coexists with multiple other bacteria in the upper aerodigestive tract. Under normal conditions, the *Candida* population is kept in relative balance to the coexisting flora. Conditions that promote disruption of this balance include the use of antibiotics and use of inhaled steroids, which decrease the local immunity of the laryngeal mucosa as well as systemic immunosuppression (Mehanna, Kuo, Chaplin, Taylor, & Morton, 2004).

NEUROLOGIC VOICE DISORDERS

Vocal Fold Paralysis/Paresis

Vocal fold paresis and paralysis both describe a loss of motion of the vocal fold. They are caused by central nervous system disorders such as Arnold-Chiari malformation, synringobulbia and stroke, and by peripheral nervous system disorders with injury of the recurrent laryngeal nerve (RLN) or superior laryngeal nerve (SLN). Vocal fold paresis indicates the partial immobility of the vocal fold's muscles from incomplete denervation of the RLN or SLN. Vocal fold paralysis indicates complete immobility of the vocal fold's muscles, which results from complete denervation of the vagus nerve or its laryngeal branches as proven by electromyography (EMG) (Figure 3–15).

There are a number of causes of vocal fold paresis, including trauma, viral illness, idiopathic, tumor, and neurologic or medical disease. Trauma is often related to surgical procedures such as thyroidectomy, anterior cervical spine surgery, cardiothoracic procedures, or from endotracheal intubation (Chandrasekhar et al., 2013; Morpeth & Williams, 2000; Strychowsky, Rukholm, Gupta, & Reid, 2014). Tumors occurring anywhere along the course of the recurrent nerve, from the skull base to the chest, may lead to vocal fold paresis (Kang et al., 2013). Rare cases of neurologic disorders such as Parkinson disease and multiple sclerosis causing vocal cord immobility have been reported in the literature (Qayyum, Mierzwa, See, Sharma, & Montgommery, 2005; Rontal, Rontal, Wald, & Rontal, 1999). If the cause of the paresis is not clear from the history (such as a recent surgery), further workup including imaging is necessary. Up to one third of patients will have idiopathic vocal fold paresis. This is a diagnosis of exclusion and is only assigned after thorough evaluation to determine the cause of the vocal fold paresis has been undertaken and proven to be negative (Dworkin & Treadway, 2009).

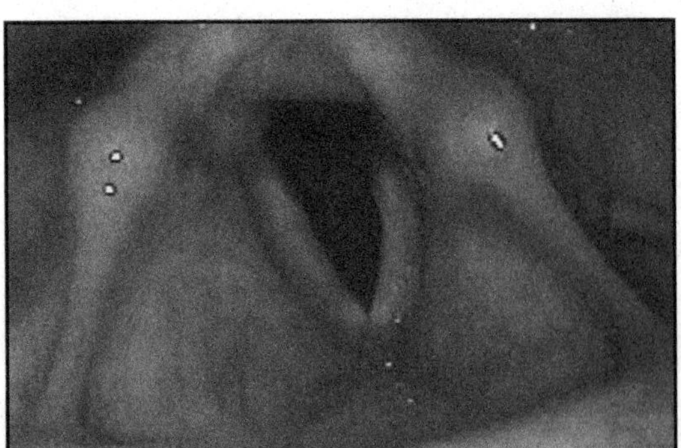

***Figure 3–15.** Left vocal fold paralysis showing foreshortening and bowing on the left vocal fold.*

Patients with vocal fold paresis or paralysis may present with a weak, breathy, hoarse, and strained vocal quality. They often complain of vocal fatigue due to incomplete glottic closure, which requires higher subglottic pressures against the incompetent glottic valve. Maximum phonation time is also reduced. Patients may also complain of dysphagia, which manifests as coughing, choking, or feeling strangled especially with liquids (Ferrand, 2012, p. 308; Flint et al., 2010, p. 843). The lower viscosity of liquids allows them to quickly traverse the glottic gap and enter the airway.

Fiber-optic laryngoscopy or stroboscopy is used to diagnose vocal fold paresis or paralysis. Adjunctive studies such as EMG and CT scan can be used in the evaluation as indicated above. Evaluations of swallowing function, including barium swallow and modified barium swallow, are ordered when there is concern for aspiration. Treatment is not necessary if the patient's voice is functional and he or she is not aspirating. Voice therapy is used to reduce hyperfunction and may improve the vocal quality. Surgical vocal fold augmentation with injection of collagen or fat or medialization thyroplasty improves glottic closure, can restore the voice, and minimize or resolve dysphagia (Misono & Merati, 2012). Laryngeal reinnervation is another procedure for rehabilitating vocal paralysis. Although there are various techniques, a common intervention involves connecting a donor nerve to the recurrent laryngeal nerve, which controls vocal fold motion. Although vocal fold motion is not restored, improved muscle bulk and vocal fold position can be achieved, leading to improved vocal fold closure and improved vocal quality. Because this process can take 4 to 6 months to provide noticeable benefit, a temporary vocal fold injection is frequently performed to improve voice while waiting for the effects of the reinnervation (Aynehchi, McCoul, & Sundaram, 2010; Paniello, Edgar, Kallogjeri, & Piccirillo, 2011).

Spontaneous recovery of vocal fold paralysis may occur if the RLN is intact. If the nerve is going to recover function, it most often occurs within 1 year following the injury or onset of paralysis (Woodson, 2008). In cases where there is no recovery of nerve function, the thyroarytenoid muscle will atrophy due to lack of neurologic stimulation. The vocal fold will assume a bowed appearance and there may be further impairment of glottic closure.

Prognosis in the singer is variable, depending on the affected nerve, position of the vocal fold, and degree of nerve impairment. See Chapter 12 for further discussion of vocal fold paralysis/paresis and singing.

Spasmodic Dysphonia

Spasmodic dysphonia (SD) is a neurologic disorder that causes involuntary laryngeal spasm that produces voice changes. Spasmodic dysphonia is a focal dystonia akin to blepharospasm or involuntary eye twitching. There are two main types of laryngeal dystonia. Adductor spasmodic dysphonia (AD-SD) causes the majority of SD and results in the vocal folds being pressed together during speaking of voiced phonemes, which leads to a strangled or strained vocal quality. Abductor spasmodic dysphonia (AB-SD) is less common and causes the vocal folds to be pulled away from one another with voiceless consonants, which leads to a breathy or weak vocal quality (Ludlow, 2011).

Botulinum toxin type A (Botox) produced by the bacterium *Clostridium botulinum* has replaced surgery for the treatment of SD. In patients with AD-SD, injection of Botox through the cricothyroid membrane into the thyroarytenoid-vocalis complex has been demonstrated to improve speaking to 60% to 100% of normal function. The duration of the effect was 3 to 4 months. Side effects following injection include breathy dysphonia for up to 2 weeks and sore throat (Flint et al., 2010, p. 839). For patients with AB-SD, injection of Botox into the posterior cricoarytenoid muscle produces improvement in symptoms, typically up to 70% of baseline. Adverse effects of Botox treatment include mild dysphagia without aspiration and mild stridor on exertion (Blitzer, Brin, & Stewart, 1998; Flint et al., 2010, p. 839). See Chapter 12 for discussion of SD and the singer.

Vocal Tremor

Tremor is an involuntary, purposeless, rhythmic movement of a part of the body. There is a 6- to 8-Hz shaking of the head, hands, and/or wavering voice, and this is termed *essential tremor*. Of those with essential tremor, approximately 10% to 20% have vocal tremor (Lebrun, Devreux, Rousseau, & Darimont, 1982). The involuntary contraction of vocal muscles can produce rhythmic variations in pitch and loudness. This fluctuation in the voice is similar to a singer's vibrato but occurs during speech as well as singing. Although pharmacologic therapies have previously been thought to be unsuccessful for tremor (Flint et al., 2010, p. 841), propranolol may be a useful noninvasive treatment for some patients with vocal tremor (Justicz et al., 2015). Surgery, including thalamotomies and implantation of thalamic nucleus stimulators, has been described but is not frequently used (Siegfried & Lippitz, 1994). Recently, Botox injection into the offending muscles has shown the most promise. The sternohyoid and sternothyroid muscles, which raise and lower the position of the larynx within the airway, have been shown to be the most tremulous. Injection of Botox into these muscles has been shown to minimize the up and down motion of the larynx, leading to a more smooth vocal quality (Gurey, Sinclair, & Blitzer, 2013). See Chapter 12 for discussion of vocal tremor and the singer.

Vocal Fold Atrophy

Atrophy of laryngeal structures (Figure 3–16) can have significant impact on the voice.

Atrophy related to loss of innervation is described in the vocal fold paralysis section above. Degenerative changes in the vocal fold epithelium, lamina propria,

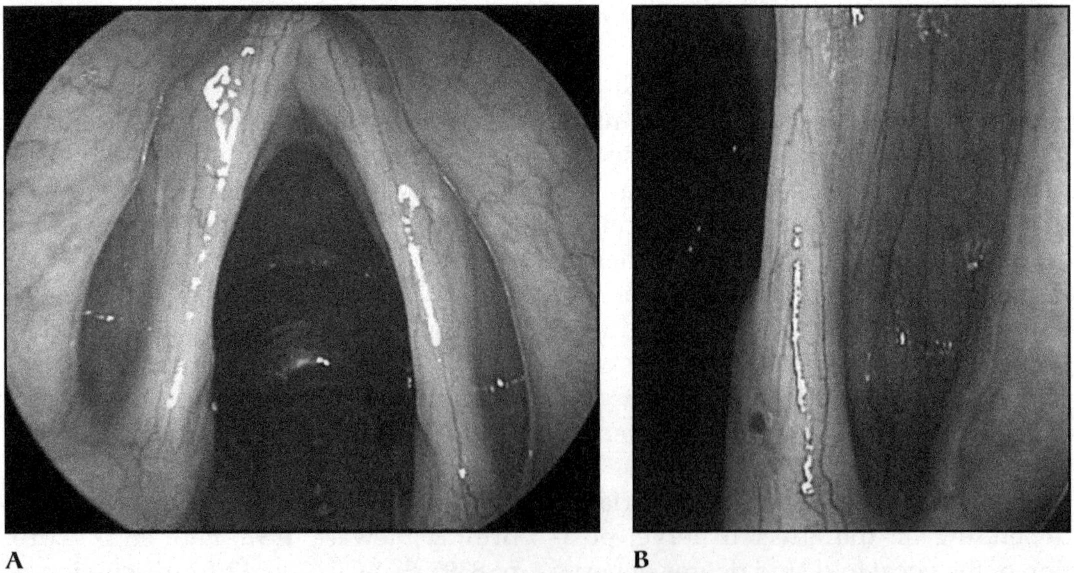

A B

Figure 3–16. ***A.*** *Bilateral vocal fold atrophy showing bowing of the vocal folds.* ***B.*** *Right vocal fold atrophy showing thinning in the vertical dimension of the vocal fold.*

and thyroarytenoid muscle occur with aging and are referred to as presbyphonia. The epithelium thickens in females and there is progressive loss of mucous glands in both sexes. The thick, dry epithelium interferes with normal vocal fold vibration. Changes in the organization of collagen and elastic fibers and the amount of hyaluronic acid in the lamina propria make it more stiff (Martins, Gonçalvez, Pessin, & Branco, 2014). Atrophy of the thyroarytenoid muscle and decreases in the speed, force, and strength of muscle contractions cause glottic incompetence (Baker, Ramig, Luschei, & Smith, 1998).

Stroboscopic exam of the aging larynx often reveals decreased vibratory motion of the vocal folds, bilateral atrophy, and glottic insufficiency. There can be compensatory hyperfunction. Jitter is more frequent in the aging population, especially in males (Benjamin, 1981). In men, the fundamental frequency increases from ages 60 to 80 (Hollien & Shipp, 1972). Vocal fold edema seen in some women is felt to be related to postmenopausal endocrine changes. This along with the lowering of the laryngeal position within the neck that occurs with aging leads to progressive lowering of the fundamental frequency and roughness of the voice in women (Mueller, Sweeney, & Baribeau, 1984). See Chapter 17 for in-depth discussion of age-related voice changes and the singer.

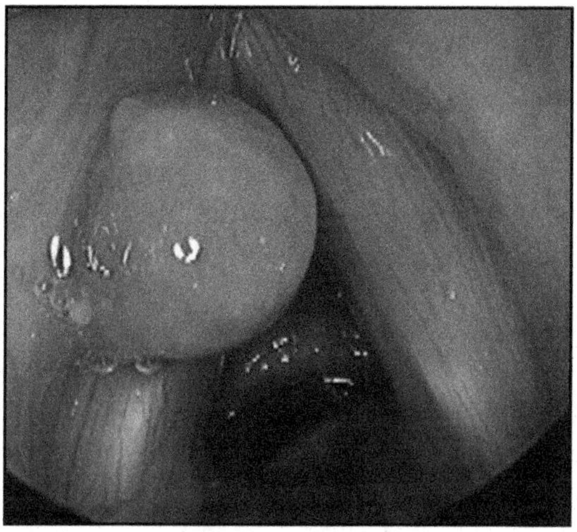

Figure 3–17. Intubation injury causing membranous granuloma left vocal fold.

TRAUMA/INJURY

Intubation Injury

Despite advances in the design of endotracheal tubes and intubation equipment, intubation-related laryngeal injury is not uncommon (Figure 3–17). Acute complications of intubation, including laryngeal mucosal injury; vocal fold hematoma, laceration, or avulsion; and arytenoid dislocation, have been reported. Postoperative hoarseness following short-term intubation (less than 4 hours) is reported to be as high as 69% (Mendels et al., 2012). Complications following long-term intubation (greater than 48 hours) are reported in approximately 90% of patients and include erythema, edema, and ulceration of the laryngeal mucosa and vocal folds in the initial stages progressing to vocal fold granuloma, pressure necrosis of the posterior commissure, interarytenoid scarring, posterior glottic stenosis, subglottic stenosis, and neuropraxia of the laryngeal nerves (Thomas et al., 1995).

There is evidence that larger endotracheal tube size correlates with worse vocal fold mobility (Colton House, Noordzij, Murgia, & Langmore, 2011). Long-term sequela of intubation is seen in approximately 10% of previously intubated patients (Thomas et al., 1995). Singers and occupational voice users should discuss the importance of their voice use with their anesthesia team and ask that experienced personnel perform the intubation and may request that a smaller endotracheal tube to be used. Although not risk free, a laryngeal mask airway (LMA) that sits above and does not pass through the vocal folds is also an alternative that can be discussed with anesthesiologists.

Patients may present with complaints of hoarseness, breathiness, globus sensation, dyspnea, and stridor in the postextubation period. Fiber-optic laryngoscopy or stroboscopy may reveal vocal fold immobility, vocal fold granuloma, and posterior or subglottic stenosis. Vocal fold immobility, vocal fold granuloma, and subglottic stenosis are addressed in other sections of this chapter. Posterior glottic stenosis will be addressed here.

The single most common cause of posterior glottic stenosis is intubation injury. The posterior glottis is the most susceptible site to intubation injury because the endotracheal tube rests in this location. Risk factors for posterior glottic stenosis include large endotracheal tubes, repeated intubation, and endotracheal tube motion. The presence of the endotracheal tube causes ulceration of the posterior glottic mucosa and cartilage. Granulation tissue forms and inflammation leads to fibrosis or scarring. Progression of the scar can cause tethering of the vocal folds with limited adduction and abduction. Surgical management is beyond the scope of this book, but all patients with respiratory compromise must undergo emergent tracheostomy (Lahav, Shoffel-Havakuk, & Halperin, 2015).

Arytenoid Dislocation and Subluxation

Arytenoid dislocation and subluxation are rare laryngeal injuries caused by endotracheal intubation (most common), laryngeal mask airway, esophagoduodeonoscopy, and external laryngeal trauma. Arytenoid dislocation is defined as displacement of the arytenoid from the cricoarytenoid joint, whereas arytenoid subluxation is displacement of the arytenoid within the cricoarytenoid joint. Although they are distinct injuries, they have similar clinical appearance and are treated in the literature as a single clinical entity. The estimated incidence of arytenoid dislocation following endotracheal intubation is less than 0.1% (Lee, Park, & Welham, 2014). Both arytenoid dislocation and subluxation lead to reduced mobility of the ipsilateral vocal fold and incomplete glottic closure, similar to what is seen with vocal fold paresis (Teng, Wang, & Lin, 2014).

Patients will often relay a history of recent endotracheal intubation or external laryngeal trauma. They will present with breathy dysphonia and may complain of dysphagia due to the incomplete glottic closure. Evaluation includes indirect fiber-optic laryngoscopy or stroboscopy, CT scan of the neck, and laryngeal EMG. EMG evaluates the integrity of the recurrent laryngeal nerve and is useful to differentiate arytenoid dislocation from vocal fold paralysis. The recurrent laryngeal nerve is expected to be fully functioning with arytenoid dislocation, whereas total disruption of nerve function is seen with vocal fold paralysis (Norris & Schweinfurth, 2011).

Treatment of arytenoid dislocation is via direct laryngoscopy and endoscopic closed reduction in the operating room. Lee et al. (2014) report immediate recovery of arytenoid motion in approximately 85% of patients and statistically significant improvements in vocal functioning in all patients. Three patients in their study did not have recovery of arytenoid motion, and this was attributed to the long interval from injury to intervention (greater than 1 year).

External Laryngeal Trauma

External laryngeal trauma is rare but potentially life-threatening if not promptly recognized and treated. The larynx is relatively exposed given its anterior and superficial location in the neck and is therefore susceptible to injury. Additionally, the laryngeal cartilage calcifies with age and lends itself to an increased likelihood of fracture when stress is applied. The estimated incidence of external laryngeal trauma is between 1 in 5,000 to 1 in 30,000 emergency room visits (Bent, Silber, & Porubsky, 1993; Schaefer, 1992). Mechanisms of injury are classified into blunt or penetrating. Blunt external laryngeal trauma may result from motor vehicle accident where the hyperextended neck is thrust forward to contact the steering wheel, forcing the larynx posteriorly against the vertebral bodies. Other mechanisms of injury include clothesline injury, sports injuries, strangling, and hanging. Penetrating trauma includes gunshot wounds and knife injuries. Blunt trauma used to far outweigh the incidence of penetrating trauma but with advances in motor vehicle safety (seat belts and air bags), this difference has been reduced (Schaefer, 2014).

Symptoms of laryngeal trauma include hoarseness, dysphagia, pain, dyspnea, and hemoptysis (Flint et al., 2010, p. 935; Schaefer, 2014). Signs of laryngeal trauma include respiratory distress, stridor, abrasion, ecchymosis, hematoma, or laceration of the anterior neck skin; bubbling from an open neck wound; subcutaneous emphysema; tracheal deviation; and exposed laryngeal cartilage (Randall, Rudmik, Ball, & Bosch, 2014; "Resident Manual of Trauma," 2012). Initial management involves securing the airway. In patients with acute or impending respiratory distress, endotracheal intubation or tracheostomy must be performed. Endotracheal intubation should not be performed in patients with suspected laryngotracheal separation. Once the airway is secured, a CT scan of the neck and direct laryngoscopy in the operating room should be performed. In patients with stable airways, examination should include indirect flexible fiber-optic evaluation of the upper aerodigestive tract as well as a CT scan of the neck. Potential findings include laryngeal fracture, arytenoid dislocation, vocal fold immobility, mucosal injury, hematoma, and edema. Patients with concerning findings on endoscopic evaluation or CT scan should be taken to the operating room for direct laryngoscopy (Schaefer, 2014). Further surgical management of laryngeal injuries is beyond the scope of this book.

All patients with significant laryngeal trauma should be followed in the outpatient setting. Prognosis depends on the extent of the injury and the structures involved. Long-term morbidity is related to laryngeal stenosis, dysphonia, and aspiration (Flint et al., 2010, p. 937). When this type of injury occurs in a singer, prognosis for recovering voice depends on the extent and severity of the injury.

MUSCLE TENSION DYSPHONIA

Muscle tension dysphonia (MTD) is a maladaptive and inefficient pattern of voice production resulting from a combination of poor breath support and unnecessary muscle tension. There is hypercontraction of the intrinsic and extrinsic laryngeal muscles as well as the facial, jaw, neck, and shoulder muscles (Van Houtte, Van Lierde, & Claeys, 2011). Muscle tension dysphonia can be primary or secondary. The cause of primary MTD is often multifactorial and includes stress-induced muscular tension, vocal overuse, and poor vocal technique in the absence of an underlying vocal fold lesion. Secondary MTD refers to tension resulting from compensatory mechanisms due to an underlying insult to vocal production (Belafsky, Postma, Reulbach, Holland, & Koufman, 2002; Lee & Son, 2005).

Symptoms of MTD may vary drastically but patients may have pain and tenderness on palpation of the anterior neck structures, hoarseness, increased vocal effort, vocal strain, pitch breaks, and reduced range. Patients may also complain of throat tightness, throat tickling, and globus sensation (Mathieson et al., 2009).

Evaluation of the patient with suspected MTD is multifaceted and includes flexible laryngoscopy or stroboscopy; observation of the patient's posture, breathing patterns, laryngeal motion with phonation, and changes in vocal quality with various movements of the tongue, jaw, or head; and palpation of the anterior neck structures (Ferrard, 2010, p. 356). Laryngoscopy or stroboscopy will reveal anterior to posterior compression of the true vocal folds and medial compression of the false vocal folds with phonation (Figure 3–18).

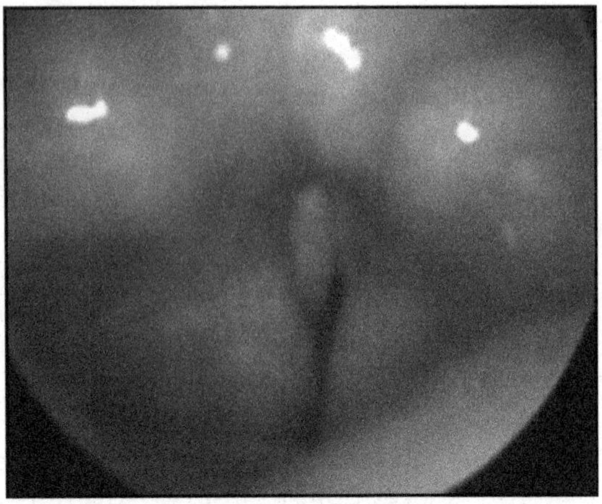

***Figure 3–18.** Muscle tension dysphonia showing adduction of the false vocal folds.*

There may be underlying vocal fold pathology in some cases. Observation of the patient's breathing pattern may reveal poor breath support (Altman, Atkinson, & Lazarus, 2005). Tenderness and tension in the anterior neck muscles and elevation of the larynx at rest suggest MTD.

The diagnosis of MTD is clinical and adjunctive studies are not necessary. Treatment is conservative and includes improved vocal hygiene and vocal retraining with a speech-language pathologist. Voice therapy, including relaxation techniques, laryngeal massage, breathing strategies, and vocal function exercises, is also effective (Mathieson et al., 2009). Improvements in voice handicap index (VHI) scores have been reported with voice therapy compared to matched control groups without voice therapy (Craig et al., 2015).

REFERENCES

Akif Kiliç, M., Okur, E., Yildirim, I., & Güzelsoy, S. (2004). The prevalence of vocal fold nodules in school-age children. *International Journal of Pediatric Otorhinolaryngology, 68*(4), 409–412.

Altman, K. W., Atkinson, C., & Lazarus, C. (2005). Current and emerging concepts in muscle tension dysphonia: A 30-month review. *Journal of Voice, 19*(2), 261–267.

Aynehchi, B. B., McCoul, E. D., & Sundaram, K. (2010). Systematic review of laryngeal reinnervation techniques. *Otolaryngology–Head and Neck Surgery, 143*(6), 749–759.

Baker, K. K., Ramig, L. O., Luschei, E. S., & Smith, M. E. (1998).Thyroarytenoid muscle activity associated with hypophonia in Parkinson disease and aging. *Neurology, 51*(6), 1592–1598.

Belafsky, P. C., Postma, G. N., Reulbach, T. R., Holland, B. W., & Koufman, J. A. (2002). Muscle tension dysphonia as a sign of underlying glottal insufficiency. *Otolaryngology–Head and Neck Surgery, 127*(5), 448–451.

Benjamin, B. J. (1981). Frequency variability in the aged voice. *Journals of Gerontology, 36*, 722–726.

Bent, J. P., Silver, J. R., & Porubsky, E. S. (1993). Acute laryngeal trauma: A review of 77 patients. *Archives of Otolaryngology–Head and Neck Surgery, 109*, 441–449.

Blitzer, A., Brin, M. F., & Stewart, C. F. (1998). Botulinum toxin management of spasmodic dysphonia (laryngeal dystonia): A 12-year experience in more than 900 patients. *Laryngoscope, 108*(10), 1435–1441.

Cancer of the larynx. (2015, May 15). Retrieved from http://seer.cancer.gov/statfacts/html/laryn.html

Chandrasekhar, S. S., Randolph, G. W., Seidman, M. D., Rosenfeld, R. M., Angelos, P., Barkmeier-Kraemer, J., . . . Robertson, P. J. (2013). American Academy of Otolaryngology-Head and Neck Surgery. Clinical practice guideline: improving voice outcomes after thyroid surgery. *Otolaryngology–Head and Neck Surgery, 148*(6, Suppl.), S1–37.

Coca-Pelaz, A., Rodrigo, J. P., Takes, R. P., Silver, C. E., Paccagnella, D., Rinaldo, A., . . . Ferlito, A. (2013). Relationship between reflux and laryngeal cancer. *Head & Neck, 35*(12), 1814–1818.

Cohen, S. M., & Garrett, C. G. (2007). Utility of voice therapy in the management of vocal fold polyps and cysts. *Otolaryngology–Head and Neck Surgery, 136*(5), 742–746.

Colton House, J., Noordzij, J. P., Murgia, B., & Langmore, S. (2011). Laryngeal injury from prolonged intubation: A prospective analysis of contributing factors. *Laryngoscope, 121*(3), 596–600.

Craig, J., Tomlinson, C., Stevens, K., Kotagal, K., Fornadley, J., Jacobson, B., Garrett, C. G., & Francis, D. O. (2015). Combining voice therapy and physical therapy: A novel approach to treating muscle tension dysphonia. *Journal of Communication Disorders, 58*, 169–178.

Dailey, S. H., & Ford, C. N. (2006). Surgical management of sulcus vocalis and vocal fold scarring. *Otolaryngology Clinics of North America, 39*(1), 23–42.

Damrose, E. J. (2008). On the development of idiopathic subglottic stenosis. *Medical Hypotheses, 71*(1), 122–125.

Dursun, G., Karatayli-Ozgursoy, S., Ozgursoy, O. B., Tezcaner, Z. C., Coruh, I., & Kilic, M. A. (2010). Influence of the macroscopic features of vocal fold polyps on the quality of voice: a retrospective review of 101 cases. *Ear, Nose, & Throat Journal, 89*(3), E12–E17.

Dworkin, J. P., & Treadway, C. (2009). Idiopathic vocal fold paralysis: Clinical course and outcomes. *Journal of the Neurological Sciences, 284*(1–2), 56–62.

Ferrand, C. T. (2012). *Voice disorders: Scope of theory and practice*. NJ: Boston, MA: Pearson.

Flint, P. W., Haughey, B. H., Lund, V. J., Niparko, J. K., Richardson, M. A., Robbins, K. T., & Thomas, J. R. (2010). *Cummings otolaryngology head and neck surgery*. Philadelphia, PA: Mosby Elsevier.

Fung, K., Lyden, T. H., Lee, J., Urba, S. G., Worden, F., Eisbruch, A., . . . Wolf, G. T. (2005). Voice and swallowing outcomes of an organ-preservation trial for advanced laryngeal cancer. *International Journal of Radiation Oncology Biology Physics, 63*(5), 1395–1399.

Garnett, J. (2014). *Subglottic stenosis in adults*. Retrieved from http://emedicine.medscape.com/article/865437-overview#a0102

Garrett, C. G., & Francis, D. O. (2014). Is surgery necessary for all vocal fold polyps? *Laryngoscope, 124*(2), 363–364.

Gökcan, K. M., & Dursun, G. (2015). Vascular lesions of the vocal fold. *European Archives of Otorhinolaryngology, 266*(4), 527–533.

Greulich, M. T., Parker, N. P., Lee, P., Merati, A. L., & Misono, S. (2015). Voice outcomes following radiation versus laser microsurgery for T1 glottic carcinoma: Systematic review and meta-analysis. *Otolaryngology–Head and Neck Surgery, 152*(5), 811–819.

Guardiani, E., Bliss, M., & Harley, E. (2010). Supraglottitis in the era following widespread immunization against *Haemophilus influenzae* type B: Evolving principles in diagnosis and management. *Laryngoscope, 120*(11), 2183–2188.

Gurey, L. E., Sinclair, C. F., & Blitzer, A. (2013). A new paradigm for the management of essential vocal tremor with botulinum toxin. *Laryngoscope, 123*(10), 2497–2501.

Harcourt, J. P., Worley, G., & Leighton, S. E. (1999). Cimetidine treatment for recurrent respiratory papillomatosis. *International Journal of Pediatric Otorhinolaryngology, 51*(2), 109–113.

Hillel, A. T., Lin, L. M., Samlan, R., Starmer, H., Leahy, K., & Flint, P. W. (2010). Inhaled triamcinolone with proton pump inhibitor for treatment of vocal process granulomas: A series of 67 granulomas. *Annals of Otology, Rhinology, & Laryngology, 119*(5), 325–330.

Hillman, R. E., Walsh, M. J., Wolf, G. T., Fisher, S. G., & Hong, W. K. (1998). Functional outcomes following treatment for advanced laryngeal cancer. Part I: Voice preservation in advanced laryngeal cancer. Part II: Laryngectomy rehabilitation: the state of the art in the VA System. Research Speech-Language Pathologists. Department of Veterans Affairs Laryngeal Cancer Study Group. *Annals of Otology, Rhinology, & Laryngology Supplement, 172*, 1–27.

Hochman, I., Sataloff, R. T., Hillman, R. E., & Zeitels, S. M. (1999). Ectasias and varices of the vocal fold: Clearing the striking zone. *Annals of Otology, Rhinology, & Laryngology, 108*(1), 10–16.

Hollien, H., & Shipp, T. (1972). Speaking fundamental frequency and chronologic age in males. *Journal of Speech, Language, and Hearing Research, 15*, 155–159.

Holmberg, E. B., Hillman, R. E., Hammarberg, B., Södersten, M., & Doyle, P. (2001). Efficacy of a behaviorally based voice therapy protocol for vocal nodules. *Journal of Voice, 15*(3), 395–412.

Hseu, A. F., Benninger, M. S., Haffey, T. M., & Lorenz, R. (2014). Subglottic stenosis: A ten-year review of treatment outcomes. *Laryngoscope, 124*(3), 736–741.

Isenberg, J. S., Crozier, D. L., & Dailey, S. H. (2008). Institutional and comprehensive review of laryngeal leukoplakia. *Annals of Otology, Rhinology, & Laryngology, 117*(1), 74–79.

Johnson, R. F., Rutter, M., Cotton, R., Vijayasekeran, S., & White, D. (2008). Cricotracheal resection in children 2 years of age and younger. *Annals of Otology, Rhinology, & Laryngology, 117*(2), 110–112.

Justicz, N., Hapner, E. R., Josephs, J. S., Boone, B. C., Jinnah, H. A., & Johns, M. M., III. (2015). Comparative effectiveness of propranolol and botulinum for the treatment of essential voice tremor. *Laryngoscope*. Advance online publication. doi:10.1002/lary.25485

Kang, B. C., Roh, J. L., Lee, J. H., Jung, J. H., Choi, S. H., Nam, S. Y., & Kim, S. Y. (2013). Usefulness of computed tomography in the etiologic evaluation of adult unilateral vocal fold paralysis. *World Journal of Surgery, 37*(6), 1236–1240.

Karkos, P. D., Thorley, D., Kaptanis, S., & Issing, W. J. (2011). Transnasal oesophagoscopy, laryngopharyngeal reflux (LPR) and oesophageal pathology: The vocal fold granuloma example and "the granulomas, LPR and Barrett's triad." *Clinical Otolaryngology, 36*(5), 516–517.

Keilmann, A., Biermann, G., & Hörmann, K. (1997). CO_2 laser versus conventional microlaryngoscopy in benign changes of the vocal cords. *Laryngorhinootologie, 76*(8), 484–489.

Klein, A. M., Lehmann, M., Hapner, E. R., & Johns, M. M., III. (2009). Spontaneous resolution of hemorrhagic polyps of the true vocal fold. *Journal of Voice, 23*(1), 132–135.

Koszewski, I. J., Hoffman, M. R., Young, W. G., Lai, Y. T., & Dailey, S. H. (2015). Office-based photoangiolytic laser treatment of Reinke's edema: Safety and voice outcomes. *Otolaryngology–Head and Neck Surgery, 152*(6), 1075–1081.

Lahav, Y., Shoffel-Havakuk, H., & Halperin, D. (2015). Acquired glottic stenosis—the ongoing challenge: A review of etiology, pathogenesis, and surgical management. *Journal of Voice, 29*(5), 646.e1–646.e10.

Lebrun, Y., Devreux, F., Rousseau, J. J., & Darimont, P. (1982). Tremulous speech: A case report. *Folia Phoniatrics (Basel), 34*(3), 134–142.

Lee, E. K., & Son, Y. I. (2005). Muscle tension dysphonia in children: Voice characteristics and outcome of voice therapy. *International Journal of Pediatric Otorhinolaryngology, 69*(7), 911–917.

Lee, S. W., Park, K. N., & Welham, N. V. (2014). Clinical features and surgical outcomes following closed reduction of arytenoid dislocation. *JAMA Otolaryngology–Head and Neck Surgery, 140*(11), 1045–1050.

Liberman, M., & Mathisen, D. J. (2009). Treatment of idiopathic laryngotracheal stenosis.

Seminars in Thoracic Cardiovascular Surgery, 21(3), 278–283.

Lira Luce, F., Teggi, R., Ramella, B., Biafora, M., Girasoli, L., Calori, G., . . . Bussi M. (2014). Voice disorders in primary school teachers. *Acta Otorhinolaryngologica Italica, 34*(6), 412–418.

Ludlow, C. L. (2011). Spasmodic dysphonia: A laryngeal control disorder specific to speech. *Journal of Neuroscience, 31*(3), 793–797.

Martins, R. H., Gonçalvez, T. M., Pessin, A. B., & Branco, A. (2014). Aging voice: Presbyphonia. *Aging Clinical and Experimental Research, 26*(1), 1–5.

Martins, R. H., Santana, M. F., & Tavares, E. L. (2011). Vocal cysts: Clinical, endoscopic, and surgical aspects. *Journal of Voice, 25*(1), 107–110.

Mathieson, L., Hirani, S. P., Epstein, R., Baken, R. J., Wood, G., & Rubin, J. S. (2009). Laryngeal manual therapy: A preliminary study to examine its treatment effects in the management of muscle tension dysphonia. *Journal of Voice, 23*(3), 353–366.

Mehanna, H. M., Kuo, T., Chaplin, J., Taylor, G., & Morton, R. P. (2004). Fungal laryngitis in immunocompetent patients. *Journal of Laryngology & Otology, 118*(5), 379–381.

Mendels, E. J., Brunings, J. W., Hamaekers, A. E., Stokroos, R. J., Kremer, B., & Baijens, L.W. (2012). Adverse laryngeal effects following short-term general anesthesia: A systematic review. *Archives of Otolaryngology–Head and Neck Surgery, 138*(3), 257–264.

Misono, S., & Merati, A. L. (2012). Evidence-based practice: Evaluation and management of unilateral vocal fold paralysis. *Otolaryngology Clinics of North* America, *45*(5), 1083–1108.

Morpeth, J. F., & Williams, M. F. (2000). Vocal fold paralysis after anterior cervical diskectomy and fusion. *Laryngoscope, 110*(1), 43–46.

Mueller, P. B., Sweeney, R. J., & Baribeau, L. J. (1984). Acoustic and morphologic study of the senescent voice. *Ear, Nose, & Throat Journal, 63*, 292–295.

Myer, C. M., III, O'Connor, D. M., & Cotton, R. T. (1994). Proposed grading system for subglottic stenosis based on endotracheal tube sizes. *Annals of Otolology, Rhinology, & Laryngology*, 103(4, Pt 1), 319–323.

Neely, J. L., & Rosen, C. (2000). Vocal fold hemorrhage associated with coumadin therapy in an opera singer. *Journal of Voice, 14*(2), 272–277.

Norris, B. K., & Schweinfurth, J. M. (2011). Arytenoid dislocation: An analysis of the contemporary literature. *Laryngoscope, 121*(1), 142–146.

Ongkasuwan, J., & Friedman, E. M. (2013). Is voice therapy effective in the management of vocal fold nodules in children? *Laryngoscope, 123*(12), 2930–2931.

Paniello, R. C., Edgar, J. D., Kallogjeri, D., & Piccirillo, J. F. (2011). Medialization versus reinnervation for unilateral vocal fold paralysis: A multicenter randomized clinical trial. *Laryngoscope, 121*(10), 2172–2179.

Pedersen, M., & McGlashan, J. (2012). Surgical versus non-surgical interventions for vocal cord nodules. *Cochrane Database Systematic Review, 6*, CD001934.

Pereira, E. R., Tavares, E. L., & Martins, R. H. (2015). Voice disorders in teachers: Clinical, videolaryngoscopical, and vocal aspects. *Journal of Voice, 29*(5), 564–571.

Petrocheilou, A., Tanou, K., Kalampouka, E., Malakasioti, G., Giannios, C., & Kaditis, A. G. (2014). Viral croup: Diagnosis and a treatment algorithm. *Pediatric Pulmonolonary, 49*(5), 421–429.

Qayyum, A., Mierzwa, K., See, M., Sharma, A., & Montgommery, P. Q. (2005). Laser arytenoidectomy for bilateral vocal fold palsy in Parkinson's disease. *Journal of Laryngology & Otology, 119*(10), 831–833.

Randall, D. R., Rudmik, L. R., Ball, C. G., & Bosch, J. D. (2014). External laryngotracheal trauma: Incidence, airway control, and outcomes in a large Canadian center. *Laryngoscope, 124*(4), E123–E123.

Resident Manual of Trauma. (2012). Retrieved from https://www.entnet.org/sites/default/files/Trauma-Chapter-8.pdf

Rontal, E., Rontal, M., Wald, J., & Rontal, D. (1999). Botulinum toxin injection in the treatment of vocal fold paralysis associated with multiple sclerosis: A case report. *Journal of Voice, 13*(2), 274–279.

Rosen, C. A., & Bryson, P. C. (2004). Indole-3-carbinol for recurrent respiratory papillomatosis: Long-term results. *Journal of Voice, 18*(2), 248–253.

Rosen, C. A., & Simpson, B. (2008). *Operative techniques in laryngology*. Berlin, Germany: Springer.

Rosen, C. A., Gartner-Schmidt, J., Hathaway, B., Simpson, C. B., Postma, G. N., Courey, M., & Sataloff, R. T. (2012). A nomenclature paradigm for benign midmembranous vocal fold lesions. *Laryngoscope, 122*(6), 1335–1341.

Schaefer, S. D. (1992). The acute management of external laryngeal trauma: A 27-year experience. *Archives of Otolaryngology–Head and Neck Surgery, 118*, 598–604.

Schaefer, S. D. (2014). Management of acute blunt and penetrating external laryngeal trauma. *Laryngoscope, 124*(1), 233–244.

Selleck, A. M., Moore, J. E., Rutt, A. L., Hu, A., & Sataloff, R. T. (2015). Sulcus vocalis (Type III): Prevalence and strobovideolaryngoscopy characteristics. *Journal of Voice, 29*(4), 507–511.

Sessions, D. G., Lenox, J., & Spector, G. J. (2005). Supraglottic laryngeal cancer: Analysis of treatment results. *Laryngoscope, 115*(8), 1402–1410.

Sidell, D. R., Nassar, M., Cotton, R. T., Zeitels, S. M., & de Alarcon, A. (2014). High-dose sublesional bevacizumab (Avastin) for pediatric recurrent respiratory papillomatosis. *Annals of Otology, Rhinology, & Laryngology, 123*(3), 214–221.

Siegfried, J., & Lippitz, B. (1994). Chronic electrical stimulation of the VL-VPL complex and of the pallidum in the treatment of movement disorders: personal experience since 1982. *Stereotactic & Functional Neurosurgery, 62*(1–4), 71–75.

Stoicheff, M. L. (1975). Voice following radiotherapy. *Laryngoscope, 85*(4), 608–618.

Strychowsky, J. E., Rukholm, G., Gupta, M. K., & Reid, D. (2014). Unilateral vocal fold paralysis after congenital cardiothoracic surgery: A meta-analysis. *Pediatrics, 133*(6), e1708–e1723.

Sulica, L. (2008). The natural history of idiopathic unilateral vocal fold paralysis: Evidence and problems. *Laryngoscope, 118*(7), 1303–1307.

Teng, Y., Wang, H. E., & Lin, Z. (2014). Arytenoid cartilage dislocation from external blunt laryngeal trauma: Evaluation and therapy without laryngeal electromyography. *Medical Science Monitor, 20*, 1496–1502.

Thomas, R., Kumar, E. V., Kameswaran, M., Shamim, A., al Ghamdi, S., Mummigatty, A. P., & Okafor, B. C. (1995). Post intubation laryngeal sequelae in an intensive care unit. *Journal of Laryngology & Otology, 109*(4), 313–316.

Torrente, M. C., Rodrigo, J. P., Haigentz, M., Jr., Dikkers, F. G., Rinaldo, A., Takes, R. P., . . . Ferlito, A. (2011). Human papillomavirus infections in laryngeal cancer. *Head & Neck, 33*(4), 581–586.

Van Houtte, E., Van Lierde, K., & Claeys, S. (2011). Pathophysiology and treatment of muscle tension dysphonia: A review of the current knowledge. *Journal of Voice, 25*(2), 202–207.

Vermund, H., Boysen, M., Brandenburg, J. H., Evensen, J., Jacobsen, A. B., Kaalhus, O., . . . Winther, F. (1990). Primary irradiation, surgery or combined therapy in squamous cell carcinoma of the larynx. A comparison of treatment results from two centers. *Acta Oncologica, 29*(4), 489–503.

What are the key statistics about hypopharyngeal and laryngeal cancers? (2015, May 15). Retrieved from http://www.cancer.org/cancer/laryngealandhypopharyngealcancer/detailedguide/laryngeal-and-hypopharyngeal-cancer-key-statistics

Woodson, G. (2008). Evolving concepts of laryngeal paralysis. *Journal of Laryngology & Otology, 122*(5), 437–441.

Yamamoto, K., Monnier, P., Holtz, F., & Jaquet, Y. (2014). Laryngotracheal reconstruction for pediatric glotto-subglottic stenosis. *International Journal of Pediatric Otolaryngology, 78*(9), 1476–1479.

Zeitels, S. M., Casiano, R. R., Gardner, G. M., Hogikyan, N. D., Koufman, J. A., & Rosen, C. A. (2002). Voice and Swallowing Committee, American Academy of Otolaryngology-Head and Neck Surgery. Management of common voice problems: Committee report. *Otolaryngology–Head and Neck Surgery, 126*(4), 333–348.

CHAPTER 4

Medical Problems and the Performing Voice

David L. Witsell and Mirabelle B. Sajisevi

MEDICAL PROBLEMS THAT AFFECT THE LARYNX

The larynx is an amazing and complex part of the human body and its normal function is critical to life. Its primary role is to allow effective exchange of oxygen and carbon dioxide; second, the larynx functions to protect the lungs during swallowing; and third, the larynx is the instrument of our voice. Medical problems often have repercussions for the larynx and its function. For purposes of clarity, "medical problems" in this chapter refers to diseases or disorders of the larynx or of other parts of our body that cause problems in the larynx. Therefore, primary treatment of some voice problems sometimes requires treating not the larynx but the part of the body that is primarily affected.

INFLAMMATION AND INFECTIONS

The human airway is divided into the upper airway and the lower airway with the division between the two occurring at the level of the larynx, specifically the vocal folds (Figure 4–1). For the performing vocalist, infections of either division of the airway can result in significant problems with voice and sound quality. The actuator of voice, the lungs, can be affected by viral, bacterial, and fungal infections that can potentially impair both inspiration and expiration.

Infections of the larynx and vocal folds typically affect mass, vibration, and closure of the vocal folds, often resulting in changes in vocal quality and pitch range. Likewise, inflammation and infections of the resonator (the throat, mouth, nose, and sinuses) can sometimes adversely affect the quality and richness of sound by altering the resonance characteristics of the performer's vocal tract. See Table 4–1 for sites of airway infections.

The upper respiratory infection (URI) is by far the most common acute condition that children and adults encounter (24 persons out of 100 annually), with adults averaging two to four URIs per year (NIAID). There are over 100 different types of rhinoviruses that cause URIs, and therefore it is difficult for our immune

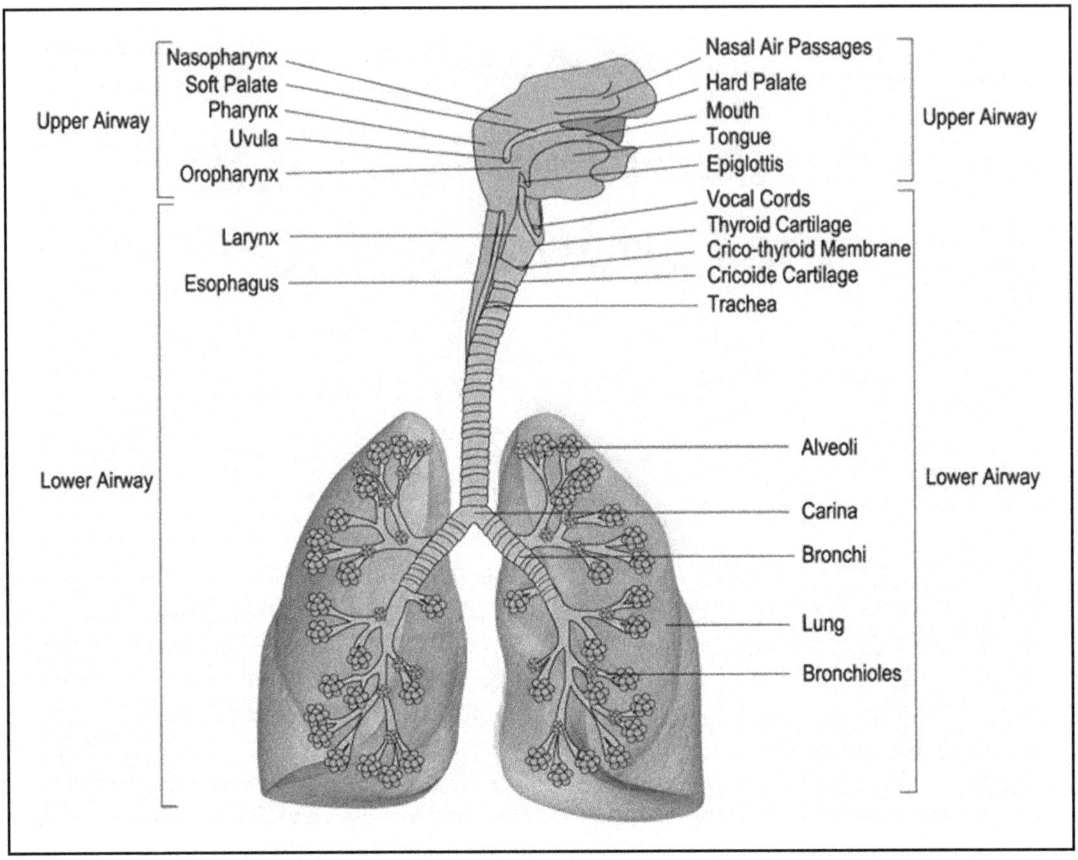

Figure 4–1. *Upper and lower airways. Reproduced with permission from EMT & Fire Training Center. Copyright © 2008. emt-national-training.com*

Table 4–1. *Sites of Airway Infections*

Upper Airway	*Example*	*Lower Airway*	*Example*
Sinuses	Sinusitis	Subglottis	Croup (children)
Nasopharynx	Adenoid infection	Trachea	Tracheitis
Mouth	Tonsillitis	Bronchus	Bronchitis
Throat	Epiglottitis	Lungs	Pneumonia

system to develop long-lasting resistance to the "common cold." The rhinovirus is spread through the air, and risk of being infected is increased by close proximity to others. In cold weather climates, this occurs in the winter when we are spending time in smaller, more crowded spaces. The rhinovirus infects the lining of the airway causing destruction of the small mucosal cells, and this in turn causes an inflammatory reaction by the body. This inflammation results in leakiness of the small capillaries in the mucosa, and swelling (or edema) ensues. When this occurs in the larynx and involves the vocal folds, the vocal folds develop increased mass and altered tension, leading to hoarseness and vocal instability, which are often experienced during the illness.

Special distinction should be made regarding the "flu." This viral infection is caused by one of three influenza viruses ("A," global infections; "B," more localized infections; "C," generally milder infections) and affects between 5% and 20% of the U.S. population annually. The flu can often infect both the upper and lower respiratory tract and results in complications (such as bacterial pneumonia or tonsillitis) more often than the usual viral infection. The flu is spread both by contact and by air. There is an antiviral for influenza on the market. Its efficacy is limited and its use is not broadly indicated, but given the potential impact of influenza infection on the voice, singers may wish to consider getting an annual flu vaccine.

Viral infections are not responsive to antibiotics, but complications from viral infections may be. The rule of thumb is that a viral infection will come on in 24 to 72 hours and symptoms should begin resolving in 5 to 6 days after clear onset. In uncomplicated URI infections, the fever tends to be low grade and associated with nasal drainage, cough, and sore throat. If symptoms persist beyond 5 to 6 days, a bacterial superinfection (due to the inflammation caused by the virus) might be occurring, and an evaluation by a health care provider may be indicated. In this case, an antibiotic may be helpful.

For details regarding the flu caused by the influenza virus, the Centers for Disease Control and Prevention is one of the best resources, providing information about whether it is in your area and what the prevailing symptoms and treatments are (http://www.cdc.gov).

Antibiotics are excellent medications for bacterial infections, but not for viral infections. Almost every medication has its side effects, and for antibiotics, the range of side effects that might affect the performer's voice is broad. Two important side effects (or side results) of using antibiotics in singers are (1) fungal infections and (2) gastrointestinal problems.

Yeast is a fungus and an inhabitant of our upper airway that aids the health and balance of the population of bacteria that live in our throats. The role and balance of yeast and bacteria are important parts of the human life cycle. Some bacteria help in the initial steps of digestion, liberating small essential molecules and vitamins that our bodies cannot otherwise absorb. Although antibiotics can be effective in killing the bad bacteria causing an infection, they are also in a way global bacterial killers that disrupt the delicate balance of good bacterial flora that help us to stay healthy. They do not kill yeast, though, which can proliferate beyond its normal balance. Yeast infections are not uncommon after antibiotic therapy (particularly long courses or after multiple different antibiotics) and can result in persistent mouth pain, taste disturbance, and hoarseness. If this occurs, an antifungal may be needed to help restore balance and improve symptoms. Fluconazole is most commonly prescribed and is effective.

Persistent hoarseness or mouth pain after the acute infection symptoms have responded to the antibiotic may indicate a yeast infection. The symptoms from a yeast fungal infection can be remarkably tenacious, persisting for months after the initial problem. Dysphonia tends to be persistent through all speaking and singing tasks, and may lead to vocal fatigue and voice strain.

Gastrointestinal problems or complaints are also part of the usual side effects from antibiotics. Diarrhea and/or bloating are the most commonly reported. GI symptoms can interfere with good abdominal breathing, which can have a negative impact on vocal technique.

Infections or inflammation of the sinuses can affect vocal quality, although often indirectly. Sinus drainage can negatively impact the source (vocal folds) by causing inflammation and irritation, and excess mucus, which may provoke throat clearing. Blockage of the sinuses can alter the singer's aural and sensory feedback system, resulting in maladaptive technical compensation. The term "sinusitis" simply refers to generalized *inflammation* of the lining of the sinuses; the term or label does not specify the *cause* of the inflammation. Sinus symptoms are usually due to viral, allergic, or reactive (particulate, ozone, pollution) irritants that have been inhaled and filtered by the nose and sinuses. Inflammation within the sinuses can cause increased nasal drainage, sinus pressure, nasal congestion, and headache. When inflammation of the sinuses is persistent, a bacterial infection can occur (only in about 2% of cases). The three major signs of a bacterial sinusitis are (1) nasal congestion, (2) opaquely colored nasal drainage, and (3) facial pain or pressure (Meltzer & Hamilos, 2011; Figure 4–2).

Antibiotics are used (and overused) commonly in the management of sinusitis. In approximately 60% of patients with bacterial sinusitis, the infection will resolve on its own, so it is *not* necessary but an *option* to use antibiotic therapy

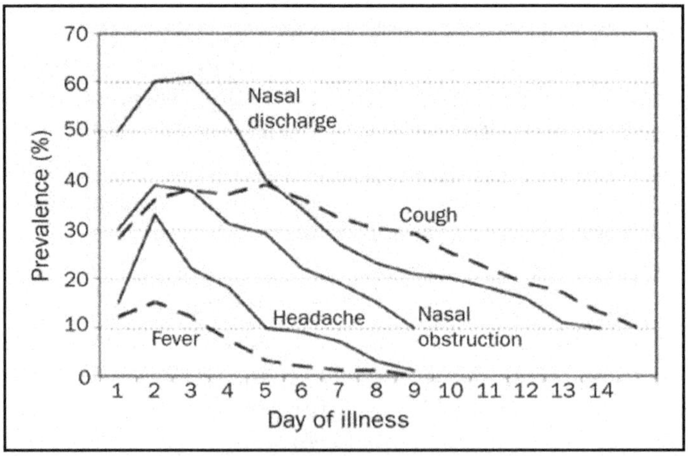

***Figure 4–2.** Normal pattern of symptom prevalence over time (days) for acute viral rhinosinusitis. Reproduced with permission from Elsevier. Meltzer, E. O., & Hamilos, D. L. (2011). Rhinosinusitis diagnosis and management for the clinician: A synopsis of recent consensus guidelines.* Mayo Clinic Proceedings, *86(5), 427–443. Copyright © 2011.*

for acute uncomplicated bacterial sinusitis if symptoms persist (Gill et al., 2006). However, the needs of the elite vocal athlete with high performance demands for whom cancellations have significant financial/career repercussions may necessitate special consideration. Busy professional singers often do not have the luxury of time to wait out an infection that is disrupting the performance schedule.

Good sinus health is the key to avoid bacterial sinus infections. Recommendations include saline irrigations twice daily, adequate topical allergy management, good hand hygiene, and compassion for oneself to allow for the body's own healing process to occur.

REFLUX

Medical problems often result in inflammation of the larynx, causing symptoms such as hoarseness, changes in pitch and dynamic range, vocal fatigue, or strain. One of the most common medical problems encountered in singers is gastroesophageal reflux disease, or GERD. When the acidic stomach contents are refluxed back through the esophagus to the level of the larynx and into the throat, the condition is called laryngopharyngeal reflux, or LPR. The upper esophagus and throat are not designed to be resistant to the effects of acidic contents and become irritated and inflamed by repeated episodes of reflux. This inflammation results in swelling of specific parts of the larynx (arytenoids and vocal folds), resulting in dysphonia.

LPR, often simply called "reflux," is a medical problem of the digestive tract that can be exacerbated or improved by anatomical and functional factors, medical treatments, and/or lifestyle habits.

Activities or situations associated with increased abdominal pressure predispose one to reflux. Obesity (particularly in those people who put on weight in the belly rather than the hips) can be a significant risk factor for reflux. Increased pressures in the abdomen can result in compressing the stomach and its contents. Normally, the lower esophageal sphincter acts like a valve that keeps stomach contents in the stomach. However, chronically high pressures in the belly can overcome the ability of this valve to stay closed and reflux ensues. Moreover, in some people, part of the stomach can be pushed into the chest through the diaphragm, resulting in what is called a "hiatal hernia." This is usually diagnosed by a swallow study and is a key sign of chronic reflux. Treatment of a hiatal hernia depends upon its size and the symptoms it is causing. Medical management and weight loss can be very helpful, but some will require surgical intervention to reduce the hernia and tighten the diaphragm to keep the stomach in the abdomen. (Lambert, Marceau, & Forse, 2005; Wilson & Hirschowitz, 1999).

Some medications can increase reflux symptoms, while others can help reduce them. Many different classes of medications can result in an increase in reflux symptoms. Antibiotics, nonsteroidal anti-inflammatories (NSAIDs, such as ibuprofen), blood pressure medications, antidepressants, and iron supplements are just a few of the categories of medications that are associated with reflux. Additionally, bisphosphonates are a class of medications that are used to treat osteoporosis and are commonly prescribed for middle aged to older women. A frequent adverse effect of this class of medications is an increase in GERD and esophagitis when not taken appropriately (Kennel & Drake, 2009).

Medications can also reduce symptoms of reflux and facilitate healing of the esophagus and throat. Calcium carbonate (Tums) can facilitate the rapid buffering of an acute and symptomatic reflux episode. H2 blockers (cimetidine, ranitidine) are another class of over-the-counter medications that can be helpful for people with reflux. This class of medications helps temporarily suppress the production of acid in the stomach by ongoing competition for the acid management job in the stomach. When you first take an H2 blocker, the higher concentration of the medication wins the fight against acid production, but as the concentration of the medicine drops, it gets dethroned by the normal acid-making manager in the stomach, and acid level can rise (~8 hours). Another class of medications, called the proton-pump inhibitors (PPIs) such as omeprazole, also compete for the acid management job, but when these medications get into the "throne," they don't leave it and acid production stops. The stomach cells must remanufacture the managing seat to resume acid production, so a prolonged response (~24–48 hours) is achieved with this class of medications (http://www.fda.gov).

The range of available medications for reflux affords an opportunity to treat reflux aggressively and appropriately. Severe reflux is treated with PPIs for long-lasting acid suppression. Mild to moderate reflux that is more predictable can be treated with the H2 blockers. Even though acid production from the stomach can be modified by these medications (helpful to most people), harmful reflux can still happen in some and this is termed "nonacidic reflux." If this is suspected, or if signs and symptoms of LPR continue despite treatments, then GI testing may be in order to understand the extent of the reflux problem and to inform further management.

Although reflux medications can be helpful in patients who truly have LPR, these medications are not helpful if the diagnosis is incorrect or incomplete. There has been a 14-fold increase in prescriptions for reflux, which has become a "catch-all" diagnosis for health care providers in the treatment of patients with hoarseness. Patients are often prescribed reflux medication when their dysphonia is in fact more complex and multifaceted. If behavioral voice therapy is indicated, reflux treatment alone will typically not resolve the voice problem. For example, muscle tension dysphonia and LPR often get confused with one another and need very different treatments (voice therapy vs. medication management) (Cohen & Garrett, 2008).

Reflux and lifestyle go hand in hand for many people. Smoking and alcohol can reduce the strength of the stomach valve; spicy foods and high fat foods, chocolate, caffeine, and some of the most wonderful treats in the world should perhaps have a label warning: "Reflux Happening Here." Large meals before bedtime can increase stomach pressure and cause reflux while sleeping (not an unusual scenario for singers dining after a performance). "Silent reflux" refers to cases in which the most obvious symptom (indigestion/heartburn) is not experienced. Signs of silent reflux include cough, mild sore or dry throat, a feeling of swelling or a lump in the throat (globus sensation), gurgling or burning sensation in the throat, or sour taste in the mouth. Singers may note increased dysphonia in the morning, need for prolonged vocal warm-up, or poor vocal quality, among other symptoms.

THYROID FUNCTION

The thyroid is a butterfly-shaped gland located right at the sternal notch with each lobe representing a butterfly's wing and the trachea and "isthmus" representing the butterfly's body. The thyroid gland is important in regulating metabolism. Hypothyroidism is the term used to describe underfunctioning of the thyroid gland so that metabolism is slowed. Fatigue, chronically feeling cold and clammy, weight gain, and swelling are signs of chronic hypothyroidism.

The larynx can be affected by hypothyroidism as well. The vocal folds can become swollen, increasing their mass and therefore lowering overall fundamental frequency and decreasing the pitch range. The chronic fatigue from hypothyroidism can also contribute to poor breath support, and decreased energy levels may affect performance. Weight gain can further exacerbate sleeping problems, potentially resulting in obstructive sleep apnea (OSA). OSA will contribute to the cycle of increasing fatigue and often depression (Ritchie & Yeap, 2015).

Hyperthyroidism is an unusual thyroid problem that has significant consequences for health and voice. Patients who are hyperthyroid have an increased metabolism and therefore might be "revved up" from their baseline normal. Signs and symptoms can include increased sweating and heat intolerance, weight loss, pressured speech, increased heartbeat, anxiety, and poor sleeping at night. With long-term hyperthyroidism, eyesight and eye position can be affected. Vocal consequences from hyperthyroidism may be related to dehydration and possibly voice overuse associated with increased anxious activity.

The diagnosis of thyroid problems uses both the signs and symptoms of hypo- or hyperthyroidism along with a blood test. The thyroid is normally regulated through TSH (thyroid-stimulating hormone) that is released by the pituitary gland at the base of the brain. A hypothyroid diagnosis is made by its signs and symptoms and a high TSH level. The pituitary secretes high levels of TSH in an attempt to drive the thyroid to make more thyroid hormone and increase metabolism. Conversely, when a person is hyperthyroid, the TSH levels dip lower and lower below normal as the pituitary dramatically decreases the amount of TSH secreted. Since there is not a thyroid shutdown mechanism per se, the pituitary's response to an elevated metabolism is to not stimulate the thyroid further.

Both conditions require medical management after a full evaluation to determine the cause. Women are more affected by thyroid problems than men are, and thyroid problems tend to run in families. People who have a positive family history of thyroid dysfunction should be screened in adulthood or if any signs or symptoms occur (Manji et al., 2006).

Benign thyroid disease may lead to vocal cord paralysis by such mechanisms as compression, stretching, or inflammation of the recurrent laryngeal nerve (Collazo-Clavell, Gharib, & Maragos, 1995).

IMMUNOLOGIC DISEASES

Immunologic diseases, or diseases that result from immune system dysfunction, can affect the voice in a number of ways. The hallmark of an autoimmune disease is that a person's own immune system loses the ability to track what is "self" and what is not. The immune system reacts to salivary tissue in Sjögren disease, resulting in a dry throat and mouth. In Wegener granulomatosis, the immune system reacts to and inflames small arteries, causing inflammation and damage to surrounding tissues. The sinuses, trachea, and lungs are often affected by this disease, and breathing problems can be either acute or chronic. Patients with scleroderma experience changes in the connective tissue of the skin and mucous membranes, resulting in decreased flexibility, while patients with sarcoidosis deposit amyloid in the tissues throughout the body, resulting in scarring and thickening of membranes (such as the vocal folds).

Immunologic diseases are generally rare but are significant health problems when they occur. The medical specialty that evaluates and manages these illnesses is called rheumatology. Rheumatologists often involve other specialists to address a specific problem or manifestation of a disease. Otolaryngologists are usually part of the care team since they have the tools and in-depth knowledge of the upper airway from the nose to the trachea.

You can visit the website for the American Autoimmune Related Diseases Association (http://www.aarda.org/autoimmune-information/list-of-diseases/) for a more comprehensive listing of these diseases and their different characteristics.

NEUROLOGIC CONDITIONS AND VOICE FUNCTION

The larynx is tightly managed and controlled by the nervous system via the recurrent and superior laryngeal nerves. These are branches of the vagus nerve that is the 10th of 12 cranial nerves. "Cranial" refers to the fact that only 12 specialized nerves of the central nervous system descend from the cranial vault directly and do not pass through the spinal cord. These cranial nerves give us our eyesight, hearing, smell, and taste. They also control the muscles of the vocal tract to shape the human voice. The recurrent laryngeal nerve is the master of vocal cord mobility and vibration, providing motor innervation for all muscles of the larynx except the cricothyroid and also providing subglottic sensory innervation.

Neurologic conditions can be grouped into central versus peripheral diseases or conditions. The term central is used when processing of intended movement is centrally affected in the brain. Examples of central neurologic conditions include strokes, spasmodic dysphonia, and Parkinson disease. In each of these three conditions, control of the vocal folds (as well as other activities such as limb movement) might be impaired. The impairment is dependent on where in the brain the problem lies. If a stroke causes damage in the outer cortex, the resulting impairment is more specific and limited than if the stroke occurs at a place where lots of areas of the brain communicate (think of it as being like the difference between a contained suburban neighborhood vs. the Jersey turnpike, which connects so many different neighborhoods).

Parkinson Disease

Parkinson disease is a central movement disorder that originates in the putamen, a busy processing center for movement. People with Parkinson disease have global impairment that is characterized as a delay in the intent to move and the action of moving. Typically, a fine tremor of the hand will be present, and when these patients walk, their feet lag behind the forward lean of their body. Vocally, people with Parkinson disease lose expressive intonations (prosody) and loudness, becoming more monotone and poorly projected. The Lee Silverman Voice Treatment can be effective in helping improve vocal projection and intelligibility (Spielman, Ramig, Mahler, Halpern, & Gavin, 2007).

Spasmodic Dysphonia

Spasmodic dysphonia (SD) is a rare disorder of connected speech. SD is better diagnosed by a clinical and perceptual evaluation than by any imaging test. The connected speech problem often disappears if the person sings or whispers, and the laugh can be robust and normal sounding. However, normal phrasing during connected speech is spastically interrupted and the interruptions increase in intensity with stress. This characteristic presentation of being able to sing normally in the face of disrupted speech initially led medical providers to assume this was a psychologic disorder. Now SD is better understood as an isolated central neurologic disorder, similar to other muscle dystonias.

Spasmodic dysphonia may be typed as adductor, abductor, or mixed. The more common SD type is the ADDuctor, in which voiced sounds are disrupted by spasms that adduct the vocal folds, resulting in a strangling sound that is peppered throughout speech at the voiced phonemes. Women are more affected than men and the disorder typically occurs in middle-aged people (>40 years old). The thyroarytenoid and vocalis muscles (the principal muscles that tense and move the vocal folds together) are the muscles that are overactive, and treatment should be directed toward reducing the spasms of these muscles.

With ABDuctor SD, the spasms cause the vocal folds to abduct on voiceless phonemes, resulting in an episodically breathy voice and poor vocal stamina. The posterior cricoarytenoid muscle normally opens the vocal folds during inspiration, but in this case it spasms during connected speech and causes the vocal folds to involuntarily open. See Figure 4–3 for location of muscles affected by SD.

Treatment of SD is accomplished with botulinum toxin (or Botox) in very small dosages injected into the small muscle group that is overactive. This is usually done as a team with laryngologist and neurologist working together. Electromyography is used to identify the correct muscle so that the toxin is precisely delivered to the target muscle. The toxin weakens the muscle resulting in smoother connected speech. Unfortunately, the Botox wears off over time, so patients have to be reinjected as the symptoms reappear, usually at intervals from 3 months to 6 months (Blitzer, Brin, & Stewart, 1998).

Vocal Fold Paralysis and Paresis

Paralysis of the left, right, or both vocal folds is most frequently a peripheral neurologic problem. This means that the intrinsic laryngeal muscles are not receiving nerve signal to control their movement. It also implies that nerve damage has occurred somewhere along the course of the recurrent laryngeal nerve (RLN) after its exit from the skull. Paralysis refers to complete denervation of the nerve, paresis to a weakening of the nerve. To know where the problem might occur, one needs to know the anatomic course of the RLN (Figure 4–4).

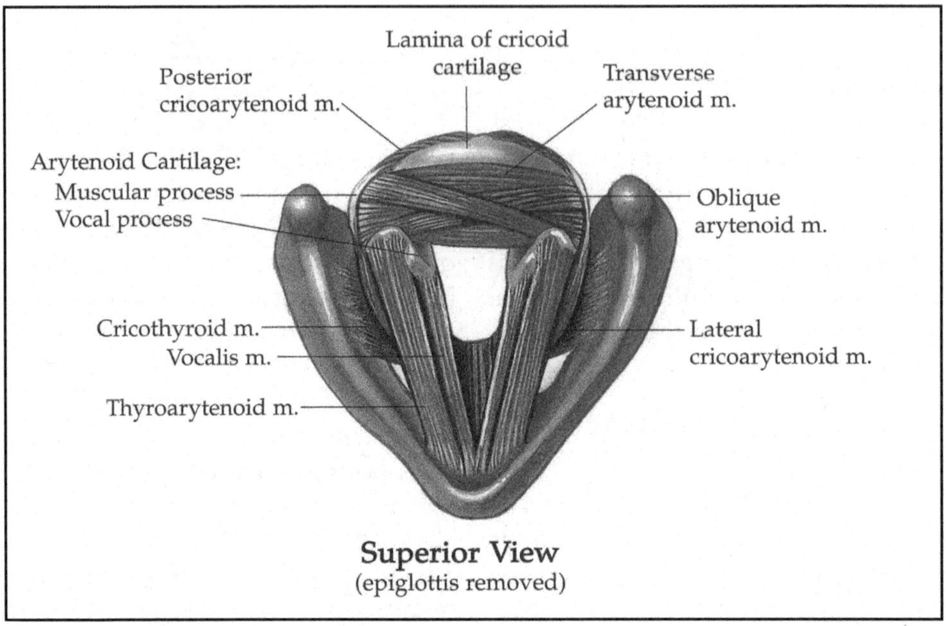

Figure 4–3. *Top view of larynx showing the intrinsic laryngeal muscles, from Larynx/Pharynx Chart. Reproduced with permission from Wolters-Kluwer Health. Copyright © 1999, 2000. The Anatomical Chart Company.*

The RLN is part of the vagus nerve, as noted previously. In human embryonic development, this branch of the vagus nerve is pulled into the chest by the aortic arch on the left and by the subclavian artery on the right. The nerve then ascends in the groove between the trachea and the esophagus and underneath the thyroid gland. This is why the RLN is named as such, because it descends with the vagus and then recurs, returning to the larynx. Any lesion along this entire course can cause vocal cord paresis (weakness) or paralysis (Rubin & Sataloff, 2007).

Vocal cord paralysis may present suddenly or gradually. It is often accompanied by a problem swallowing liquids that makes the patient feel like he or she is choking. The voice becomes weak and breathy, and the person fatigues very quickly from talking and/or singing. Pitch range is reduced.

Evaluation of vocal cord paralysis usually involves a complete head and neck exam, laryngoscopy and/or videostroboscopy, and a computed tomography (CT) scan of the neck from the base of the skull to the arch of the aorta. A laryngeal EMG study (performed by a laryngologist and neurologist) can help distinguish between a central and a peripheral neurologic problem and can offer prognostic information.

Vocal cord paralysis can be a sign of something very serious such as lung cancer or thyroid cancer. It can also be a complication of surgery or of prolonged anesthesia. In such cases, the signs and symptoms of vocal cord paralysis appear shortly after the procedure (Misono & Merati, 2012). See Table 4–2 for examples of surgeries in which damage to the RLN might occur.

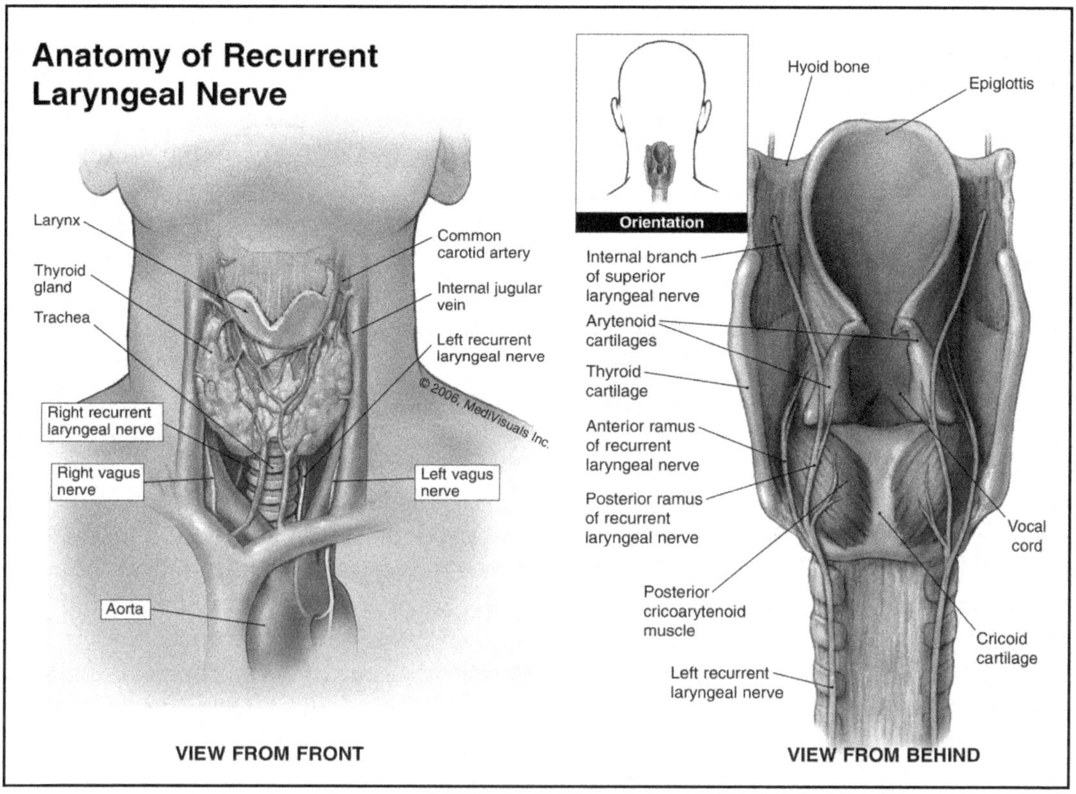

Figure 4–4. *Anatomy of the recurrent laryngeal nerve. Reproduced with permission from MediVisuals, Inc. Copyright © 2006.*

Table 4–2. *Surgeries That Have a Risk of Injury to the Recurrent Laryngeal Nerve*

Neck Surgery Complication	***Chest Surgery Complication***
Thyroid surgery	Pulmonectomy (removal of lung)
Cervical fusion surgery	Heart surgery
Carotid artery surgery	Aorta surgery
Cervical esophagus surgery	Mediastinoscopy (chest lymph node biopsy)

Idiopathic (and/or viral) vocal cord paralysis is the term that is used when a specific origin of recurrent laryngeal nerve injury is not known. This can occur in 10% to 40% of cases and is more common on the left, likely due to the longer length of the left RLN. In cases of viral vocal cord paralysis, symptoms may gradually appear over several days as the upper respiratory illness subsides. This is because the initial inflammation and swelling of the vocal folds associated with the upper respiratory infection may promote adequate closure and vibration.

Once the swelling resolves, the glottic gap created by the immobile vocal cord becomes more symptomatic, resulting in breathiness and vocal fatigue (Myssiorek, 2004). In 30% to 50% of cases, the patient may not notice a significant change in their speaking voice due to adequate compensation by the opposite side.

Vocal cord paralysis can be managed conservatively or aggressively, depending on the cause of the injury and expected recovery of the nerve. Spontaneous recovery of the nerve can occur within a year of the injury, as long as the nerve sheath is intact (as in viral cases). The recovery can be complete (back to normal) or partial (vocal cord paresis), in which case the person has some impairment of their speaking and/or singing voice due to a persistent weakness on the affected side (Figure 4–5).

Conservative management for vocal fold paresis begins with patience and voice therapy to help the person to compensate for the weakness in a healthy way. Pacing voice use is also an essential strategy for a good outcome. All too often, compensation for the weakness is accomplished by "pushing harder." This can be a maladaptive strategy and could potentially result in additional damage to the structure of the vocal cord. Keep in mind that the nerve will repair itself by 1 mm (about 1/16 of an inch) every week beginning at the site of injury, so long-term planning and realistic expectations for performing are needed. Seeing a laryngologist with a voice therapist is the foundation for good voice recovery (Schwartz et al., 2009).

In cases where the vocal cord is permanently paralyzed, surgical options can help move the affected vocal cord to

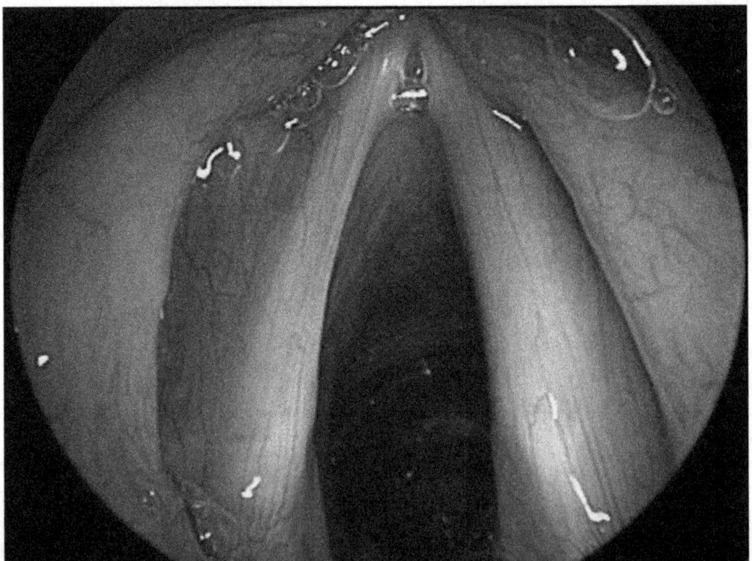

Figure 4–5. *Laryngoscopic view of the vocal folds showing mild atrophy of paretic left vocal fold. Copyright © 2015, Duke University Medical Center.*

a more favorable position and improve vocal projection and quality. This is called a "medialization thyroplasty" and is most often performed with the patient awake so that the voice can be "tuned." This procedure can be done in a number of different ways (injection vs. through a small incision) with different materials (collagen, Gore-Tex, Silastin, etc.) depending on the situation. Additionally, a nerve transfer can be accomplished from the ansa-hypoglossal nerve to the recurrent nerve in select patients with an excellent result (Crumley & Izdebski, 1986).

The superior laryngeal nerve (SLN) is also a branch of the vagus nerve. The external branch of the SLN supplies motor function to the cricothyroid (CT) muscle while the internal branch provides sensation to the mucosa at and above the vocal folds. Complete or partial denervation to the SLN (SLN paralysis or paresis) can impair the ability to lengthen the vocal folds, which can significantly affect pitch control and range. The CT muscle also moves the vocal folds to the paramedian position, and thus paresis may contribute to vocal fatigue.

Neurodegenerative Diseases

Neurodegenerative diseases can also affect vocal cord movement and voice function. Examples of these include amyotrophic lateral sclerosis (ALS or Lou Gehrig's disease) and pseudobulbar palsy. Both of these disorders are generally accompanied by other signs and symptoms, including articulation and swallowing problems and emotional lability. Another disorder, called myasthenia gravis, is caused by antibodies that block transmission between the nerve and muscle at the neuromuscular junction. This disorder results in rapid muscle fatigue that can recover after rest.

The complex presentation of neurologic diseases that can have voice manifestations requires multidisciplinary care and specialized treatments. Management of these problems always begins with a comprehensive evaluation by skilled clinicians who can understand the symptoms and put them into a diagnostic framework.

MEDICATIONS AND THE VOICE

Tremendous advances in human health have been fostered by scientific inquiry and discovery. Illnesses can be cured or managed, many cancers are removed and eradicated, and functional deficits are improved. Medications, whether synthesized or extracted from plants or other natural resources, are a mainstay of health in the United States. Nearly all human medications modify an action, a reaction, function, or dysfunction within the human body, either by intended primary action and/or by secondary actions that may be an unintended consequence of the drug or its metabolite. The unfortunate reality is that medications are *not* entirely specific, and while they may treat a problem very nicely, inevitably they affect other systems or organs of the body. Side effects of medications are a particular challenge to manage, especially in singers and as we age and accumulate a longer and longer list of daily remedies (Table 4–3).

The Food and Drug Administration in the United States requires rigorous multistep testing and proof that the benefits of the drug outweigh the risks of taking it. The road to drug approval is

Table 4–3. *Medications, Their Common Usage, and Their Common Side Effects*

Class/Type	Example	Use	Side Effects
Allergy nose (sprays)	Fluticasone Budesonide	Reduces congestion and allergic reactions	Nose bleeds, throat Irritation, headache
Analgesics (nonnarcotics), antipyretics	Ibuprofen Naproxen Acetaminophen	Relieves mild pain and reduces fever	Gastric irritation, nausea, ringing in the ears
Antibiotics	Amoxicillin Levofloxacin	To treat infections	Bloating, taste disturbance, yeast infections, rash
Anticholinergic medications	Dramamine Scopolamine Oxybutin Ipratropium Glycopyrrolate	COPD, bladder problems, asthma, motion sickness, postnasal drip, drooling	Urine retention, dry mouth, blurred vision, dry nose and throat
Antidepressants	Fluoxetine Nortriptyline Bupropion	Improves mood	Drowsiness, dry mouth, blurred vision, constipation
Antihistamines (oral tablets)	Benadryl Loratidine Cetirizine	Reduces congestion and allergic reactions	Mucosal dryness (dry mouth, dry eyes, constipation), drowsiness and dizziness
Anxiolytics	Diazepam Klonopin	Reduces nervousness Improves tremors	Sedation, dizziness, memory problems
Cholinergic medications	Cevimeline Pilocarpine Pyridostigmine	Sjögren syndrome, dry mouth Glaucoma Myasthenia gravis	Arrhythmias, worsened asthma or breathing, sweating
Corticosteroids	Prednisone	Reduces inflammation Modulates immune response	Anxiety, insomnia, water retention, increased appetite
Decongestants	Pseudoephedrine	Reduces congestion	Tiredness, dry mouth, constipation
Diuretics	Furosemide	Reduces water retention	Dehydration, low blood pressure, blood potassium elevation
Inhalers	Albuterol Fluticasone	Opens airways in the lungs	Altered heart rate, dry mouth, fungal laryngitis
Muscle relaxants	Cyclobenzaprine	Relieves muscle cramping	Drowsiness, dry mouth, blurred vision, constipation
Neurotoxin	Botulinum toxin	Spasmodic dysphonia Spasticity Drooling	Weakness, rash, swallowing problem

Table 4–3. *continued*

Class/Type	Example	Use	Side Effects
Pain medications (narcotics)	Oxycodone Codeine	Reduces pain perception	Drowsiness, dry mouth, blurred vision, constipation
Reflux	Omeprazole Tagamet	Reduces acid secretion	Headache, bloating, B vitamin deficiency, poor calcium absorption

very expensive, upwards of $800,000 to $2 billion once it is in human clinical trials. This approval is expensive because a company must show that a drug is both *safe* for human use and *efficacious* at the prescribed dose. Through this approval process, side effects are meticulously documented within the context of the study. After approval, postmarketing surveillance of the drug use and side effects occurs. You can and should report any significant medication side effect through the manufacturer or through your health care provider (http://www.fda.gov).

For the vocal athlete, medications are best understood by the way they target or adversely interact with the upper (nose, throat, and larynx) and lower (trachea and lungs) airways. Any medication that causes a change in the upper or lower airway environment has the potential to positively or adversely affect the vocal tract. The most frequent concern is whether the medication causes dryness of mucosa or change in the tenacity and/or viscosity of mucus. Either may decrease the efficiency of vocal cord vibration and predispose the singer to vocal quality changes and increased vocal fatigue.

Several classes of medications are of particular interest. These include antibiotics and reflux medications (discussed earlier), antihistamines, corticosteroids, inhalers for lung problems, and finally stimulants (including caffeine). Additional information on the effects of medication and voice can be found at this link to the National Center for Voice and Speech (http://www.ncvs.org/rx.html).

Allergies and Antihistamines

Allergies to pollen, dust, and dust mites are very common and take a toll on the health care system of the United States. What does "being allergic" mean? Allergy is a term commonly used to describe the end result of what is a very complicated immune and biochemical pathway. The end result of this complicated pathway is a constellation of signs and symptoms that include sneezing, nasal congestion, itchy eyes or throat, and often a watery nose. Specific white blood cells (eosinophils and mast cells) are responsible for initiating the biochemical cascade that results in the allergic response.

In the case of allergies, there is a problem with cataloguing the first time the immune system encounters the allergen. Because this is an *immune system cataloguing error*, to be allergic requires that the person has encountered the allergen before and filed it incorrectly as invader rather than an uninteresting bystander. This is different from viruses and infections that are catalogued correctly, conferring immunity to the invader through a specific antibody taken from the existing antibody arsenal. Unfortunately, this cataloguing error can occur at any time, so a person can become allergic at any point in his or her life.

Once an allergy response is triggered, a biochemical alarm is released and immune cells gather and release *histamine* that causes leaks to develop in the tiny capillaries in the surrounding area leading to inflammation. In the case of allergic rhinitis (nasal allergies), the nose becomes congested and leaky at the same time, restricting airflow and resulting in copious postnasal drip. Often the eyes and throat are involved as well, and the inflammatory response can result in a rough and paradoxical dry feeling in the throat and eyes and vocal fold edema.

Allergic reactions take nearly 18 hours to resolve. Therefore, people with allergies should adopt a daily management strategy, since they are likely to come into contact with that allergen very frequently, as in the case of pollen or house dust. This is why allergy medicines work best as preventative strategies rather than in the moment. Oral decongestants to treat nasal congestion can be helpful for short-term relief but can also elevate blood pressure and cause mucosal drying, which may have a negative effect on voice.

One key to management of allergies is knowledge about what you are allergic to and avoidance of those things. This can be more difficult for singers on tour because they have less control over their environment. A clean bedroom and bed linens are a must. Hardwood floors usually collect less dust and can be helpful to reduce chance of exposure. Traveling with your own pillow can be helpful. Allergy testing may be beneficial in identifying which allergens the patient is sensitive to. Many people can identify situations or seasons where they predictably have problems and can treat the allergies seasonally. Desensitization via allergy shots or sublingual immunotherapy may be considered if symptoms are not adequately controlled with medications and environmental adaptations.

Antihistamines are the medication class that is used to treat allergies. There are antihistamines that have a side effect of sedation (Benadryl) and others that do not sedate (loratidine) because they do not cross over the blood-brain barrier. Both classes decrease mucus production and can cause a drier mouth and throat. These allergy pills are best used in people who need a more systemic approach to allergy control because they have allergic reactions in the nose, throat, eyes, and lungs or experience an allergic rash.

Nose sprays can be of particular help when the main symptoms are in the nose and throat. Nasal steroid sprays (fluticasone, budesonide) can be very helpful in controlling the allergic response. A newer antihistamine nasal spray (azelastine) is also available and can be used in addition to a nasal steroid spray, as they complement each other. The advantage of the nasal sprays is that they work topically, usually are not systemically drying, and have minimal (if any) systemic side effects. Steroid sprays can cause a minor nosebleed and antihistamine sprays can have a bad taste.

Of note, once-a-day medications, whether pills or sprays, need to be taken on a regular basis rather than as needed. It will take about 3 to 5 days for these medications to get to a consistent therapeutic level. They prevent the allergic cascade and if they are effective, patients may stop using them, thinking that their allergies are gone. This is the worst time to stop them! A consistent allergy management regimen must be maintained to optimize the beneficial results (Dykewicz et al., 1998).

Corticosteroids

Corticosteroids are a powerful class of medications that are used by health care providers to help control inflammation. They mimic other hormones in the body and when taken at therapeutic doses can have dramatic beneficial effects. Taken over time, corticosteroids can result in side effects that are also dramatic. Examples include bone density loss, fluid retention, and redistribution of fat in the body with the face becoming rounded in appearance (called "moon facies"). Additionally, since corticosteroids modulate and suppress the immune system, infections from yeast and other opportunistic organisms or bacteria can occur.

Many otolaryngologists and laryngologists use corticosteroids in acute situations when a performer has developed hoarseness due to inflammation and swelling of the vocal folds. It is essential that the vocal folds be checked prior to prescribing these medications to ensure that the hoarseness is not an impending sign of a vocal cord hemorrhage. Three to six days of oral steroid treatment are common, and treatment usually starts at a high dose and rapidly tapers thereafter. The onset of corticosteroid benefit is between 3 and 6 hours and can last several days, so these medications should be taken according to the patient's need for maximum benefit (Table 4–4).

These medications are powerful and should be used with caution in people with diabetes, psychiatric problems, heart problems, and insomnia.

Corticosteroids are also used in sudden idiopathic neuropathies such as recurrent laryngeal nerve paralysis, facial paralysis, sudden hearing loss, and other problems where the underlying theory is that swelling and inflammation around the nerve are causing damage or dysfunction. Limited evidence exists to substantiate the positive benefit of using corticosteroids in these illnesses, so careful consideration should be placed on the use of this class of medications (Cohen, Dinan, Roy, Kim, & Courey, 2014; Cope & Bova, 2008).

Inhalers for Lung Problems

Asthma and chronic obstructive pulmonary disease (COPD) are primary reasons for health care providers to place a patient on inhaled medications. The goal is to improve lung function and airflow by reducing the reactivity of the lungs and reducing inflammation and excess secretions. Asthma and COPD are primarily problems with exhalation of air, in which air gets trapped in the lungs and results in

Table 4–4. *Corticosteroid Duration of Action*

Short Acting	*Intermediate Acting*	*Long Acting*
Hydrocortisone	Prednisone	Dexamethasone
Cortisone acetate	Triamcinolone	Betamethasone

decreased exchange of oxygen and carbon dioxide. Since the larynx is powered by breath support, vocal stamina and quality are lost when these illnesses become exacerbated. Because the problem is in the lungs, breath support for vocal function will be lost regardless of the breathing technique (clavicular vs. abdominal).

Inhalers have different mechanisms of action. The corticosteroid inhalers (fluticasone) reduce inflammation in the lung tissues, while other inhalers work specifically on mucus secretion (tiotropium bromide) in the lungs or on the smooth muscles surrounding the bronchioles (albuterol). These medications are very effective but also have consequences that are relevant to the vocal athlete (Chung, Caramori, & Adcock, 2009), as discussed below.

The powder form of these medications can cause local irritation and dryness. Patients on asthma inhalers should be instructed to rinse the mouth with water, gargle, and spit after each use. Fungal infections of the larynx can happen due to both the delivery method and the action of the inhaled medication. Hoarseness, painful phonation, or impairment of vocal range can occur gradually or suddenly. A laryngologist can usually determine if a fungal (yeast) infection is present on examination and may recommend treatment with an antifungal. Unfortunately, some people will have recurrent problems with fungal laryngitis and will need ongoing management or a medication change if possible (Ishizuka et al., 2007). The balance between managing asthma and optimizing voice can sometimes be challenging.

Albuterol inhalers are used as "rescue" inhalers to treat bronchospasm. This medication works by causing the tiny airway muscles to relax, opening up the airways to both inhalation and exhalation. This medication has a relatively short duration and may need to be redosed throughout the day. A beta-blocker called propranolol is sometimes taken for stage fright and will render this rescue inhaler ineffective. Propranolol is contraindicated in patients with asthma because of this interaction.

Stimulants, Including Caffeine

The medical indications for stimulants are limited. They include attention-deficit hyperactivity disorder (ADHD), narcolepsy, and obesity complicated by obstructive sleep apnea. Stimulants work by increasing the levels of dopamine in the brain and chronic use can alter natural dopamine synthesis. The effects of increased dopamine are increased wakefulness, awareness, and concentration for those patients with ADHD. Stimulants can lead to mania and increased anxiety and can also have effects outside of the brain such as increased blood pressure and heart rate. Dryness of the mouth can occur as well. Prescribed stimulants (Ritalin) have a high potential for abuse. They are Schedule I drugs in the United States and are highly controlled.

Caffeine is a stimulant and the active component of many energy drinks and diet formulas. It is the stimulant naturally found in teas and coffee. A moderate amount of caffeine is considered to be 200 mg and is the average adult intake per day. Caffeine reaches peak blood levels in 1 hour after consumption. Studies have shown that moderate caffeine intake improves aerobic performance in recreational and elite athletes (Spreit, 1995).

Caffeine is commonly thought to be a diuretic that can lead to dehydration. The truth is a bit more complicated. Caffeine is a weak diuretic, but the body adjusts to its effects and excessive water loss is not a concern, so daily intake of a usual amount of caffeine does not cause dehydration. If caffeine is taken at high doses (greater than 250 mg), a significant short-term diuretic effect will occur, but not to the extent that it disrupts sodium and potassium balance in the blood. More water will be lost than taken in and one might experience some mild thirst. Intermittent consumption of caffeinated beverages can increase anxiety and arousal. This causes the body's own nervous system to be more sensitive to natural adrenaline. Adrenaline in turn can decrease salivary flow and result in dryness of the respiratory tract. For the vocal athlete, this drying effect from higher doses of caffeine can be enough to increase the effort of singing and should be considered in the overall health of the performer (Maughan & Griffin, 2003). See Table 4–5 for examples of the quantity of caffeine in common drinks and snacks.

Table 4–5. ***Caffeine Content of Common Soft Drinks and Snacks***

Item	*Size (oz)*	*Caffeine (mg)*
Tea	5	40–80
Coffee	5	60–150
Cola drinks (Coke/Pepsi)	12	43–45
Mountain Dew	12	55
7-Up, Sprite, root beer	12	0
Coffee yogurt/ice cream	8	40–60
Milk chocolate	1	1–15
Dark chocolate bar	1	20

HORMONAL CONSIDERATIONS

The endocrine system and changes in the body's hormonal environment can have a significant impact on the voice. One explanation for this is the presence of estrogen, androgen, and progesterone receptors in the laryngeal tissues. As a result, the hormone changes that occur during puberty, the menstrual cycle, and menopause result in changes in the larynx and ultimately the voice.

Females may develop dysphonia due to fluctuations in hormones related to the menstrual cycle (Figure 4–6). Premenstrual voice syndrome (PMVS), also known as premenstrual dysphonia, affects one third of menstruating females and is characterized by vocal fatigue, decrease in vocal range, and loss of vocal power. The changes responsible for this syndrome are unknown but are thought to be related to edema caused by elevated estrogen levels. Indeed, videostroboscopies performed on women in the premenstrual portion of their cycle demonstrate vocal fold swelling resulting in disturbances in muscle function and vibratory patterns. Interestingly, observers are often unable to detect any difference in voice quality of singers during the premenstrual phase. However, singers are able to identify which of their own recordings were taken during their premenstrual phase and perceive a negative impact on vocal quality (Kadakia, Carlson, & Sataloff, 2013; Oberlander, 2010).

In the luteal phase of the menstrual cycle, a relatively high proportion of progesterone is present in the beginning of the phase. Progesterone results in more viscous secretions, leading to decreased vibratory efficiency (Kadakia et al., 2013).

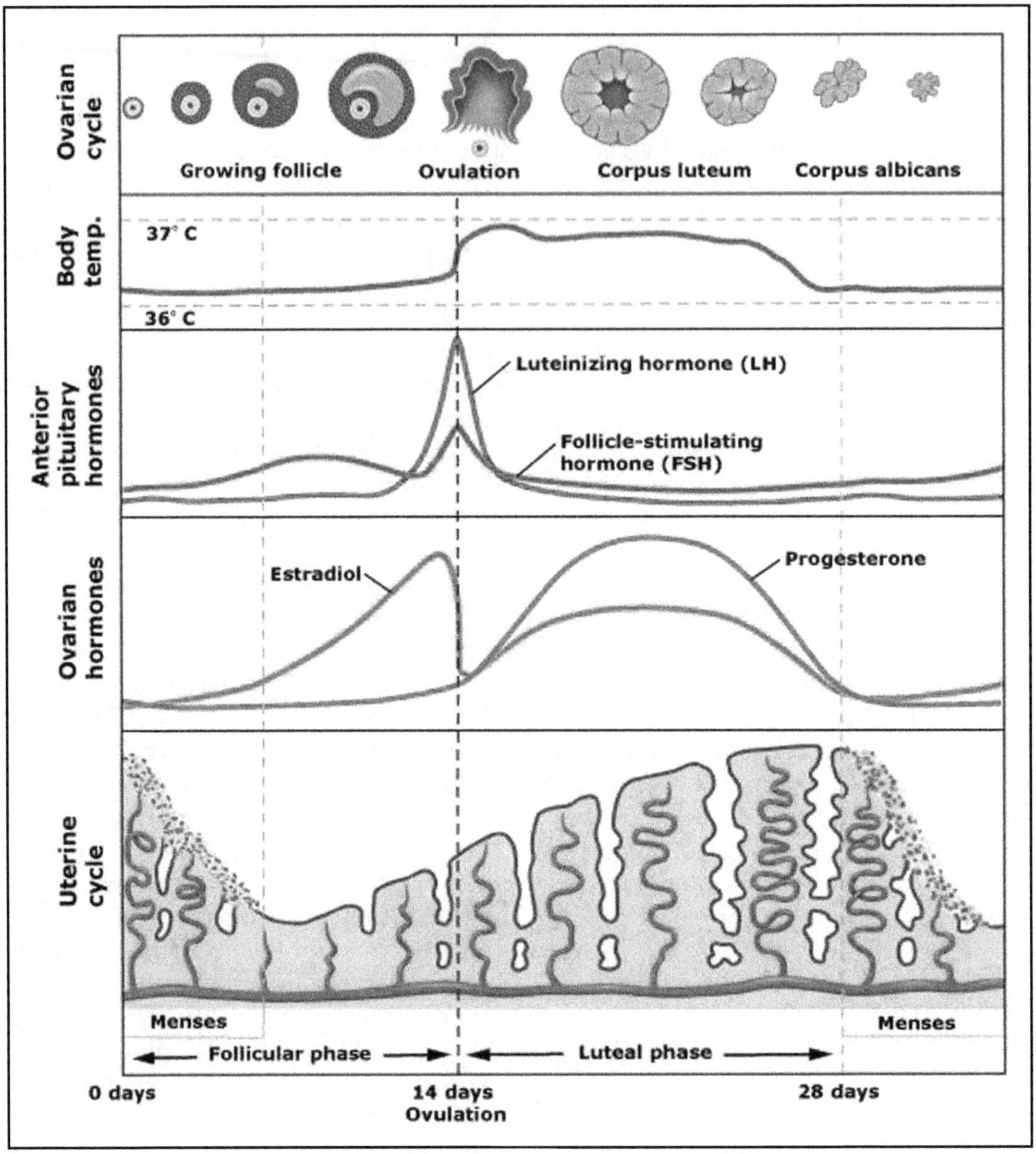

Figure 4–6. *The cyclical changes that occur during the normal menstrual cycle in women. Reproduced with permission from Encyclopaedia Britannica.*

The end of the phase is characterized by a sharp drop in both estrogen and progesterone. Continuous changes in the concentrations of sex hormones have been hypothesized to also interfere with laryngeal neuromotor control (La, Sundberg, Howard, Sa-Couto, & Freitas, 2012). Oral contraceptive pills (OCPs), which stabilize hormone variation across the menstrual cycle, are one proposed treatment to decrease the changes in vocal function. In one study, singers on OCPs rated higher on voice perception scores and mood (Oberlander, 2010; Ryan & Kenny, 2009). This study also concluded that it is important to educate singers that their own perception regarding their vocal quality may not coincide with perception of quality by others (Ryan & Kenny, 2009).

Pregnancy results in numerous changes that affect the voice. The increase in estrogen, progesterone, and testosterone, particularly in the last trimester, results in water absorption into Reinke's space. This may lead to voice aperiodicity, lowering of fundamental frequency, and uncontrolled timbral changes. Elevated phonation threshold pressures and collision threshold pressures have been demonstrated, suggesting that pregnancy affects vocal fold motility. Increased progesterone leads to decreased lower esophageal tone and gastric motility, resulting in gastroesophageal reflux. Abdominal breath support may be affected by the enlarging uterus, resulting in compensatory muscle tension in the neck, head, throat, and tongue muscles. Consideration should be given to discontinuation of singing if abdominal breath support becomes significantly compromised; however, many singers have been able to continue singing up to their due date without adverse consequences, and therefore the decision to stop singing should be made on an individual basis. The strain associated with the birthing process may result in injury to the vocal folds. Therefore, singers should be evaluated postpregnancy if postpartum dysphonia is noted (Kadakia et al., 2013; La & Sundberg, 2010).

Menopause marks another time when significant changes in hormone levels occur. There is a significant decrease in estrogen, although ovaries continue to secrete androgen (Kadakia et al., 2013). The resulting changes in laryngeal mucosa lead to vocal fatigue, decreased power and range, and lower fundamental frequency. Hormone replacement therapy has been found to improve voice quality and counteract vocal changes caused by menopause (D'haeseleer, Depypere, Claeys, Baudonck, & Van Lierde, 2012); however, its use has been associated with increased risk of coronary artery disease, stroke, venous thromboembolism, and breast cancer. Therefore, consultation with an endocrinologist and laryngologist is recommended when considering this treatment option (Heman-Ackah, 2004). Androgens have been recommended by some physicians to counteract the decreased libido and hot flashes associated with menopause; however, androgens can cause deepening of the female voice that is irreversible and therefore should be avoided in singers. The effects of aging may also become evident after menopause and include atrophy of laryngeal muscles and stiffening of the cartilages and vocal folds (Kadakia et al., 2013). It may be difficult to distinguish age-related changes from hormone-related changes. See Chapter 17 for in-depth discussion of effects of aging and menopause on the singing voice.

Males are also subject to voice changes related to hormones. There is a complex interaction of testosterone and DHT (dihydrotestosterone) at puberty, resulting in rapid increase in mass of the laryngeal framework, increased muscle and ligament bulk, and thus markedly decreased pitch (Kadakia et al., 2013)—typically by about one octave (Colton & Casper, 1996). During adolescent voice change, the voice begins with a husky quality and unsteady pitch with oscillating tones. The pitch can fluctuate day to day but the trend is toward lower, more stable tones. The average time from onset to completion of adolescent voice change is 3 to 6 months (Aronson & Bless, 2009).

Some adolescent males experience a form of muscle tension dysphonia known as puberphonia or mutational falsetto, in which the preadolescent higher pitched voice persists after puberty. The patient typically presents with a high-pitched voice, breathy vocal quality, poor projection, and often with frequent pitch breaks (Andrews, 1999; Colton & Casper, 1996). In essence, the voice becomes "stuck" in the falsetto (cricothyroid dominant) mechanism. Some feel that this may occur as a reaction to the normal vocal instability of the adolescent male voice. The speaker unconsciously "holds onto" the voice that is more familiar and more stable (Colton & Casper, 1996). Puberphonia typically resolves with voice therapy, in which the clinician guides the speaker to "discover" and maintain appropriate thyroarytenoid dominant vocal register.

In summary, hormone fluctuations that occur in males and females have significant impact on the voice. Knowledge of these changes is important to help with evaluation, counseling, and treatment.

VOCAL CORD DYSFUNCTION/ IRRITABLE LARYNX

Normal respiration is characterized by abduction of the vocal folds on inspiration and slight adduction on expiration (Forrest, Husein, & Husein, 2012). Upon phonation, the vocal folds adduct to position the vocal folds near midline (Woodson, 2015). Exhalation causes subglottic pressure to increase until the vocal folds are displaced laterally. This resultant decrease in pressure, along with elastic forces on the vocal fold and Bernoulli effect, causes the vocal folds to return to midline and the cycle is repeated (Woodson, 2015). Vocal fold dysfunction (VFD), also known as paradoxical vocal fold motion (PVFM), is a respiratory condition where intermittent paradoxical closure of the vocal folds occurs during respiration (Frank-Ito, Schulz, Vess, & Witsell, 2014). Other terms for this condition include paradoxical vocal cord dysfunction and episodic laryngeal dyskinesis.

Episodes of PVFM typically last seconds to minutes, are experienced around the upper respiratory tract (sensation of tightness in the throat or throat closing), and occur primarily during inspiration (Frank-Ito et al., 2014). This results in symptoms similar to that of airway obstruction such as choking, cough, dysphonia, and shortness of breath. PVFM is often is misdiagnosed as asthma. Using a computer model, a study of airflow dynamics suggests that an episode of PVFM can reduce airflow rate by more than 50%, create disturbed flow with high velocity in the glottis, and negatively impact aerodynamics beyond the larynx. Flexible fiber-optic laryngoscopy is important in the diagnosis of this condition to rule out other causes of airway obstruction and visualize the paradoxical vocal fold motion (Forrest et al., 2012); however, due to the intermittent nature of the disorder, false-negative exams may occur. In this situation, provocation techniques can be performed to elicit PVFM, such as exposing the patient to noxious stimuli while laryngosocopy is performed. For some patients, PVFM is primarily associated with exertion, particularly for elite athletes. In such cases, induced exertion (such as walking or running on a treadmill) may be used to elicit symptoms. Clinical history and pulmonary function tests are also important diagnostic elements, in addition to flexible laryngoscopy (Frank-Ito et al., 2014).

PVFM can be categorized into primary and secondary. The etiology of primary PVFM is thought to be psychologic, which was found to represent 70% of cases in a prospective study (Forrest et al., 2012). Psychologic testing revealed the majority of these patients to have a classic conversion disorder, which is characterized by deficits in voluntary motor or sensory functioning without a physiologic basis or organic cause. The symptoms are not intentionally produced and are thought to arise in response to a stressful situation (Owens & Dein, 2006). However, a small minority of patients appeared to be malingering (Forrest et al., 2012).

Causes of secondary PVFM consist of medical disorders and can further be divided into neurologic conditions that are based on an abnormal motor response or hypersensitivity reactions (Forrest et al., 2012). Some neurologic etiologies of PVCM include spasmodic dysphonia and multiple sclerosis, but these are rare causes. Laryngeal hypersensitivity plays a far more common role in secondary PVFM, and patients often have more chronic symptoms compared to primary PVFM. Patients with laryngeal hypersensitivity who have symptoms attributable to laryngeal tension (such as dysphonia or laryngospasm with or without globus or chronic cough), visible and palpable evidence of tension, and the presence of a sensory trigger are classified as having irritable larynx syndrome (ILS). It is hypothesized that patients with ILS have a central nervous system (CNS) change that leaves sensorimotor pathways in a hyperexcitable state and therefore inappropriately reactive to stimuli (Morrison, Rammage, & Emami, 1999). Gastroesophageal reflux disease, postviral illness, emotional distress, and habitual postural muscle misuse are suggested as causative agents that result in this CNS hyperreactivity (Figure 4–7).

The treatment of PVFM is dependent on the underlying etiology. For primary PVFM, speech therapy focusing on breathing exercises that improve laryngeal control, cough interruption strategies (such as coughing through tightly pursed lips to reduce forceful vocal fold collision), strategic avoidance of PVFM triggers, relaxation techniques, and stress reduction are recommended. For exercise-induced PVFM, treatment may involve practicing laryngeal control strategies under gradually increasing levels of exertion. If these measures fail, then consideration can be given to referral for

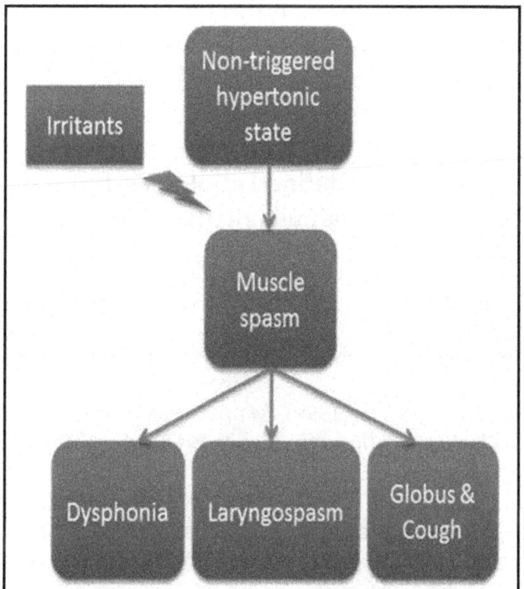

***Figure 4–7.** Irritable larynx syndrome. Adapted from Morrison, M., Rammage, L., & Emami, A. J. (1999). The irritable larynx syndrome.* Journal of Voice, *13(3), 447–455.*

psychologic counseling and additional measures such as cognitive-behavioral therapy (Forrest et al., 2012). Comorbid conditions that contribute to PVFM such as asthma, reflux, and chronic sinusitis must be addressed as well. Patients with asthma have a predisposition to developing PVFM, possibly related to the use of inhalers, and physicians should maintain a high level of suspicion for PVFM in poorly controlled asthmatics (Forrest et al., 2012). Conversely, many patients with PVFM are misdiagnosed as having asthma, and methacholine challenge may be appropriate to clarify the diagnosis and guide treatment. In patients with secondary PVFM, management should include decreasing the suspected laryngeal irritants. For example, patients with reflux should be given proton-pump inhibitors, while those with allergies and postnasal drainage should be treated with antihistamines or nasal steroids. For patients with chronic cough related to laryngeal hypersensitivity, neuromodulating agents such as amitriptyline can be considered (Cohen & Misono, 2013). PVFM can be challenging to treat, due to its varied and sometimes vaguely defined etiologies, but with persistence it can usually be managed.

REFERENCES

Andrews, M. L. (1999). *Manual of voice treatment: Pediatrics through geriatrics* (2nd ed.). San Diego, CA: Singular.

Aronson, A. E., & Bless, D. M. (2009). Normal voice development. In T. Hiscock (Ed.), *Clinical voice disorders* (pp. 14–16). New York, NY: Thieme Medical.

Blitzer, A., Brin, M. F., & Stewart, C. F. (1998). Botulinum toxin management of spasmodic dysphonia (laryngeal dystonia): A 12-year experience in more than 900 patients. *Laryngoscope, 108*(10), 1435–1441.

Chung, K. F., Caramori, G., & Adcock, I. M. (2009). Inhaled corticosteroids as combination therapy with beta-adrenergic agonists in airways disease: Present and future. *European Journal of Clinical Pharmacology, 65*(9), 853–871.

Cohen, S. M., Dinan, M. A., Roy, N., Kim, J., & Courey, M. (2014). Diagnosis change in voice-disordered patients evaluated by primary care and/or otolaryngology: A longitudinal study. *Otolaryngology–Head and Neck Surgery, 150*(1), 95–102.

Cohen, S. M., & Garrett, C. G. (2008). Hoarseness: Is it really laryngopharyngeal reflux? *Laryngoscope, 118,* 363–366.

Cohen, S. M., & Misono, S. (2013). Use of specific neuromodulators in the treatment of chronic, idiopathic cough: A systematic review. *Otolaryngology–Head and Neck Surgery, 148*(3), 374–382.

Collazo-Clavell, M. L., Gharib, H., & Maragos, N. E. (1995). Relationship between vocal cord paralysis and benign thyroid disease. *Head and Neck, 17*(1), 24–30.

Colton, R. H., & Casper, J. K. (1996). *Understanding voice problems: A physiological perspective for diagnosis and treatment.* Baltimore, MD: Lippincott Williams & Wilkins.

Cope, D., & Bova, R. (2008). Diagnosis and management of rhinitis: Complete guidelines of the Joint Task Force on Practice Parameters in Allergy, Asthma and Immunology. *Laryngoscope, 118*(9), 1556–1560.

Crumley, R. L., & Izdebski, K. (1986). Voice quality following laryngeal reinnervation by ansa hypoglossi transfer. *Laryngoscope, 96*(6), 611–616.

D'haeseleer, E., Depypere, H., Claeys, S., Baudonck, N., & Van Lierde, K. (2012). The impact of hormone therapy on vocal quality in postmenopausal women. *Journal of Voice, 26*(5), 671.e1–671.e7.

Dykewicz, M. S., Fineman, S., Skoner, D. P., Nicklas, R., Lee, R., Blessing-Moore, J., . . . Schuller, D. (1998), Diagnosis and management of rhinitis: Complete guidelines of the Joint Task Force on Practice Parameters in Allergy, Asthma and Immunology. *Annals of Allergy, Asthma & Immunology, 81*(5), 478–518.

Forrest, L. A., Husein, T., & Husein, O. (2012). Paradoxical vocal cord motion: Classification and treatment. *Laryngoscope, 122*(4), 844–853.

Frank-Ito, D. O., Schulz, K., Vess, G., & Witsell, D. (2014). Changes in aerodynamics during vocal cord dysfunction. *Computers in Biology and Medicine, 57,* 116–122.

Gill, J. M., Fleischut, P., Haas, S., Pellini, B., Crawford, A., & Nash, D. B. (2006). Use of antibiotics for adult upper respiratory infections in outpatient setting: A national ambulatory network study. *Family Medicine, 38*(5), 349–354.

Heman-Ackah, Y. D. (2004). Hormone replacement therapy: Implications of the women's health initiative for the perimenopausal singer. *Journal of Singing, 60*(5), 471–475.

Ishizuka, T., Hisada, T., Aoki, H., Yanagitani, N., Kaira, K., Utsugi, M., . . . Mori, M. (2007). Gender and age risks for hoarseness and dysphonia with use of a dry powder fluticasone propionate inhaler in asthma. *Allergy Asthma Proceedings, 28*(5), 550–556.

Kadakia, S., Carlson, D., & Sataloff, R. T. (2013). The effect of hormones on the voice. *Journal of Singing, 69,* 571–574.

Kennel, K. A., & Drake, M. T. (2009). Adverse effects of bisphosphonates: Implications for osteoporosis management. *Mayo Clinic Proceedings, 84*(7), 632–638.

La, F. M., & Sundberg, J. (2010). Pregnancy and the signing voice: Reports from a case study. *Journal of Voice, 25*(4), 431–439.

La, F. M., Sundberg, J., Howard, D. M., Sa-Couto, P., & Freitas, A. (2012). Effects of the menstrual cycle and oral contraception on singers' pitch control. *Journal of Speech, Language, and Hearing Research, 55,* 247–261.

Lambert, D. M., Marceau, S., & Forse, R. A. (2005). Intra-abdominal pressure in the morbidly obese. *Obesity Surgery, 15,* 1225–1232.

Manji, N., Carr-Smith, J. D., Boelaert, K., Allahabadia, A., Armitage, M., Chatterjee, V. K., . . . Franklyn, J. A. (2006). Influences of age, gender, smoking, and family history on autoimmune thyroid disease phenotype. *Journal of Clinical Endocrinology and Metabolism, 91*(12), 4873–4880.

Maughan, R. J., & Griffin, J. (2003). Caffeine ingestion and fluid balance: A review. *Journal of Human Nutrition and Dietetics, 16*(6), 411–420.

Meltzer, E. O., & Hamilos, D. (2011). Rhinosinusitis diagnosis and management for the clinician: A synopsis of recent consensus guidelines. *Mayo Clinic Proceedings, 86*(5), 427–443.

Misono, S., & Merati, A, L. (2012). Evidence-based practice: evaluation and management of unilateral vocal fold paralysis. *Otolaryngologic Clinics of North America, 45*(5), 1083–1108.

Morrison, M., Rammage, L., & Emami, A. J. (1999). The irritable larynx syndrome. *Journal of Voice, 13*(3), 447–455.

Myssiorek, D. (2004). Recurrent laryngeal nerve paralysis: Anatomy and etiology. *Otolaryngologic Clinics of North America, 37*(1), 25–44.

Oberlander, E. (2010). Premenstrual syndrome and its effects on laryngeal functionality: An approach for singers and pedagogues. *Journal of Singing, 67*(1), 27–34.

Owens, C., & Dein, S. (2006). Conversion disorder: The modern hysteria. *Advances in Psychiatric Treatment, 12*(2), 152–157.

Ritchie, M., & Yeap, B. B. (2015). Thyroid hormone: Influences on mood and cognition in adults. *Maturitas, 81*(2), 266–275.

Rubin, A. D., & Sataloff, R. T. (2007). Vocal fold paresis and paralysis. *Otolaryngologic Clinics of North America, 40*(5), 1109–1131.

Ryan, M., & Kenny, D. T. (2009). Perceived effects of the menstrual cycle on young female singers in the Western classical tradition. *Journal of Voice, 23*(1), 99–108.

Schwartz, S. R., Cohen, S. M., Dailey, S. H., Rosenfeld, R. M., Deutsch, E. S., Gillespie, M. B., . . . Patel, M. M. (2009). Clinical practice guideline: Hoarseness (dysphonia). *Otolaryngology–Head and Neck Surgery, 141,* S1–S31.

Spielman, J., Ramig, L. O., Mahler, L., Halpern, A., & Gavin, W. J. (2007). Effects of an extended version of the Lee Silverman voice treatment on voice and speech in Parkinson's disease. *American Journal of Speech-Language Pathology, 16*(2), 95–107.

Spreit, L. L. (1995). Caffeine and performance. *International Journal of Sports Nutrition, 5,* S84–S99.

Wilson, L. J., Ma, W., & Hirschowitz, B. I. (1999). Association of obesity with hiatal hernia and esophagitis. *The American Journal of Gastroenterology, 94,* 2840–2844.

Woodson, G. E. (2015). Laryngeal and pharyngeal function. In M. A. Richardson, P. W. Flint, B. H. Haughey, V. J. Lund, J. K Niparko, K. T Robbins, . . . M. M. Lesperance (Eds.). *Cummings otolaryngology: Head and neck surgery* (6th ed., pp. 831–833). Philadelphia, PA: Elsevier.

CHAPTER 5

Vocal Hygiene for Singers

Vocal hygiene refers to taking care of the voice (like dental hygiene means taking care of the teeth) and also taking care of the body in order to support the voice. The body is the support system and "carrying case" for the vocal instrument and a number of seemingly unrelated health considerations can have a direct effect on the voice. Good vocal hygiene is important for optimizing vocal health for anyone, but especially for singers, given the athletic nature of their vocal activities. Mastering vocal hygiene is vitally important for recovery from a vocal injury, and for many singers, this element will be a critical part of the rehabilitation plan. The information in this chapter is summarized in an educational handout in Appendix 5–A.

HYDRATION

The vocal folds are bathed in mucus, which acts as an important lubricant to protect them from the heat and friction of vibration. If the mucus remains thin and slippery, it will fulfill its lubricating role well. However, dehydration can contribute to increased viscosity of the mucus, making it thick and gooey, undermining its lubricating function. The importance and benefits of both internal and external hydration for vocal health have been well documented. Poor hydration increases phonatory effort and phonation threshold pressure (PTP, the minimum amount of subglottic pressure needed to initiate vocal fold vibration) (Leydon, Sivasankar, Falciglia, Atkins, & Fisher, 2009; Verdolini, Titze, & Fennell, 1994; Verdolini et al., 2002).

Recommendations for adequate fluid intake vary. In *Dietary Reference Intakes: The Essential Guide to Nutrient Requirements,* Otten, Hellwig, and Meyers (2006) recommend 3.7 liters per day of total beverages for adult males and 2.7 liters per day of total beverages for adult females. Many people are chronically dehydrated, and for them, increasing fluid intake to over 3 liters may seem like a daunting task. I typically recommend 2 liters per day of noncaffeinated and nonalcoholic beverages (see below for discussion of caffeine and alcohol). If you are working with a singer who finds achieving adequate hydration challenging, set small goals and celebrate small improvements. For people who just don't like drinking water, you can suggest flavoring the water or drinking herbal teas (hot or cold). Urine color is a useful indicator of adequate hydration. "Sing wet and pee pale" is a common endorsement among voice teachers, and an apt one.

Some people feel that drinking ice-cold water is contraindicated for singing, as the larynx and esophagus share a common wall and the water temperature may affect the entire area. The idea is that once muscles are warmed up, you don't want to do anything to make them cold again (think of a pitcher keeping his jacket over his arm between innings or dancers wearing leggings during breaks). Although there is merit to this argument, the cold water is not in fact making direct contact with the muscles primarily in question (i.e., the intrinsic and extrinsic laryngeal muscles). I am usually much more interested in getting the water *into* the singer than worrying about the temperature. If having the water ice-cold makes it more likely the singer will drink it, I count that as a hydration win.

Surface hydration can have short-term benefits for vocal function (Leydon et al., 2009; Verdolini et al., 1994). Many singers find steam inhalation both soothing and vocally beneficial. This can be accomplished by simply inhaling the steam from a hot beverage (killing two birds with one stone, assuming the individual drinks the liquid), by inhaling shower steam, or by using a personal steamer. Room humidifiers or vaporizers can be helpful too, especially if the indoor environment is dry. I always caution singers to be religious about cleaning such devices to avoid sending irritants and bacteria into the room.

Caffeine

Caffeine has long gotten a bad rap in the realm of vocal health, as it is a diuretic and thought to be dehydrating. The diuretic effect of caffeine kicks in at about 250 mg (see Chapter 4 for further discussion and Table 4–5 for relative caffeine levels in various beverages). However, Maughan and Griffin, (2003) report that regular caffeine consumers develop a tolerance to its effects, including the diuretic effect. Recent studies have examined effects of caffeine on voice in quantities ranging from about 100 to 400 mg (Erickson-Levandoski & Sivasankar, 2011; Franca, Simpson, & Schuette, 2013). These studies found that caffeine did not have a significant effect on vocal acoustics, PTP, or phonatory effort.

In the grand scheme of substances that have potential to harm the voice, the evidence for caffeine as a vocal villain appears weak. Voice rehabilitation is loaded with admonitions and prohibitions, and there are so many changes singers must make to get their voices back on track. I am disinclined to make another big "no-no" out of caffeine consumption related to hydration (although caffeine can be a reflux trigger, and singers who have GERD should be counseled accordingly). If the singer doesn't drink a lot of water, I usually present it as a negotiation: Try to keep the caffeine under 250 mg, and get the water up to the recommended level.

Alcohol

Alcohol is also a diuretic and can therefore be dehydrating. Interestingly, Hobson and Maughan (2010) concluded that the dehydrating effect of alcohol is blunted when the body is in a hypohydrated state (specifically for beer). I don't think this makes a strong argument in favor of drinking alcohol for hydration, though, as the dehydrated state one would need to be in for the effect to occur is obviously vocally undesirable. For some, alcohol can be a reflux trigger. As with caffeine, I typically advocate for moderation in alcohol consumption, taking my cue from most healthcare providers who recommend limiting oneself to no more than one to two drinks per day.

My counseling around alcohol is usually focused on the behavioral risks and the potential for unwise voice use when in an inebriated state. When inhibitions are lowered and judgment is impaired, the singer is much less likely to be mindful of how much, how loudly, and how intensely her or she is using the voice, especially when in a social setting that is loud and boisterous. Furthermore, alcohol affects coordination, so when singers use alcohol while performing, vocal technique may be compromised.

Moisturizing Throat Sprays

Many singers swear by lubricating throat sprays, such as Singer's Saving Grace, Entertainer's Secret, or Vocal-Eze. Roy, Tanner, Gray, Blomgren, and Fisher (2003) looked at the effect of three potential laryngeal lubricants (water, mannitol, and Entertainer's Secret Throat Spray) on PTP, an indicator of efficient phonation and phonatory effort. They found that while mannitol did reduce PTP, the benefit lasted only 20 minutes. Water and Entertainer's Secret had no significant effect on PTP. Based on this apparent lack of efficacy, I don't recommend these products to singers. However, if they are in the habit of using them and perceive them to be helpful, I see no harm in continuing, although I do usually check the ingredients of the specific product to make sure it does not contain alcohol or other contraindicated substances.

While I see no harm in singers using this type of product, I am careful to ascertain why they feel they need it. If there is chronic throat irritation, it is important to get at the source and not just try to cover it up. The irritation could be a result of allergies, reflux, or poor hydration, any of which would be better treated medically or behaviorally.

Medications That Cause Mucosal Dryness

Medications and effects on the voice were covered in Chapter 4. However, the topic bears reviewing here as some medications—particularly over-the-counter allergy and cold treatments—can be systemically drying, and therefore can affect the voice. I am always careful not to recommend that singers take or discontinue medications, as that is outside my scope of practice. However, for singers who are using oral antihistamines and decongestants regularly, I usually consult our laryngologists or advise singers to consult their physicians to see if a topical treatment (such as a nasal steroid or antihistamine spray) is an option. See Chapter 4 for additional information about optimal treatment for chronic congestion or postnasal drip for singers.

The Milk Myth

"Don't ever have dairy products when you're going to sing" is a tried-and-true tenet of singing mythology. It appears to be just that: a myth. There is no research that suggests an increase in laryngeal mucus viscosity associated with dairy products. On the contrary, there is some research that has found that dairy products do nothing to increase production or viscosity of mucus (Thiara & Goldman, 2012). Part of the reason for this myth may have to do with the fact that milk is a relatively viscous beverage. When you drink a glass of milk, you can see the residue clinging to the inside of the glass after it is empty. It will similarly coat the inside of the mouth and throat immediately after drinking, which may be perceived as a mucus-like sensation. Some people have a dietary intolerance for dairy products that may cause gastrointestinal symptoms. Despite the lack of evidence, many singers still swear that dairy makes them have an increased sensation of mucus in the throat. I usually say, "If that's how it feels to you, and if it feels better when you don't consume dairy, then heed what your body is telling you and avoid it."

SELF-CARE

Since the body is the carrying case and support system for the vocal instrument, one's general health can have a significant impact on the voice. Getting adequate rest, nutrition, and exercise are important contributors to overall health. Achieving this can be challenging depending on individual circumstances and is especially hard for singers who are on the road a lot. In such cases, you may need to strategize with the singer to optimize self-care habits.

Most singers recognize that having an upper respiratory infection, cold, or flu can cause an acute alteration of voice. Strenuous use of the voice (such as singing) under these conditions can potentially lead to a more chronic injury, especially if it occurs repeatedly. Avoiding getting sick in the first place is the best way to circumvent the problem. Singers should practice good handwashing habits, using soap and water or alcohol-based hand sanitizers before eating and before touching eyes, nose, or mouth.

Mental wellness is an important aspect of the singer's self-care. Singing can be a stressful act and, depending on the singer's personal circumstances, professional status, and singing environment, stress can become a major component in the singer's overall health. If you suspect that the singer is struggling to achieve mental wellness, provide appropriate resources and referrals. This will be discussed in greater depth in Chapter 8.

INHALED SUBSTANCES

Cigarette Smoking

Smoking cigarettes indisputably puts singers at risk for vocal fold damage (Branski, Zhou, Kraus, & Sivasankar, 2011). Cigarette smoking causes laryngeal cancer and can also cause the voluminous swelling of polypoid corditis. Either will have a significant negative impact on the voice. In short, smoking and singing don't mix. This goes for second-hand smoke as well.

Electronic Cigarettes

Unfortunately, many people who are smokers believe that e-cigarettes are not harmful. At this point, the jury is still out. Pisinger and Dossing (2014) reviewed 76 studies on e-cigarettes but weren't able to draw any firm conclusions on safety due to the many problems they found with the studies (methodology, study size, conflicts of interest). However, many e-cigarettes contain propylene glycol (also used in stage smoke), which is a laryngeal irritant (see below under "Stage Smoke"). I advise singers that until we know more about the safety of e-cigarettes, they should avoid the risk and quit smoking altogether.

Marijuana

Although smoking marijuana does not present the same cancer risk as smoking tobacco, marijuana is addictive, the inhaled smoke is a laryngeal irritant, and inhalation of burning particles can potentially cause thermal injury. Some believe that vaporized marijuana decreases the thermal and irritant risk. I provide this information to my patients, along with the same advice about the potential for unwise vocal behavior any consciousness-altering substance may engender (see below under "Use of Recreational Drugs").

Stage Smoke

Stage smoke is not limited to theatrical productions and concerts, it may also be used in religious services that feature a theatrical worship style. There are a number of different organic and inorganic products used to create stage smoke. The most common are glycol-based products. These chemicals are very irritating and potentially toxic (Herman & Rossol, 2006). If you are working with a singer who performs in environments where stage smoke is used, it will be important to consider whether the exposure may contribute to laryngeal irritation and the overall voice problem. If so, it may be necessary to have a conversation with the relevant production staff to explore whether the type and duration of exposure can be limited.

USE OF RECREATIONAL DRUGS

Any substance that alters the singer's consciousness will have a negative impact on coordination, and on the ability to be aware of voice use and use good judgment. Obviously, drug use has health and lifestyle implications that extend beyond the issue of vocal health. If you suspect that a singer you are working with has a drug or alcohol problem, provide him or her with information on getting appropriate help. This must be handled carefully and sensitively. If the singer has the impression that you are being judgmental, he or she may discontinue rehabilitation. Try to express your concerns in a genuine and compassionate manner, and couch the risks in the context of the singer's overall vocal wellness and singing rehabilitation goals.

LARYNGEAL BEHAVIORS

Throat Clearing

Throat clearing is traumatic to the vocal folds. The violent adduction associated with this behavior creates a risk for tissue damage and may become self-perpetuating. The throat clear causes vocal fold irritation, and the irritation stimulates the urge to clear the throat. Often, the throat clearing is done in an attempt to clear mucus from the vocal folds. This, too, becomes a vicious cycle: The throat clear traumatizes the vocal fold tissue, and the body sends more mucus to protect the tissue.

The discussion of the dangers of throat clearing provides a great opportunity to reinforce the importance of hydration. The mucus is supposed to be there.

When it is thin, slippery, and lubricating, we don't perceive it. It is only when the viscosity of the mucus increases that it starts to feel irritating. So, improving hydration can decrease the need to clear.

No matter what starts it, once throat clearing is a chronic behavior, it crosses the line into habit. In order to eliminate it, the throat clear will need to be replaced with a new habit, and this takes time. A study by Lally, van Jaarsveld, Potts, and Wardle (2009) found that it took subjects 18 to 254 days to form new habits, with the average being about 66 days. It may be necessary to repeatedly remind the singer of this. I often describe the urge to throat clear as being like the urge to scratch an itch—you have to consciously suppress it. Replacing it with a new behavior such as swallowing or taking a sip of water can help and supports hydration goals. You can also recommend a "gentle" throat clear, using air to blow the mucus off the folds. There should be no voicing when this is done correctly.

Lozenges

Singers often find it helpful to use lozenges or hard candy to keep the mouth moist. This is fine, as long as the lozenges don't contain irritating or anesthetizing ingredients. Menthol and eucalyptus (common cough drop ingredients) are irritating to the throat and should be avoided. Benzocaine is a topical anesthetic found in a number of throat lozenges that can have the effect of masking throat pain. If the throat pain is related to muscle tension, allergic irritation, reflux, or dehydration, the solution is to address the underlying problem, not cover it up. Mint is a muscle relaxer that can exacerbate reflux. For people who feel the need to use lozenges, I usually recommend those containing glycerin, slippery elm, or pectin. There are a number of products featuring these ingredients on the market.

Yelling and Screaming

Yelling and screaming are also included in the list of phonotraumatic vocal behaviors that should be avoided. Sometimes this type of voicing is required for performers, particularly for actors. We will discuss techniques for "safe" yelling in Chapter 13. However, if the singer is engaging in this type of voice use for interactions (such as yelling across the house to call the kids to the dinner table), athletic or other spirit events, cheerleading, or regularly speaking in environments that are so loud one has to yell to be heard, appropriate adaptation is indicated. This might mean finding an alternative to yelling in the house (using a bell or whistle to call the kids, or even calling or texting them via cell phone), using a noisemaker at athletic or spirit events, using amplification in noisy environments, moving to a quieter location to speak, or communicating through writing in noisy environments if necessary. Although it is possible to teach appropriate vocal coordination for cheerleading, this is an activity that is vocally taxing. If singing is a priority and the singer has an injury, it may be necessary to put cheerleading on the back burner or discuss nonvocal involvement (such as lip synching) with the cheerleading coach, at least in the short term.

Whispering

Many people believe that whispering counts as voice rest. If the whisper is accomplished with very low intensity, no vocal fold contact, and no supraglottic strain, this might be true. The problem is that the inherent low intensity of whispering renders it a poor option for communication, and in an effort to be heard, people usually use excessive laryngeal strain (and in some cases, vocal fold adduction) when whispering. The degree to which individuals strain during whispering is quite variable (Rubin, Praneetvatakul, Gherson, Moyer, & Sataloff, 2006). Fleischer, Kothe, and Hess (2007) found varying patterns of glottal and supraglottal configuration during whispering, including partial or total contact of membranous vocal folds. They concluded that because the vocal folds weren't vibrating, whispering may be viable for postoperative communication purposes. However, the results certainly suggest supraglottic and isometric vocal fold tension that may promote hyperfunctional voice. In my opinion, it is much better to target efficient voice use or take a brief "voice nap" than to resort to whispering.

REFERENCES

Branski, R. C., Zhou, H., Kraus, D. H., & Sivasankar, M. (2011). The effects of cigarette smoke condensate on vocal fold transepithelial resistance and inflammatory signaling in vocal fold fibroblasts. *Laryngoscope*, *121*(3), 601–605.

Erickson-Levandoski, E., & Sivasankar, M. (2011). Investigating the effects of caffeine on phonation. *Journal of Voice*, *25*(5), E215–E219.

Fleischer, S., Kothe, C., & Hess, M. (2007). Glottal and supraglottal configuration during whispering. *Laryngorhinootologie*, *86*(4), 271–275.

Franca, M. C., Simpson, K. O., & Schuette, A. (2013). Effects of caffeine on vocal acoustic and aerodynamic measures of adult females. *Codas*, *25*(3), 250–255.

Herman, H., & Rossol, M. (2006). Artificial fogs and smokes. In R. T. Sataloff (Ed.), *Vocal health and pedagogy. Volume II: Advanced assessment and practice*. San Diego, CA: Plural.

Hobson, R. M., & Maughan, R. J. (2010). Hydration status and the diuretic action of a small dose of alcohol. *Alcohol and Alcoholism*, *45*(4), 366–373.

Lally, P., van Jaarsveld, C. H. M., Potts, H. W. W., & Wardle, J. (2009). How are habits formed: Modeling habit formation in the real world. *European Journal of Social Psychology*, *40*(6), 998–1009.

Leydon, C., Sivasankar, M., Falciglia, D. L., Atkins, C., & Fisher, K. V. (2009). Vocal fold surface hydration: A review. *Journal of Voice*, *23*(6), 658–665.

Maughan, R. J., & Griffin, J. (2003). Caffeine ingestion and fluid balance: A review. *Journal of Human Nutrition and Dietetics*, *16*(6), 411–420.

Otten, J. J., Hellwig, J. P., & Meyers, L. D. (Eds.). (2006). *Dietary reference intakes: The essential guide to nutrient requirements*. Washington, DC: National Academies Press.

Pisinger, C., & Dossing, M. (2014). A systematic review of health effects of electronic cigarettes. *Preventive Medicine*, *69*, 248–260.

Roy, N., Tanner, K., Gray, S. D., Blomgren, M., & Fisher, K. V. (2003). An evaluation of the effects of three laryngeal lubricants on phonation threshold pressure (PTP). *Journal of Voice*, *17*(3), 331–342.

Rubin, A. D., Praneetvatakul, V. L., Gherson, S., Moyer, C. A., & Sataloff, R. T. (2006). Laryngeal hyperfunction during whispering: Reality or myth? *Journal of Voice*, *20*(1), 121–127.

Thiara, G., & Goldman, R. D. (2012). Milk consumption and mucus production in children with asthma. *Canadian Family Physician*, *58*(2), 165–166.

Verdolini, K., Min, Y., Titze, I. R., Lemke, J., Brown, K., van Mersbergen, M., . . . Fisher, K. (2002). Biological mechanisms underlying voice changes due to dehydration. *Journal of Speech, Language, and Hearing Research*, *45*(2), 268–281.

Verdolini, K., Titze, I. R., & Fennell, A. (1994). Dependence of phonatory effort on hydration level. *Journal of Speech, Language, and Hearing Research*, *37*(5), 1001–1007.

APPENDIX 5–A

Vocal Hygiene for Singers

Vocal hygiene refers to taking care of your voice (like dental hygiene means taking care of your teeth) and also taking care of the body in order to support the voice. Good vocal hygiene is important for optimizing vocal health for anyone, but especially for you as a vocal athlete. Mastering vocal hygiene is vitally important for your recovery from a vocal injury and long-term vocal health.

HYDRATION

The vocal folds are bathed in mucus, which acts as an important lubricant to protect them from the heat and friction of vibration that occurs when you talk or sing. The mucus should be thin and slippery to be lubricating. Dehydration can make the mucus thick and gooey.

1. Try to drink at least 64 ounces of water per day. You may need even more if you are very physically active. Urine color during waking hours can be a good indicator of how well you are hydrated. "Sing wet and pee pale." If you just don't like drinking water, try flavoring it or drinking herbal teas, hot or cold.
2. Steam inhalation can get droplet moisture to the vocal folds. This can be accomplished by simply inhaling the steam from a hot drink, by inhaling shower steam, or by using a personal steamer. Room humidifiers or vaporizers can be helpful too, especially if the indoor environment is dry. Be religious about cleaning these devices to avoid sending irritants and bacteria into the room.

CAFFEINE

Caffeine is a diuretic and can be dehydrating if consumed in large quantities. Try to keep caffeine consumption to no more than 250 mg per day. Use the chart below to estimate the amount of caffeine in various beverages.

Item	Size (oz)	Caffeine (mg)
Tea	5	40–80
Coffee	5	60–150
Cola drinks (Coke/Pepsi)	12	43–45
Mountain Dew	12	55
7-Up, Sprite, root beer	12	0
Coffee yogurt/ice cream	8	40–60
Milk chocolate	1	1–15
Dark chocolate bar	1	20

MOISTURIZING THROAT SPRAYS AND LOZENGES

1. To date, there has been no research that demonstrates lasting benefits

of lubricating throat sprays, such as Singer's Saving Grace, Entertainer's Secret, or Vocal-Eze. However, if you find throat sprays helpful, it's okay to use them. Just check the ingredients to make sure they don't contain alcohol, which can irritate your throat.

2. Lozenges are okay as long as they don't contain irritating or anesthetizing ingredients. Menthol and eucalyptus (common cough drop ingredients) are irritating to the throat and should be avoided. Benzocaine is a topical anesthetic found in a number of throat lozenges that can have the effect of "masking" throat pain. Look for lozenges containing glycerin, slippery elm, or pectin.

ALLERGY AND COLD MEDICATIONS

Oral antihistamines and decongestants can dry out the throat and make your mucus thicker. If you have allergies or a cold, ask your doctor whether a topical treatment (such as a nasal steroid or antihistamine spray) is an option.

THROAT CLEARING

Throat clearing is traumatic to the vocal folds and can lead to a vicious cycle: The throat clear traumatizes the vocal fold tissue, and the body sends more mucus to sooth the tissue. Improving hydration will keep your mucus thin and decrease the need to clear. Try taking a sip of water or swallowing when you feel the urge to clear. If the throat clear is a habit, it will take time to get over it. Be patient and suppress the urge.

YELLING AND SCREAMING

Yelling and screaming should be avoided, as this type of voice use can cause vocal strain and may lead to voice injury. This might mean that you need to find an alternative to yelling in the house (use a bell or whistle to call the kids, or even call or text them via cell phone). Other strategies for reducing yelling include using a noisemaker at athletic or spirit events, using amplification in noisy environments, and moving to a quieter location to speak or communicating through writing when you are in noisy environments. Cheerleading is an activity that is vocally taxing. If singing is a priority for you and you have a vocal injury, you might need to put cheerleading on the back burner or talk to your coach to see if nonvocal involvement (such as lip synching) may be an option, at least in the short term.

WHISPERING

Whispering can cause strain in your throat. If you feel the need to conserve your voice, practice efficient vocal exercises or take a short "voice nap."

CIGARETTE SMOKING

Smoking cigarettes causes vocal fold damage and can cause laryngeal cancer. Smoking and singing don't mix! The jury is still out on whether electronic cigarettes are safe. However, many e-cigarettes contain propylene glycol (also used in stage smoke), which is a laryngeal irritant. Until we know more about the safety of e-cigarettes, you should avoid the risk and quit smoking altogether.

ALCOHOL AND DRUG USE

1. Alcohol is a diuretic and can be dehydrating. This doesn't mean you have to abstain from drinking, but you should use moderation.
2. Street drugs can cause damage to the vocal folds, depending on the drug used and the delivery method. Smoking marijuana can cause thermal (heat) injury to the vocal folds.
3. Any substance that alters your consciousness will have a negative impact on your vocal coordination as well as your ability to use good judgment about how much and how intensely you're using your voice, so you should avoid alcohol and other substance use when performing or speaking in noisy environments.

SELF-CARE

1. Your body is the carrying case and support system for your vocal instrument. Make sure you get enough rest and exercise, and eat well.
2. Having an upper respiratory infection, cold, or flu can affect your voice, and singing when you have a cold can potentially lead to a more chronic injury, especially if it occurs repeatedly. Practice good handwashing habits, using soap and water or alcohol-based hand sanitizers before eating and before touching eyes, nose, or mouth.

CHAPTER 6

Preparing the Singing Voice Rehabilitation Plan

Once the voice problem has been accurately diagnosed, it is time to begin developing your rehabilitation plan. This plan will not only serve as your guide through the rehabilitation process—creating scaffolding and structure to ensure regular progress and desirable outcomes—but will also facilitate your discussions with the singer, providing a shared framework so that the singer will understand the rationale underlying the rehabilitation plan, the rehabilitation goals, and expectation for results.

The human voice is a very complex phenomenon. The larynx, whose basic bodily functions are protecting the airway and impounding air in the thorax to assist with heavy lifting or bearing down (as in elimination or childbirth), interacts with the respiratory system and vocal tract under the control of the nervous system via the vagus nerve (the nerve that is also vital for respiratory, cardiac, digestive, and adrenal function, among others) to produce voice. We "hijack" these bodily systems to produce voice for communication and at an even higher and more athletic level for singing, which brings us art, entertainment, worship, culture, heritage, identity, joy, comfort—in short, voice and singing are the bedrock of our humanity.

Obviously, voice production is immensely complex—a problem in any and all of the core bodily systems may contribute to a problem with voice. Thus, the rehabilitation process must be designed to ensure that all underlying factors are appropriately addressed. In this chapter, we explore what those factors are, the boundaries and overlap of habilitation and rehabilitation, a suggested framework for developing and organizing the rehabilitation plan, and considerations for your interactions with the singer.

A HYBRID PROFESSION REQUIRES A HYBRID MENTALITY

Historically, the teaching of singing has been largely supported by the experience, intuition, and knowledge of the singing teacher. The voice lesson encounter is highly interactive and responsive—with an "apprentice-master" model (LeBorgne & Rosenberg, 2014). The singer sings, and the teacher responds with an instruction that may include imagery, mechanical adjustment, body movement, positional change, interpretive or expressive gesture, or one of a number of other elements. The singer sings again, attempting to incorporate the instruction into the execution, and the process continues, gradually moving the singer toward the sound ideal.

Although voice teachers inevitably make an informal assessment of the singer on first hearing, there has typically not been an institutional or professional requirement or even expectation that such assessment should be systematically documented. Voice teachers have not been expected to develop written goals to address everything that goes on in the lesson or to formally measure and document progress toward goals at every lesson. Most voice teachers use some form of documentation in their teaching, however, the format and content are largely designed by and completed at the discretion of the teacher, although in some cases, the form and content of documentation are dictated by an educational institution.

Until relatively recently, voice teachers typically were not expected to possess a deep knowledge of the science of singing. They may have had a cursory understanding of vocal anatomy but often did not have a thorough understanding of the physiology of the voice, acoustics of singing, neuroanatomy of voice, or the complex interaction of body systems (respiration, phonation, resonance) that must coordinate optimally to achieve the desired sound. In fact, many voice teachers have deliberately shunned such knowledge, perhaps fearing that it would confuse and inhibit singers (Bozeman, 2007; Helding, 2007; Titze, 2008). Teaching was considered more art than science. Fortunately, due in large part to the work of a number of pioneering vocal pedagogues in the 20th century, this is changing. The science of singing is becoming more and more an expected component of voice pedagogy, especially in the *teaching* of pedagogy. Ward (2013) surveyed over 500 voice teachers and reports that most use a combination of science and imagery in their teaching.

The practice of clinical speech-language pathology, on the other hand, has been steeped in understanding the scientific underpinnings of all aspects of speech, language, and swallowing. With the emergence and heightened emphasis on evidence-based practice, the expectation that any clinical intervention must have a demonstrated and citable basis in science and research has deepened continuously over the years. Clinicians are expected to make an assessment that compares quantifiable results to proven norms, to make a prognosis for improvement that has a clinical basis, and to develop an evidence-based intervention plan with measurable goals that is designed to address specific areas of deficit and gradually move the subject ever closer to the normal range. When the goals are achieved—or when the subject ceases to make progress—the clinician is expected to discharge him or her from services. This phenomenon is largely driven by the fact that speech-language pathology services fall within health care that is covered by insurance or within educational special services, both of which require evidence-based documentation throughout the process of evaluation and treatment. Because of this background and culture, the speech-language pathologist may dismiss or discount intervention strategies for which they cannot find a research basis—interventions that a voice teacher may empirically and experientially deem effective based on observation of consistent positive results in their teaching.

Remember that singing voice rehabilitation is a hybrid profession—the fusion of voice pedagogy and clinical voice rehabilitation. In my opinion (and based on my experience), the successful singing voice rehabilitation specialist must stand with one foot solidly in each camp, marrying the practical and intuitive voice teacher with the scientific clinician. He or she must be thoroughly up to date on current research in singing voice science and voice rehabilitation, and must use and apply this knowledge in the rehabilitation process. Furthermore, the rehabilitation plan must be driven by the underlying injury and by a prognosis for recovery that is consistent with the body of evidence regarding the typical course of the injury. However, he or she must also respond to each singer on an individual basis and be capable of skillfully supplementing evidence-based treatment with standard voice pedagogy techniques (and occasionally novel techniques that are idiosyncratically successful) even in the absence of specific and citable research to support use of such techniques. Having said that, the knowledgeable singing voice rehabilitation specialist should be able to clearly articulate a rationale for every successful intervention strategy employed based on the underlying principles of biomechanics and acoustics of voice, motor learning, and shaping behavior. I have observed this to be an effective approach in the work of many notable colleagues in this profession and in my own work with thousands of singers.

FIVE ELEMENTS OF SINGING VOICE REHABILITATION

As you begin the rehabilitation process with the singer, consider all of the elements or factors that may potentially contribute to the voice problem so that you can determine which will need to be addressed in the rehabilitation plan (Figure 6–1). These elements include the following:

- Medical factors
- Vocal hygiene
- Vocal coordination and conditioning
- Vocal pacing
- Emotional factors

Emotional Factors

Although last enumerated in the above listing, I place this category of contributing factors first in this discussion. Whatever their nature, emotions are a cog in the rehabilitation mechanism that can dramatically affect all the other elements.

For some singers, there will not be a pressing emotional component to the voice problem, but in all likelihood, the prevailing majority will have some degree of emotional response to the voice problem, and the nature and intensity of this response can play a large role in how well the singer is able to take action and participate in the recovery process. The emotional reaction can range from mild anxiety over the financial or functional repercussions of the voice problem to an overwhelming crisis of identity.

Emotional concerns may reflect the singer's self-blame for the injury, feeling "damaged" or defective, or feeling he or she is not a "whole" person as a result of the voice problem. Income and livelihood or participation in worship or spiritual activity may be threatened by the voice problem, creating stress and anxiety. If the vocal load has to be reduced, the singer may feel he or she is letting other people down or not fulfilling professional obligations. Singers may also feel overwhelmed

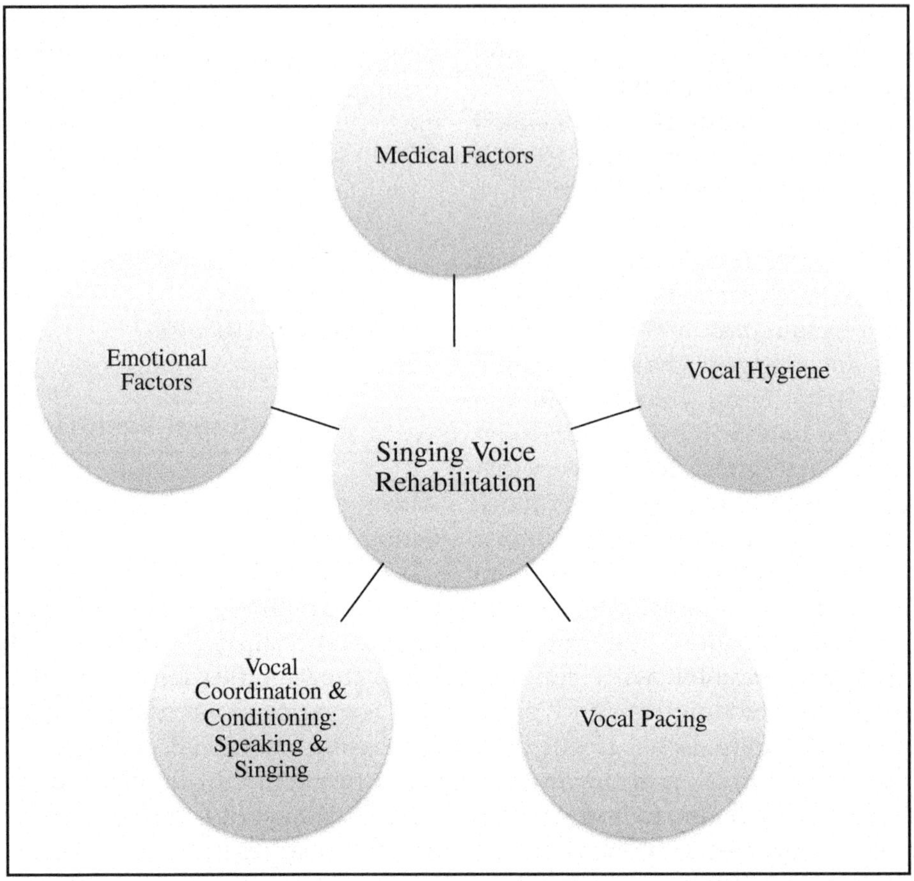

Figure 6–1. ***Elements that contribute to voice problems. All relevant elements should be considered in developing the singing voice rehabilitation plan and should be reviewed on a regular basis.***

by all that they will need to do to get the voice back on track—attend rehabilitation sessions (which likely will include a financial and time investment), adjust amount of voice use, consider voice priorities, and make lifestyle changes to address medical and vocal hygiene concerns. There may be emotional resistance to making the necessary changes.

In some cases, the singer's emotional state may signify an obstacle to achieving rehabilitation goals. The devastation he or she feels may create a sort of inertia—paralyzing the singer in such a way that the prospect of addressing all the necessary ingredients for recovery seems insurmountable. For others, the emotional response may serve as a catalyst, spurring them to a high level of motivation and providing an incentive to tackle each facet of the rehabilitation plan. For successful outcome, you will need to be able to discern and understand the emotional underpinnings of the voice problem for each individual singer and respond accordingly. Your role in supporting the emotional needs of the singer will be discussed in depth in Chapter 8.

Medical Factors

Numerous medical factors can have an impact on vocal function. These have been addressed in detail in Chapters 3 and 4. As a singing voice rehabilitation specialist, you will need to develop a solid familiarity with medical problems that can affect the voice and their appropriate treatment. This is an area where you will need to rely on your clinical foundation. Your resources must be scientific and evidence based, and must be deep enough to understand the full ramifications of medical conditions and their treatment. A cursory overview will not be enough. You will also need to keep abreast of current research to ensure that your knowledge is up to date and accurate.

In many cases, the ideal treatment for a medical problem in a singer may be different than for a nonsinger, underscoring the importance of having a voice-knowledgeable physician (ideally a laryngologist) on the voice care team. Keep in mind that neither speech-language pathologists nor singing teachers are qualified to treat medical problems. You should be very careful about doling out medical advice, particularly relative to medications. To do so without the involvement of a physician not only creates a liability risk for you but also may jeopardize the desired outcome.

Vocal Hygiene

Improving vocal hygiene is often a key component in recovery from a voice disorder. It will be important for you to include optimizing vocal hygiene as a part of the rehabilitation plan. For detailed review of vocal hygiene factors, see Chapter 5.

Vocal Coordination and Conditioning: Speaking and Singing

In order to recover from a vocal injury, the singer must optimize coordination of the entire vocal system—respiration, phonation, resonance—for speaking and singing. In the world of voice habilitation, we would refer to this as "vocal technique," and this term can certainly be applied in the context of rehabilitation. However, *vocal technique* doesn't entirely capture the interface of injury and ability in the way that *coordination* does. The singer may have an excellent foundation in vocal technique. However, technique can be undermined by injury, resulting in maladaptive compensation that may manifest itself as muscle tension (in any of the vocal subsystems), obstructive body alignment, decreased ability to optimize the interaction of airflow and glottal closure, or poor coordination of vocal fold vibration and the vocal tract. Thus, for the *trained* singer, the rehabilitation objective is not so much establishing vocal technique but adapting technique to effectively compensate for the underlying structural alteration.

Another scenario is that of the relatively untrained singer who has never had (or never taken) the opportunity to develop vocal technique under conditions of vocal health and who now has a vocal injury. Voice rehabilitation in this case will indubitably involve establishing the groundwork for vocal technique as one would in a voice habilitation setting, but this foundational work will be taking place in the context of injury with the same inherent necessity for achieving optimal and adaptive compensation as described above for the trained singer.

A broad spectrum exists between these extremities in terms of amount, appropriateness, and quality of training. Regardless of his or her training background or skill, it will be incumbent on you to lead the singer to a level of coordination that will both support the resolution of the injury and long-term vocal health.

The singer must also achieve the highest level of vocal *conditioning* possible to promote restoration of whatever function has been compromised by the injury. Exactly what function(s) will be targeted will vary depending on the singer and the injury but might include range, stamina, quality, and ease of phonation.

Nowhere in the singing voice rehabilitation process is the provider's dual background in pedagogy and clinical knowledge more important than it is here. Without thoroughly understanding the nature and physiologic implications of the underlying injury, even the most accomplished voice teacher may be stymied by the interaction of the altered anatomy and vocal technique, and his or her attempts may prohibit recovery or even exacerbate the problem. The intervention of the clinically trained speech-language pathologist who does not have adequate experience in building technique in a healthy instrument will be equally ineffective.

Throughout the course of voice rehabilitation, vocal coordination and conditioning will be addressed by developing a systematic vocal exercise regimen for the singer that encompasses both speaking and singing that is customized to his or her vocal injury, style of singing, and skill level and that can be transitioned to repertoire. Guidelines and resources for developing an appropriate exercise regimen that is tailored and personalized are addressed in depth in the corresponding section of this book (Chapters 9–13).

Vocal Pacing

The basic premise of vocal pacing is this: How much is the singer using the voice, how intensely, and in what situations? Uncovering the answers to these questions will reveal what adjustments are necessary to achieve a vocal load that facilitates resolution of injury and is sustainable for the long-term health of the singer. Mastering vocal pacing is without question one of the most important concepts and components of the voice rehabilitation process. The relatively large portion of this book that is devoted to this topic proportionately reflects my observation and experience regarding how central and indispensable vocal pacing is to recovering from a voice problem and to maintaining vocal health.

Athletes are well schooled in the importance of balancing activity and rest for successful performance and injury prevention. This principle is no less important for the vocal athlete. In all likelihood, a significant portion of the rehabilitation process for the singers you work with will be devoted to discovering and maintaining this balance. The nature of the underlying injury will guide you in formulation of appropriate and specific objectives. For example, the vocal pacing goals for a singer with mild vocal fold edema or muscle tension dysphonia will be different than for a singer recovering from an acute vocal fold hemorrhage or microflap surgery. Singers with vocal fold atrophy may in fact need more vocal exercise, not less.

It can be very challenging for the singer to implement the adjustments in voice use that are needed, whether decreasing or increasing the load. Modifying ingrained habits is not easy for any of us. Optimizing vocal pacing can require significant lifestyle changes, the necessity of which may give rise to resistance on the part of the singer, which may be compounded if a sense of obligation is attached to some or all vocal demands. Leading singers to make wise vocal pacing choices (the operative concept being "choices") will require significant skill and counseling on your part so that they are prepared and empowered for change. We examine a variety of approaches for achieving this in the relevant chapters.

Contributing Factors Overlap and Connect

Not every singer will have a problem in each of the five areas enumerated herein, but this paradigm can provide a useful framework as you make an inventory of what you and the singer will address in the rehabilitation goals. Consider also that any of these elements may have an impact on any other. For example, if the singer has allergic rhinitis (a medical factor) and inadequate hydration (a vocal hygiene factor), the associated edema and irritation of the respiratory tract may result in vocal fold edema or irritation, which will have an impact on how well the vocal folds vibrate. This may then lead to maladaptive compensatory effort on the part of the singer, which will affect the singer's ability to achieve optimal coordination and conditioning. Suboptimal coordination and conditioning will lead to decreased vocal stamina, which will reduce (or inhibit increasing) the tolerable vocal load—a vocal pacing factor. If vocal pacing is out of balance, the singer may have to cancel performances, resulting in loss of income, which may lead to additional stress and anxiety about the voice problem: an emotional factor (Figure 6–2).

Without addressing the underlying medical and vocal hygiene problems, it will be difficult to realize the desired level of technical proficiency, maximize vocal stamina, or resolve the emotional stress. Conversely, resolution in one area can promote resolution in another. Thus, you must not only assess which factors are in play but also constantly reassess whether all of the contributing factors are being adequately managed.

HOW IS SINGING VOICE REHABILITATION DIFFERENT FROM VOICE LESSONS?

As noted previously, singing voice *habilitation* refers to building vocal technique in a healthy instrument and to the normal development and enhancement of vocal skill. Singing voice *rehabilitation* refers to application of vocal technique and addressing contributing factors to restore a function that has been lost. Grasping this fundamental principle is essential for distinguishing voice *lessons* from voice *rehabilitation* (or *therapy*, in the clinical setting). If the singing voice rehabilitation specialist is appropriately prepared, he or she should be able to address the entire voice in a holistic fashion—encompassing all the contributing elements enumerated above in a systematic and integrated fashion—to lead the singer to a condition of restored vocal health.

Singing requires exquisite athleticism and coordination. Any singer will

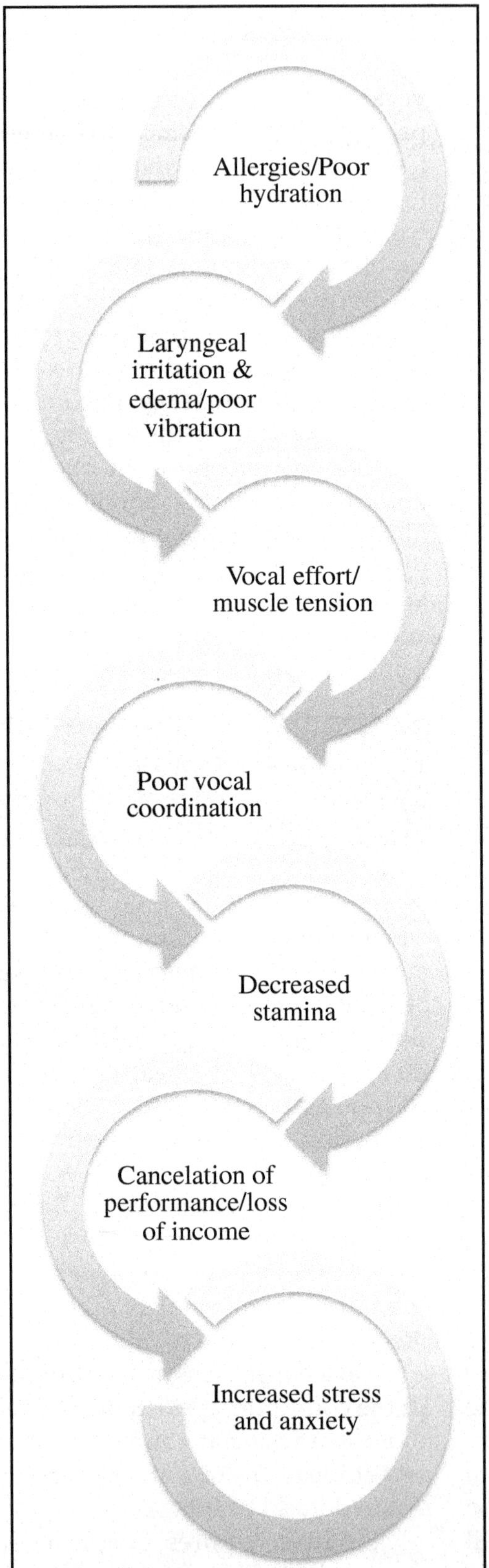

***Figure 6–2.** Contributing factors overlap and connect. A problem in one area may contribute to or exacerbate a problem in another.*

have "deficits" in what he or she is able to achieve. The expectation is that through instruction and/or experience, the singer will continually develop and enhance his or her skills to achieve a higher and higher level of precision and skill. For a singer with a voice injury, the deficit may be part of the baseline, or it may arise and persist as a result of compensating for an injury. The singing voice rehabilitation specialist must be able to distinguish deficits associated with a normal emerging voice from those that result from a voice disorder.

Why is this distinction important? First of all, although there is considerable overlap relative to the elements included in voice lessons and voice rehabilitation, the content diverges in important ways. If the provider's training and background is not suitable to span this divergence, he or she must be prepared to refer to an appropriate provider when reaching the fork in the road. In other words, we all need to know the limits of our scopes of practice.

For example, voice rehabilitation cannot be accomplished without addressing the coordination of the vocal instrument for speaking voice. Most voice teachers do not have adequate training in habilitation or rehabilitation as it relates to the speaking voice. Therefore, the nonclinical provider must seek to ensure that the voice care team includes a speech-language pathologist with expertise in voice to address that aspect of the recovery. Ideally, this should occur in tandem with singing voice rehabilitation, not sequentially (American Speech-Language-Hearing Association [ASHA], 2005). Conversely, repertoire considerations such as developing suitable programs, set-lists, or audition books is typically not a part of the clinical singing voice rehabilitation process. Even if it were an appropriate component of rehabilitation, the clinical singing voice rehabilitation specialist may not be sufficiently knowledgeable about repertoire for every style of singing. The singer should be referred to someone (a voice teacher or coach) with the right expertise in such cases.

The distinctions between voice lessons and voice rehabilitation are sometimes quite subtle but are clear enough to provide some general "rules of thumb." Both singing teachers and singing voice rehabilitation specialists work on developing a vocal exercise regimen for warm-up and technical proficiency, but in the context of singing voice rehabilitation, the design of the exercise regimen is focused on supporting recovery from the injury. In the voice lesson, preparation of repertoire is a strong focus and is addressed in depth, while in rehabilitation, repertoire is used therapeutically to ensure transfer of skills learned in exercises and to confirm that healthy vocal production is being utilized in the context of performance. Artistic interpretation, musicianship, facilitation/recommendations for artist management, audition preparation, languages, and diction are primarily the domain of the voice lesson and are addressed only tangentially in singing voice rehabilitation when they intersect with recovery and vocal health concerns.

There is a second reason that distinguishing habilitation from rehabilitation is important. If one is working in a clinical setting and billing insurance for rehabilitation, the singer must be discharged from services when the clinical goals have been met. To continue forward from this point is not only unethical, but it also endangers the future of insurance coverage for clinical voice rehabilitation. Therefore, we must be scrupulous in adhering to the line between habilitation and rehabilitation.

For singing voice rehabilitation specialists who do not work in a clinical setting, there may be less need for a bright and discernable line between rehabilitation and habilitation, as the ethical question relative to billing insurance does not apply. In such cases, it is essential that the provider ensure that the voice care team includes professionals who will competently address the medical, speaking voice and vocal pacing components of recovery. Of course, it goes without saying that the nonclinical provider's knowledge of voice disorders must be thorough and deep enough to design an exercise regimen that is guided by the injury and resultant functional impairment.

PARTING IS SUCH SWEET SORROW: WHEN TO DISCHARGE FROM SINGING VOICE REHABILITATION

How will you know when you have reached the line where rehabilitation ends and habilitation continues? You are working with singers to build and enhance technique which will optimize coordination of voicing subsystems and promote resolution of the injury. If you're doing your job right, the singer will continue to improve technically and often (although not always) the voice quality will also continue to improve. In this sense, aren't they continuing to make progress? Shouldn't you continue treatment as long as they are making progress? The answers are, respectively, yes and no. Once the singer has returned to his or her preinjury status (or baseline), the transition to habilitation and enhancement of vocal skills has begun. You will determine when this has happened primarily based on the results of videostroboscopy at appropriate intervals, results of objective measures (such as pre-post acoustic testing, administration of perceptual assessments, and patient self-assessment tools such as the VHI-10 and SVHI-10), and by ongoing assessment of function, including vocal stamina, pitch and dynamic range, vocal quality, and ease of phonation. Having a recording of the singer prior to injury will be very helpful in assessing when he or she is back to baseline. It is important to note that, depending on the severity of the injury, the singer may not completely return to preinjury status. In such cases, you can determine whether you think he or she has reached maximum improvement by measuring relevant components over a period of several sessions. If measurements are stable in the face of constant outside factors (e.g., medical factors are adequately controlled, vocal pacing has been optimized, vocal hygiene has been maximized, benefits of surgical intervention have been achieved or ruled out, etc.), it is time to consider discharging the singer.

Sometimes when you recommend discharge, you may encounter resistance from the singer despite having met the clinical criteria for discontinuing treatment. There can be a number of reasons for this. The singer may have developed a sense of emotional dependency on you and/or the rehabilitation sessions, or may fear regressing or relapsing once the sessions have ended. If the singer has made a lot of technical advances during the rehabilitation process, he or she may come to view the rehabilitation sessions as an avenue to ongoing vocal development (as in voice lessons). When this happens, you will need to reiterate the distinction between voice habilitation and voice rehabilitation, review the progress the singer has made (rehabilitation goals have been met or function has been maximized), and, in the case of clinical singing voice rehabilitation, delineate your ethical obligation to adhere to discharge protocol. It can be helpful to reassure the singer that he or she can always consult you again in the future should a relapse or reinjury occur.

Making Appropriate Referrals for Transition to Voice Habilitation

Finishing voice rehabilitation doesn't have to be the end of the singer's technical or vocal health endeavors. As with any athlete, ongoing training with an appropriate teacher is highly desirable and you should encourage the singer to continue his or her vocal development through voice lessons. Getting to know the voice teachers in your area will help you in making referrals. It is important to match the singer with a teacher whose teaching experience is style-appropriate, and it is advisable to promote communication between yourself and the teacher (if the singer is willing). This will ensure that the teacher is apprised of the singer's history. Some clinical singing voice rehabilitation specialists continue to work with their therapy patients in a private lesson capacity after discharging from therapy. In my opinion, this does not present a conflict of interest as long as the clinician is also an accomplished vocal pedagogue with appropriate experience and skills to address the singer's chosen style and long-term voice training needs.

Recurrence or Reinjury

It is not at all unusual for the singer to experience a relapse or reinjury after having been discharged. A number of factors may contribute to reinjury or recurrence of the problem, such as a change in the singer's vocal load or changing medical factors. Resuming rehabilitation with appropriate goals may be necessary to get the singer's voice back on track again. As long as the results of the reevaluation support the recommendation, this is a perfectly appropriate plan of action.

PREPARING FOR THE VOICE REHABILITATION SESSION: INTERACTIONS, STRUCTURE, AND CONTENT

Interactions

Preparing the Singer for Change

For a successful singing voice rehabilitation outcome, it is of critical importance to quickly and clearly ensure that the singer understands the overall treatment plan, confirm that your goals are aligned, address any confusion or doubts about whether the rehabilitation process will be effective, and establish that the process will be a partnership in which you will collaborate with the singer to restore vocal health. All of this will help to create a bond of trust between yourself and the singer and, if at all possible, should be achieved in the first session. If you can accomplish this, you will significantly increase the likelihood that the singer will "buy in" to the process and commit to the long-term plan.

Motivational interviewing has been demonstrated to be an effective interaction style in a variety of therapeutic contexts, including voice therapy (Behrman,

2006). Behrman (2006, p. 218) enumerates the key elements of the model pertaining to therapist-patient interaction as expressing empathy, developing discrepancy (encouraging the patient to make his or her own arguments for change), "rolling with resistance" (allowing rather than suppressing resistance), and supporting self-efficacy (the individual's belief in his or her ability to change a behavior), and she examines dialogue styles that support these principles. These include asking open-ended questions, affirmation of statements or actions, reflective listening, summarizing, and eliciting change talk (helping "the patient transition from ambivalence and resistance to expressing the need for change and developing a plan of action"). From an experiential perspective, I can affirm that this type of patient-centered approach is very effective in establishing a positive connection with the singer and empowering the singer to make the necessary but difficult changes for voice recovery.

At the first session, review the rehabilitation plan with the singer. Start by affirming the things the singer is already doing that support vocal health, then indicate the areas that seem to be contributing to the voice problem. Briefly describe how these factors will be addressed in the rehabilitation process and encourage the singer to participate in this plan for change. It is critical that you ascertain whether your goals are aligned with the singer's. For example, you may identify impairment of vocal range and stamina, inadequate vocal pacing, and poor hydration as targets of the rehabilitation plan. The singer may be primarily concerned about painful phonation. If this is the case, it will be important to "connect the dots" and discuss with the singer how each element of the rehabilitation plan will contribute to an overall reduction of painful phonation (and in all likelihood, the singer will end up with improved range and stamina to boot!).

As discussed earlier in this chapter, the vocal mechanism is extremely complex. Provide the singer with a brief, simplified overview of how the voice works. This doesn't need to be an in-depth lecture on vocal anatomy, physiology, and acoustics—just enough of the basics to illustrate the underlying mechanics and the interconnectedness of the subsystems. Outlining the elements of singing voice rehabilitation and how they apply to the singer will help to further establish a framework, distilling the complex components into a concrete construct. It might be helpful to have a visual illustration, as in Figure 6–3.

This diagram has also been provided in the form of a handout to which you may add specific targets for each singer (see Appendix 6–A).

The first session is a good time to reiterate to the singer that you will be collaborating to achieve the desired outcome. A statement like, "We're going to do this together," or "I'm going to help you reach your vocal health goals" can be very reassuring to the singer and can quickly help establish the bond of trust that is necessary for successful outcome.

Behrman (2006) provides an excellent example of a "change plan worksheet" to encourage the singer to take ownership of and actively participate in developing the rehabilitation plan. Topics include what changes the patient wants to make and for what reasons, the steps the patient will take in making change, how the patient will seek support from other people, how the patient will know if the plan is working, what things might interfere with the plan, and what the patient will do if the

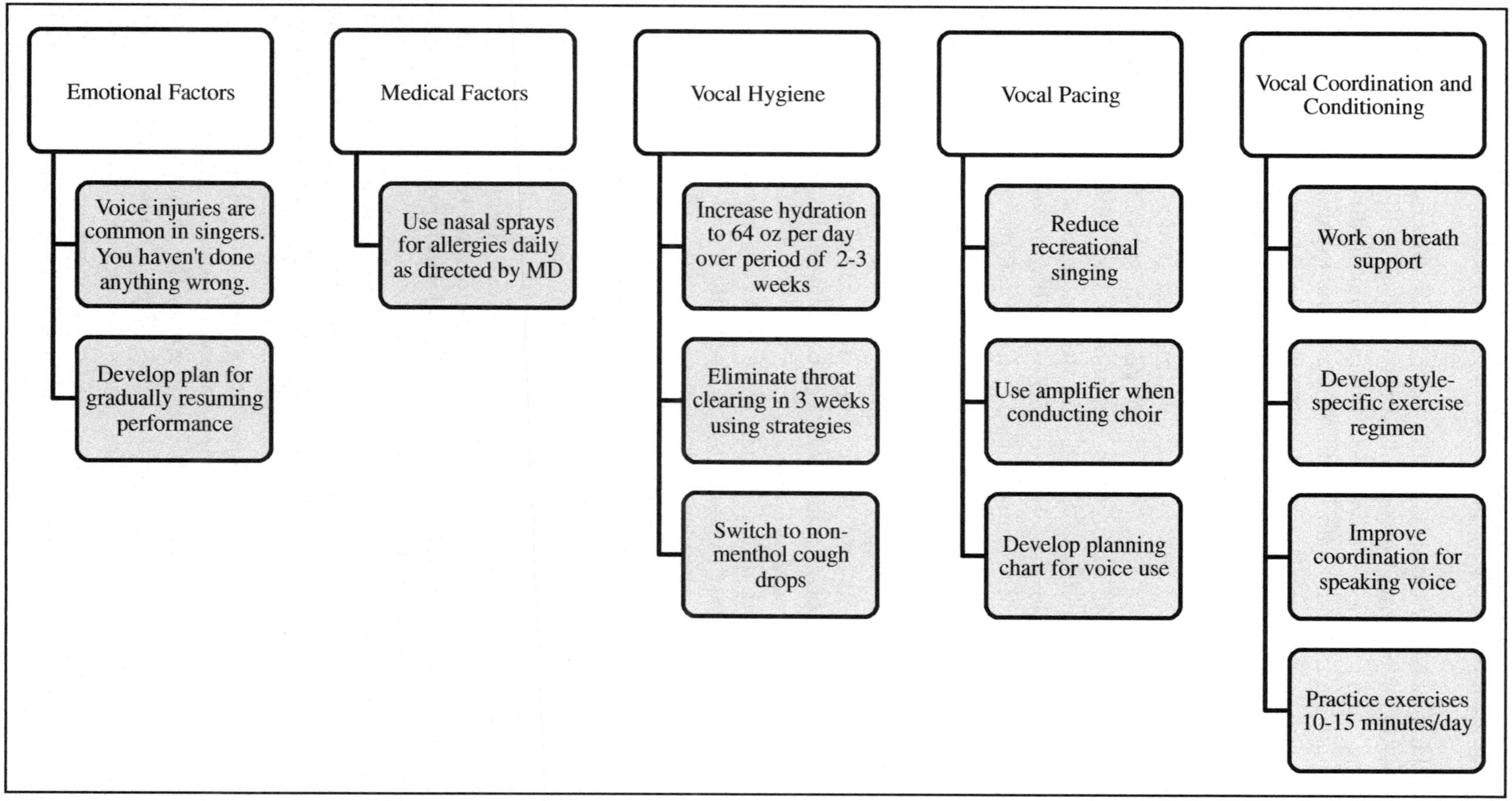

Figure 6–3. *Outline of sample rehabilitation plan for singer education.*

plan isn't working. She lists specific, open-ended statements for patients to respond to, encouraging them to take an active role in developing the treatment plan and stating it in their own words, which supports self-efficacy. See the full article for an example of a completed change plan worksheet.

Feedback

Feedback in the voice rehabilitation session may be intrinsic or extrinsic. With *intrinsic feedback*, the singer uses his or her senses to self-assess. Examples of this might include positioning the singer in front of a mirror to help monitor posture (visual feedback), playing back a recording of the singer speaking or singing to elicit self-assessment and determine whether the sound produced was aligned with what the singer intended (auditory feedback), or having the singer self-monitor sensation of body position or movement (proprioceptive or kinesthetic feedback). *Extrinsic* feedback is the information you provide to the singer to let him or her know how well or accurately the task was performed. We will focus on the effects of feedback on motor learning when we explore shaping voice in Chapter 9.

I introduce the topic of feedback at this juncture to encourage you to maintain a positive valence in the verbal feedback and cuing you provide to the singer. Research has demonstrated that use of positive language in interactions is more effective than negative language in eliciting change and/or promoting positive relationships (Beaman & Wheldall, 2000; Fredrickson & Losada, 2005). Frederickson and Losada (2005) recommend a ratio of at least three positive statements to one corrective statement. Gottman, Coan, Carrere, and Swanson (1998) found that the ratio of positive to negative statements in interactions predicted divorce in married couples and identified a ratio of 5:1 as "the magic ratio" in successful relationships.

I believe the importance of using positive language is especially true when working with singers, who typically have an internal critical voice and who may have been subjected to negative comments in the context of voice lessons, auditions, and/or performance reviews, often leading to defensiveness and fear relative to singing. The singer's trust in you will depend on realizing that he or she will not be judged in the rehabilitation environment. Words like "wrong" and "bad" and all their pejorative progeny will undermine the effectiveness of your intervention and may inhibit the singer, who is already in a vulnerable state. Instead, try to use language that is descriptive and specific. For example, you might say, "That sounded clearer," or "That didn't sound as projected as it did the last time," "I hear some strain there," or "That sounded very free."

When you introduce a new task or exercise, try to minimize responding to the first few attempts the singer makes. If you immediately apply a correction to the initial attempts, the singer may feel inhibited as you proceed, and this hesitation may persist every time you introduce a new exercise or task. Exercising restraint in expressing your immediate response also establishes to the singer that it is safe to experiment without being judged for every sound, spoken or sung. Give the singer the opportunity to try it a few times. This allows you to see what patterns emerge relative to self-awareness, self-assessment, and/or self-correction. If he or she demonstrates these skills, you can reinforce the awareness and insight. A helpful way to create a partnership in rehabilitation can be to review the performance of a particular task together and elicit a self-assessment *before* you give any feedback. Recording the session can be useful in achieving this, enabling you to stop, play back what just happened, and assess it together. This practice also has the benefit of allowing you to determine the accuracy of the singer's self-assessment and to gradually promote greater accuracy, ensuring that home practice will be optimally successful.

Structure

There are many ways to structure the singing voice rehabilitation plan and individual sessions—perhaps as many different ways as there are providers! Rather than looking for a "golden rule" for how to organize the session, I encourage you to seek a structure that ensures relevant factors are addressed, that fits your teaching/intervention style, and—most important—fits the learning style of the singer you are working with. If there is an overarching caveat, it is to avoid becoming entrenched in a single format. The more flexible and responsive you can be to what is present and calling out for attention in any given session, the more effective your intervention will be.

Number and Frequency of Rehabilitation Sessions

Voice rehabilitation programs are typically one to two 30- to 60-minute sessions per week for 4 to 8 weeks. This range can be regarded as a rough guideline. Having sessions occur at weekly intervals allows the singer to have enough time to process and practice the material covered in the previous session while ensuring you are able to assess the accuracy of execution (avoiding habituation of inaccurate execution) and address any questions or confusion that may arise during the interval. In the case of traumatic injury and especially following phonosurgery, weekly sessions make it possible for you to determine whether recovery is progressing on schedule or whether something may have happened that suggests reinjury. In such cases, repeat stroboscopy may be indicated to ascertain whether an adjustment in the treatment plan is needed.

A number of circumstances can influence the number and frequency of sessions and may dictate an adjustment in the rehabilitation plan. Singers with more severe disorders, complex contributing factors, or difficult surgery recovery may require more sessions, possibly spanning several months. Scheduling flexibility and availability (on the part of both the provider and the singer), distance that must be traveled for rehabilitation sessions, and the singer's financial resources may necessitate wider time intervals between sessions. Some singers just may need a little more time in between sessions to thoroughly digest what was covered and to have adequate opportunity to practice. On the other hand, there are some situations in which a more intensive regimen is indicated, perhaps several sessions per week or even daily for a short period. This may be especially appropriate when you need to cover a lot in a short amount of time, as in cases where singers are traveling a great distance for rehabilitation. In the clinical setting, insurance coverage may limit the number and possibly even the frequency of sessions.

Sometimes rehabilitation begins, only to be interrupted due to the singer's family or work demands, illness, or other circumstances that "trump" immediate attention to the voice problem. When this happens, it may be necessary to suspend rehabilitation until the limiting factors have been resolved. As you gain experience, your ability to predict the arc of rehabilitation will become more accurate and assured.

Supporting Home Practice

What happens in the voice rehabilitation session is only a small part of the recovery process. Of equal (or possibly greater) importance is what happens in between the sessions. You can help the singer succeed in the ensuing period by providing concrete instructions, resources, and tools to facilitate "homework" and by clearly emphasizing the importance of home practice from the very beginning. You might consider a statement such as, "Your independent practice of the rehabilitation exercises will have a significant impact on your vocal progress, and may expedite the number of sessions you will need," thus empowering the singer with the potential to influence the duration of rehabilitation and successful outcome.

I strongly recommend use of recording during the treatment session. This might be done using your own studio or therapy room equipment, providing the singer with a CD or digital recording to listen to between sessions, or the singer may simply record the session on his or her own device or smartphone. Providing the singer with a recording will facilitate home practice by ensuring all the exercises have been documented in the preferred order, in the recommended keys,

Practicing in the Car

Many of the singers I work with practice their vocal exercise routines while driving. I grudgingly concede that this has benefits in terms of multitasking and having relative privacy in which to explore exercises in an uninhibited fashion. However, there are obvious negative implications associated with the impossibility of achieving optimal alignment for singing while seated in the car, the inevitable divided attention (the singer is not allocating full attention to the demands of driving or to the mechanics of singing) and the Lombard effect resulting from the ambient noise generated by a car in motion and surrounding traffic. While I always discuss these disadvantages with singers and urge them to carve out time when they can practice under more optimal circumstances, I have come to accept that for some, it's either practice in the car or don't practice at all, and if that is the case I will fall on the side of getting the practice into the singer's regular routine. One important caveat that I share with every singer when introducing SOVT with straws of any size: No straw in the car. Were the airbag to go off, or even if the singer stopped suddenly and hit the steering wheel, having a pointy projectile in the mouth could have disastrous consequences. Switch to another SOVT sound that doesn't require external props.

using the recommended phonemes, syllables, or words. The recording can also include any discussion undertaken in the session, such as education, ideas for vocal pacing, and your specific instructions for how to practice.

You can also support the singer's completion of "homework" by providing written summaries, outlines, forms, handouts, or any other printed or digital material. Get to know the singer's learning and organizational style as soon as you can so that you can customize the support of home practice. Be sure to ask the singer in the following session if the format was helpful, or if there is a more effective way to help him or her complete the home practice.

Recording the Singing Voice Rehabilitation Session: Whole or In Part?

I have experimented with recording the session as a whole or in part and have arrived at the personal conclusion that it is best to record the whole thing. The benefit of partial recording is that you can record just the exercises you want the singer to practice so that he or she only has a short segment to listen to. A concise recording could potentially increase the likelihood that the singer will practice the exercises. Recording the session in its entirety obviously will yield a much longer product—possibly so long that the singer won't bother to listen at all because he or she doesn't have 30 to 60 minutes to devote to it. This could have a negative effect on practice compliance. However, I have found on numerous occasions that when I record only part of the session, something significant happens in the part of the session that isn't recorded, such as an especially fruitful vocal pacing brainstorming session, an important breakthrough of insight or change, or supportive conversation regarding the singer's struggle with emotional factors. For this reason, I have continued to record the entire session. If I record onto a CD, I create a new track each time we start something new so that the singer can easily skip the sections that don't need review. With digital files, it is easy to edit out the parts that don't need multiple hearings. My rationale for including the whole session is also driven by feedback I have received from the singers I work with, who frequently state how valuable it is to listen back to sessions again and again, how they often hear or understand something we discussed in a different or more meaningful way with subsequent or repeated listening, or experience an insightful realization about their speaking voice habits by listening to themselves in spontaneous conversation.

Keep in mind that if you record the entire session, what you say and the way you say it will be repeated over and over again to the singer as he or she listens. This is another reason to keep your language in the session positive and provides opportunities for your instructions and interactions to penetrate deeply. Remember to stop the recording during the session if anything of a particularly sensitive nature arises that you or the singer would not want to be captured forever.

Content

Be Thorough, but Adaptable

Regardless of the structure you decide on, it will be important to ensure that all applicable elements of voice rehabilitation are addressed during the overall process—emotional factors, medical factors, vocal hygiene, vocal pacing, and vocal coordination/conditioning.

At times you may systematically address all relevant elements in a single session—starting out with a review of the voice journal and any emotional concerns that have arisen since you last met, collaborating with the singer to identify a few new strategies to add to the vocal pacing plan, checking the status of vocal hygiene goals and making sure medications are being taken as directed, and then devoting time to reviewing and expanding vocal exercises for speaking and singing. In other cases, some elements may need to be addressed only minimally or not at all. For example, if a singer already has excellent vocal hygiene, there is no need to target this domain in the rehabilitation process—you can simply reinforce the good habits. For other singers, there may not be any medical factors in play.

There will likely be times when you devote entire sessions to a single element, such as vocal pacing, or the singer's emotional response to the voice injury. There may be sessions in which the singer is feeling particularly frustrated or discouraged, shares an upsetting experience related to the voice, or has a lot of questions and concerns about how and when he or she can expect to be better. It could potentially take a whole session to unpack and discuss the issues. There may be entire sessions devoted exclusively to vocal exercise and transferring skills to repertoire during which you may not spend time on the other components of the rehabilitation plan. When this happens, don't worry that you're not addressing all the goals in the session—you are responding to what is present and most needed at that particular moment in time. Have a plan for what you want to cover, but also be prepared to adapt if the specific situation calls for it. I always have a plan for each session before starting, but I have found it helpful to begin by saying to the singer, "Is there anything you want to be sure we get to today?" This helps me ensure that the goals I have "roughed out" for the session are aligned with what the singer immediately needs and helps avoid having an issue of critical importance to the singer arise at the very end when there may not be adequate time to address it.

Before we leave this topic, I offer one caveat: Sometimes the people you work with may perseverate on a particular subject or facet of the voice problem to the exclusion of other critical elements and to the point that it becomes an obstacle to achieving rehabilitation goals. The gifted interventionist is able to discern a pressing concern that requires attention from a recurrent distraction and can gently steer the singer back to the overall plan.

Here's an example: "Bill" is a singer who reports "constant" sensation of mucus in the throat and need to clear the throat, despite multiple laryngeal exams that have revealed normal viscosity of mucus in the pharynx and larynx, and despite your repeated counseling that the sensation of irritation is likely related to muscle tension and inadequate hydration. At the third session, he appears to be launching once again into a prolonged expostulation on the topic. You might say something along these lines, "I understand how frustrating it is to feel that irritation in your throat all the time. I want to be sure I've explained the strategies for avoiding throat clearing clearly, so we'll go over them again at the end of the session. In the meantime, I have some vocal exercises that will really help you with that irritated sensation. Why don't we try working on these for the next 15 minutes or so, and then see if you're still feeling the mucus in your throat? I'll just get you a glass of water, and we'll get started." In this manner, you validate Bill's concerns, let him know that you are not discounting the impact and reality of the sensation, invite him to engage with you in an immediate plan for resolution, let him know he will have a chance to bring it up again later, and subtly reinforce your hydration recommendations.

It takes time and experience to develop the discernment to know when to firmly stick to the plan, when to flexibly deviate from it, and how to do it all in such a way that the singer feels supported and understood. Consider that the rehabilitation plan is based on factors that are dynamic, not static. Thus, modifying the plan (even within a single session) can make the intervention more effective and expedited. This ability is fed by and also feeds your knowledge and proficiency. If you are open to adapting, each singer you work with will guide you in perfecting this skill.

Attendance, Concordance, and Dropout

Some singers will diligently attend all sessions as scheduled, exhibit a high level of motivation and commitment throughout the rehabilitation process, make steady progress toward rehabilitation goals, and experience full recovery. Celebrate and enjoy these instances! Unfortunately, in many cases, obstacles to completing rehabilitation will arise, which may or may not be possible to overcome. This may be manifested by frequent cancelations, inadequate home practice, inability to follow recommendations for medical management or vocal hygiene, poor progress toward rehabilitation goals, or intractability of injury, to name just a few. Sometimes the singer may drop out of rehabilitation altogether. When this happens, look first to yourself to determine whether some element of the rehabilitation design or interactions during the session may be contributing to the singer's apparent inability to "stick to the program."

Compliance and *adherence* are terms that are often used (particularly in a medical or clinical context) to describe this "stickiness." Such terms tend to put the burden of action on the person receiving the treatment, medication, teaching, and so on. The "Concordance Model" (Bissell, May, & Noyce, 2001) suggests a different paradigm, one in which all participants in the process—in our case the singer, singing voice rehabilitation specialist, voice teacher, speech-language pathologist, physician, and anyone else involved in singing voice rehabilitation—work as a team, collaborating to achieve the best possible outcome. Titze and Verdolini Abbott (2012) advocate for application of this model to both voice habilitation and rehabilitation, and I wholeheartedly recommend it to you as well. If you view the rehabilitation process from this perspective, it will become a partnership between you and the singer.

Sometimes, in spite of your best efforts and high-quality care, singers will drop out of rehabilitation. A number of

Titze and Verdolini Abbott (2012, pp. 248–249) provide a helpful list of steps that can be taken to maximize concordance, the singer's "buy-in" and sense of ownership in the rehabilitation process. In addition to providing knowledge about the health condition, establishing a warm and supportive mode of interaction and ensuring that verbal interactions are adapted to the need of the patient, they recommend that you do the following:

- "Help cultivate an internal (self-determining) focus and readiness for change
- Give written instruction, or even execute a contract
- Provide self-monitoring aids, and follow-up
- Build social support for the client (family, friends)
- Hook them early, but also advise against the 'quick fix'"

possible factors may be at work in these cases, such as insurmountable financial, travel, or time impediments or psychological factors. Some singers may just not be ready to make the commitment to rehabilitation, perhaps because they don't perceive the voice problem as having a significant enough impact, lack the maturity to commit to the rehabilitation process, or because the lifestyle adjustments that are necessary for recovery are perceived as too difficult or constraining. If you have singers who are not attending sessions regularly, who cancel sessions frequently, or have dropped out entirely, be sure to follow up with them with a friendly and supportive phone call or e-mail to see if you can identify obstacles that may be overcome. If they decide not to continue their sessions, let them know that they may resume rehabilitation later if it becomes more feasible and that you are available to discuss any questions or concerns that arise in the future. Always leave the door open to restart if circumstances change.

Hapner, Portone-Maira, and Johns (2009) reported a dropout rate of 65% in voice therapy, although their study was not limited to professional voice users. Duarte de Almeida, Rodrigues Santos, Barreto Bassi, Caldas Teixeira, and Cortes Gama (2013) reported a lower dropout rate of 35.2% among teachers. No studies have specifically looked at therapy completion among singers.

Hapner et al. (2009) examined diagnosis, severity of dysphonia, severity of perceived handicap, and demographic variables (age, gender, and ethnicity) as possible factors contributing to therapy completion. Results indicated that "none of these factors were significantly related to completion/dropout from therapy." In a later study, Portone-Maira, Wise, Johns, and Hapner (2011) found that patients who attended a greater number of sessions and had a shorter time interval between otolaryngology referral and speech-language pathology evaluation were more likely to complete voice therapy.

REFERENCES

American Speech-Language-Hearing Association. (2005). *The role of the speech language pathologist, the teacher of singing, and the speaking voice trainer in voice habilitation* (Technical report). Rockville, MD: American Speech and Hearing Association Ad Hoc Joint Committee with the National Association of Teachers of Singing and the Voice and Speech Trainers Association. Retrieved from http://www.asha.org/members/deskref-journals/deskref/default

Beaman, R., & Wheldall, K. (2000). Teachers' use of approval and disapproval in the classroom. *Educational Psychology, 20*, 431–446.

Behrman, A. (2006). Facilitating behavioral change in voice therapy: The relevance of motivational interviewing. *American Journal of Speech Language Pathology, 15*(3), 215–225.

Bissell, P., May, C. R., & Noyce, P. R. (2001). From compliance to concordance: Meeting the needs of patients? *International Journal of Pharmacy Practice, 9*(SI), 7.

Bozeman, K. (2007). A case for voice science in the voice studio. *Journal of Singing, 63*(3), 265–270.

Duarte de Almeida, L., Rodrigues Santos, L., Barreto Bassi, I., Caldas Teixeira, L., & Cortes Gama, A. (2013). Relationship between adherence to speech therapy in patients with dysphonia and quality of life. *Journal of Voice, 27*(5), 617–621.

Fredrickson, B., & Losada, F. (2005). Positive affect and the complex aspects of human flourishing. *American Psychologist, 60*(7), 678–686.

Gottman, J. M., Coan, J., Carrere, S., & Swanson, C. (1998). Predicting marital happiness and stability from newlywed interactions. *Journal of Marriage and the Family, 60*(1), 5–22.

Hapner, E. R., Portone-Maira, C., & Johns, M. M. (2009). A study of voice therapy dropout. *Journal of Voice, 23*, 337–340.

Helding, L. (2007). Science and the vocal art, part one: In search of common ground. *Journal of Singing, 64*(2), 141–150.

LeBorgne, W. D., & Rosenberg, M. (2014). History of classical voice pedagogy. In W. LeBorgne & M. Rosenberg (Eds.), *The vocal athlete* (pp. 197–212). San Diego, CA: Plural.

Portone-Maira, C., Wise, J. C., Johns, M. M., III, & Hapner, E. R. (2011). Differences in temporal variables between voice therapy completers and dropouts. *Journal of Voice, 25*(1), 62–66.

Titze, I. (2008). An appeal for patience and long-suffering by singing teachers in their assessment of the value of voice science. *Journal of Singing, 64*(5), 593–594.

Titze, I. R., & Verdolini Abbott, K. (2012). *Vocology: The science and practice of voice habilitation*. Salt Lake City, UT: National Center for Voice and Speech.

Ware, R. (2013). The use of science and imagery in the voice studio—A survey of voice teachers in the United States and Canada. *Journal of Voice, 69*(4), 413–417.

APPENDIX 6–A

Rehabiliation Plan for Singer Education

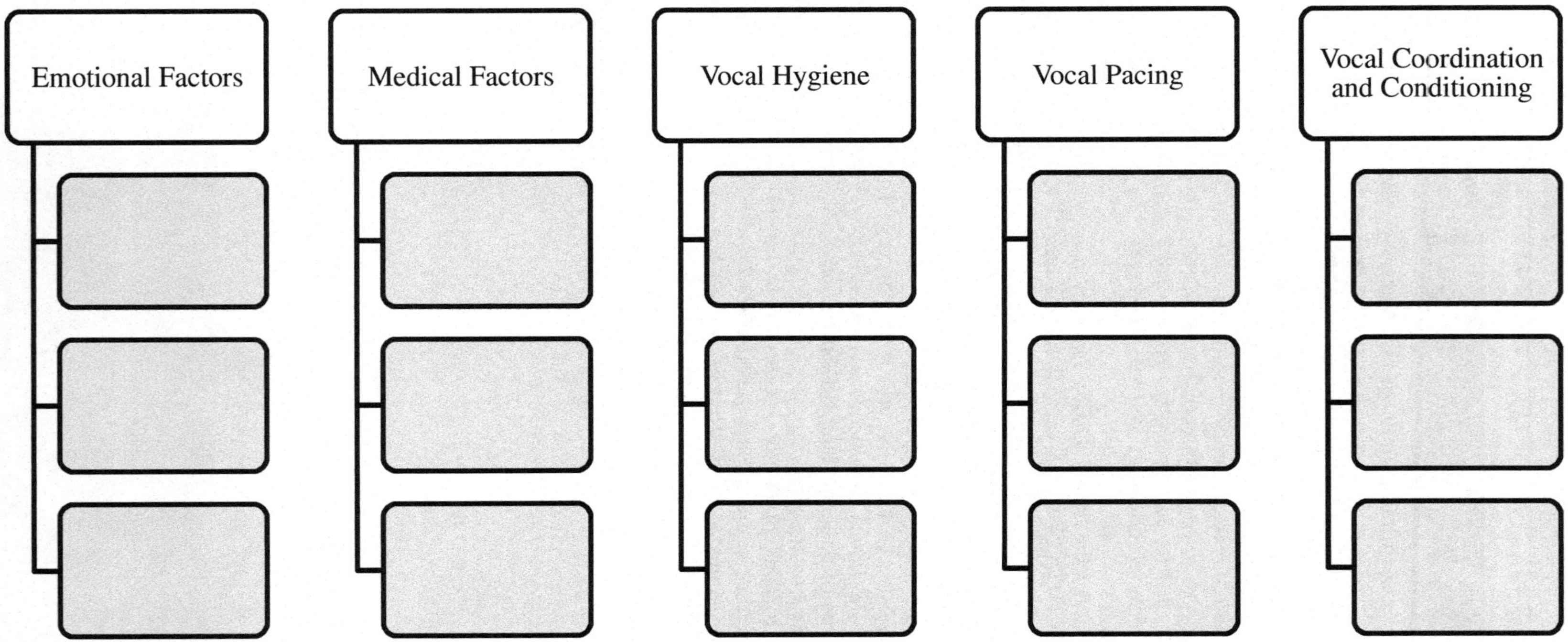

CHAPTER 7

Taking a Closer Look: Specific Populations and the Rehabilitation Plan

The specific vocal demands, training history, and vocal health needs of singers can vary extensively depending on their professional status, singing situations, style, and genre. Therefore, the rehabilitation plan for a lead singer in a rock band will be different than for an opera singer, and different for a music educator than for a college student. Familiarity with the vocal demands, singing environments, and typical voice use for different types of singers will be critical in order for you to provide precise and effective recommendations and intervention. A number of the types of singers you will most likely encounter in your practice will be explored in this section. For purposes of this chapter, our focus will primarily be on classical, musical theater, and contemporary commercial music (CCM) singing. CCM singing refers to Western singing styles that are outside classical or musical theater genres and may include rock, pop, country, gospel, bluegrass, blues, jazz, contemporary Christian, R&B, and folk, among others (LoVetri, 2008). Additional considerations for classical versus CCM singing are delineated in Chapter 10.

Obviously, exhaustive inclusion is beyond the scope of this text. Whenever you encounter a singer whose style or genre is not familiar to you, it will be incumbent on you to research the typical environments, performance practices, rehearsal patterns, performing schedules, expectations of participants/directors, singing culture, and any other relevant factors associated with the chosen style of singing. As an example, the first time I worked with a singer of Carnatic (Indian classical) music, I devoted hours to learning not only about the musical aspects of this type of singing but also the typical training background, practice habits, duration of performances, posture during performances, and mode of interaction with other musicians during rehearsal and performance, among other aspects of the tradition. This knowledge was critical in order for me to determine applicable vocal pacing recommendations, develop suitable exercises, and avoid imposing culturally inappropriate expectations.

CUSTOMIZING THE SINGING VOICE REHABILITATION PLAN

Regardless of style, genre, or professional status, the rehabilitation plan should encompass all the factors outlined in the preceding chapter. Ensuring the singer has excellent vocal hygiene habits is an important first step in the vocal rehabilitation plan, as are assessing vocal skill, reviewing warm-up routine, and speaking voice use. We will explore vocal coordination/conditioning and vocal pacing in depth in the corresponding sections of this book, and you should study those sections thoroughly in preparing your singing voice rehabilitation plans. In this chapter, we will touch on considerations related to those factors that are particular to specific singing populations.

Assess Performance Habits

Carefully review the singer's typical performance habits. If videos of performances are available, review them together to assess technique, strenuousness of performance, singing range in a typical performance, speaking voice efficiency on and off stage, use of sound equipment, movement during performance, and any other factor that you think may be addressed to promote vocal health. Playing an instrument, microphone position, or conducting can affect posture and may need to be adjusted to achieve improved vocal efficiency.

Regular Vocal Exercise and Practice Routine

The singer may or may not be in the habit of regularly completing vocal exercises and applying vocal technique to repertoire. If not, establishing a practice routine may become a primary focus when planning goals for the rehabilitation process. If the singer does not have adequate training, the rehabilitation process may include quite a bit of voice *habilitation*. As you develop the vocal exercise regimen for the singer, provide guidance as to how the singer may incorporate this regimen into the daily routine to build vocal technique, stamina, range, and overall conditioning. You may start with a relatively brief practice time—10 to 15 minutes per day—and gradually expand the duration and content as guided by the singer's stamina, priorities, and goals. Entering practice time into a voice calendar, chart, or phone reminder can serve both to remind the singer to complete practice and document when and how often practice has been completed. See Chapters 11 and 12 for strategies for customizing rehabilitation exercises and Chapter 14 for strategies for planning voice use and practice time. Chapter 14 also includes vocal pacing handouts for specific singing populations.

Lifestyle Considerations

For singers who travel frequently to perform, life on the road may challenge the practice of good self-care—particularly relative to sleep, nutrition, and exercise. These elements should be included in rehabilitation goals as needed, as should optimizing vocal hygiene.

SINGING POPULATIONS

Relevance of Professional Status

The term "professional singer" is a bit ambiguous. There are differing opinions regarding the criteria for classification as "professional." Some may only consider singers who receive all their income from performing to be "professional." Others may weigh how selective the performing situation is (e.g., a soloist appearing with the New York Philharmonic vs. with a regional symphony or community choral society). Still others would measure professionalism by the level of public recognition or celebrity the singer achieves. For purposes of this discussion, we will consider this category to include any singer who has income from performing and for whom a voice problem jeopardizes income and/or professional status.

Voice problems for elite, celebrity singers certainly constitute an emergency. Not only do their reputations and incomes hang in the balance, but also the livelihoods and interests of all the other professionals involved in their performances (including presenters, directors, agents, instrumental musicians, crew, etc.). However, a voice problem is no less urgent, distressing, or significant to singers for whom performing represents only a portion of total income *or* for passionate amateur performers. This may include performers in community theater or opera productions, weekend rock-band singers, church or synagogue soloists, or singers who supplement their performing income with an academic or private studio teaching career or other "day job."

Classical Singers

Classical singing typically refers to singers of Western classical music, including opera, concert, oratorio, chamber music, art song, and choral music.

Training and Education

Most classical singers have had vocal training. Those performing at a high level usually have extensive training—perhaps multiple degrees in vocal performance—and are knowledgeable and articulate in discussing technical aspects of singing. Even singers who are occasional performers ordinarily have had some private instruction. Classical singers usually receive education regarding principles of vocal health, although it is important to probe this information as depth and accuracy of knowledge can vary widely.

Singing Activities and Vocal Pacing Considerations

Performance schedules for concert and opera are usually fairly well spaced, often with a day off between performances, and professional classical singers usually have far fewer performances per week than musical theater or CCM singers. However, the singer may be involved in a number of different performing activities that overlap or become concentrated at times, presenting a challenge for vocal pacing. For example, the singer may have a professional choral position in addition to theatrical, concert, worship, or recital engagements. Since classical singers rarely use amplification, the intensity of singing required to project over an orchestra in a large concert hall or theater can be very high. In addition, the amount of time that goes into preparing for performance may be greater than for other types of singing. Recovery time between performances is essential. Many times, it is the overlapping of performance, rehearsal, preparation for upcoming engagements, auditions, voice lessons, coaching, and teaching that causes voice use to be out of balance for the classical singer. Examining the vocal load allotted to individual practice and rehearsal time may be even more revealing than the performance schedule, and optimizing vocal pacing related to the singer's preparation time will likely be very fruitful.

Musical Theater Singers

Training and Education

As with classical singers, the musical theater singer typically has had at least some vocal training, although there are musical theater singers with minimal training who perform at very high professional levels, particularly for shows that employ contemporary singing styles. Assessing technical knowledge and skill is a must.

Musical theater singers are expected to be accomplished in legit, belting, and CCM styles. Depending on how thoroughly and appropriately singers have been trained, they may or may not have a sound technical basis for all the singing they do (LoVetri & Weekly, 2003; Weekly & LoVetri, 2009). For this reason, it is vital that vocal exercise regimens for this population address both classical and belt technique.

The performing life of musical theater singers includes speaking for the stage (an activity for which they may or may not have adequate training or technique), which may need to be addressed as part of the rehabilitation process.

Singing Activities and Vocal Pacing Considerations

It is not unusual for musical theater singers to be in rehearsal for one show at the same time they are in production for another, and they may have audition, voice lesson, and individual practice schedules that rival those of classical singers. The musical theater singer faces the additional challenge of having performances that are comparable in length and intensity to those of classical singers, but with much more strenuous schedules. For Broadway singers and in most regional theaters, eight performances per week is the norm. For musical theater singers who work on a more part-time or intermittent basis, the long-term schedule will not be as intense but will likely follow a similar pattern for the periods of time when they are engaged in performances. Even with amplification (not always provided), the singing demands of the musical theater singer can be daunting, and optimizing vocal pacing will be an important aspect of the rehabilitation plan.

Contemporary Commercial Music (CCM) Singers

CCM singing is no longer limited to clubs, bars, and concert venues. As noted above, musical theater/Broadway singers are expected to be proficient in singing a variety of contemporary styles, and numerous hit musicals feature this style of singing. Worship environments, including churches and synagogues, often feature this type of singing. And the burgeoning a cappella group scene is yet another setting in which CCM singing is proliferating.

The spectrum of experience/professional level for CCM singers is very broad, ranging from the "weekend warrior" who may jam in a garage band with the occasional public performance to elite professionals with extensive and demanding tour and recording schedules. Providing rehabilitation exercises and vocal pacing education that is customized to the singer's particular demands is critical for optimal outcome.

Training and Education

CCM singers may have little or no vocal training, or if they have training, it may not be style appropriate (e.g., they may have received classically oriented training that doesn't align with what they sing) (LoVetri

& Weekly, 2003; Weekly & LoVetri, 2009). They may not have a warm-up routine or vocal exercise regimen that is appropriate for their voices. Education regarding vocal hygiene, vocal pacing, and other aspects of vocal health may be incomplete or inaccurate, and the singer may be less cognizant of the vocal impact of lifestyle factors such as smoking and drinking than classical and musical theater singers.

For this population, your work on improving vocal coordination and conditioning may need to begin with the basics of vocal technique, particularly for singers who have little or no vocal training. It is of utmost importance that exercises are appropriate for contemporary singing technique and that the singer understands that adequate warm-up before performances is crucial.

Singing Activities and Vocal Pacing Considerations

CCM singers may be solo singer-songwriters, soloists who perform with prerecorded backup tracks, or they may sing in a band or a cappella vocal group. They may perform in bars and clubs, private parties, concert halls, and outdoor music festivals or at sports events or places of worship. They may tour or their performances may be primarily local. They often engage in recording activities.

Performing schedules for CCM singers are variable. For many, performances are frequent, long, and intense. Set length can range from 45 minutes to several hours. Many not only have performances on back-to-back days but multiple performances on the same day. Unlike singers in musical theater or opera performances, a lead singer in a band may sing fairly constantly throughout the show, and there is usually no one who can "cover." If the CCM singer can't go on, the entire performance often has to be cancelled. For professionals, cancellation has significant financial and reputation consequences. At the highest level, a single canceled performance can represent losses in the multiple millions of dollars (Waddell, 2014). This can lead the singer to feel pressured to go ahead with a performance when not in optimal vocal condition, which may contribute to or exacerbate a vocal injury.

Use of Sound Equipment. CCM singers almost always use amplification, but the quality of their sound equipment and skill at using it may or may not be adequate. Optimizing use of sound equipment is a critical component in maintaining vocal health and promoting recovery from injury. For singers who don't have good sound mixing and good monitors, there is often a tendency to oversing because they can't hear themselves accurately. In many cases, the singer uses the sound equipment and sound engineering available at the venue that may or may not be of good quality, yielding unpredictable results. If your knowledge of sound equipment is adequate, you can advise singers to help them optimize results (Edwards, 2014). See Chapter 18 for more detailed information about use of sound equipment.

Worship Soloists

Worship soloists include church soloists, cantors, praise and worship leaders, or anyone who acts as a soloist in the context of a worship service or activity.

According to Pew Research Center (2015), over 70% of Americans are affiliated with Christian faiths, and nearly 6% with non-Christian faiths (22.8% are unaffiliated). Virtually all religions of the world include singing or chanting as a part of worship activities (Ellingson,

1987; Gellman & Hartman, 2002) and you may work with singers who are Christian, Jewish, Hindu, Buddhist, Muslim, or from other world or indigenous religious traditions. It is likely that for many of the singers you work with, singing will play a significant role in their spiritual lives.

The typical style of singing, amount of training, and vocal load of the worship soloist can be quite variable. Those who sing primarily in classical style usually have had at least some training, and many are professionals for whom worship singing is part of a load that may also include concert, opera, theater, music education, or teaching singing. Some singers may have been trained in classical singing but engage in worship singing in contemporary styles. Others may have no training at all. Depending on the singer's specific vocal demands, singing style, and professional status, you may find it helpful to draw on resources from the other sections in this chapter.

Worship Style, Training, Performance Activities, and Vocal Demands

Exhaustive review of singing activities in all religions is beyond the scope of this text, however, it may be helpful to understand the typical vocal demands and worship style for some of the singers you are most likely to encounter in your practice. The range of styles for worship soloists is very broad, as are training history, frequency of performance, performing environment, and use of sound equipment. Refer to the relevant sections on classical and CCM singers for considerations and recommendations.

Gospel Singing. There are many types of gospel singing, and the particular stylistic characteristics and vocal demands of individual gospel singers differ from one to another. Robinson-Martin (2009) identifies at least four broad categories of gospel performance style: Traditional, Southern, Inspirational, and Contemporary. Worship services typically include singing by soloists and ensembles, feature contemporary elements such as a praise band, and are often led by a praise and worship leader.

Key elements of gospel singing may include improvisational runs, expressive use of moans, growls, and other emotional vocalization. Gospel singing is very spiritual: there is a desire and expectation that the singer will act as a vessel of the Holy Spirit, resulting in a performance that is emotional and energetic (Robinson-Martin, 2009). This intention of achieving "Anointing" and serving to spread the word of God through singing has ramifications for vocal pacing in that the singer may feel that being mindful of quantity and intensity of singing (as well as being aware of vocal technique) may interfere with their role as a vessel.

Historically, gospel singers have learned technique intuitively through immersion and imitation rather than pedagogical instruction. Gospel choirs learn music by repetition, not using written notation. Thus, performance is always from memory (Garnett, 2009; Hall, 2011; Hopkins, 2015). This method of rote learning means that the singer has to sing the part over and over again to learn it thoroughly and prepare for performance. This can present challenges in optimizing vocal pacing, but use of recordings and "mental practice" can help to ensure the singer is adequately prepared while still conserving voice (see Chapter 14).

Contemporary Worship. Contemporary worship is increasingly common in Christian services. In contemporary worship, a praise and worship leader plans and directs the musical aspects of the worship service, which features components found in popular music genres, including CCM singing, use of a rock- or pop-style instrumental ensemble, sound engineering, and sometimes staging, lighting, and other theatrical elements (Harris, 2012; Moss, 2001). The duties of praise and worship leaders differ considerably from those of traditional choir directors and church soloists. The praise and worship leader is typically a singer who is at the forefront in leading worship during services, often in collaboration with the minister or pastor. Praise and worship leaders act as soloists and may play an instrument to accompany themselves or others. The worship leader is often in charge of leading/directing and performing with a band, chorus, and/or small vocal ensemble and leading the congregational singing. It is not unusual for the praise and worship leader to have pastoral counseling and administrative duties as well (Harris, 2012; Moss, 2001).

Jewish Cantors. Jewish cantors act as the musical leader of the congregation in the Jewish synagogue. The vocal demands of cantors can be extremely high. They typically sing in services one to two times per week, as well as at special events such as weddings and funerals. They also have a variety of vocal demands outside of services, including preparing young congregants for their Bar or Bat Mitzvahs, teaching classes (ranging from preschool to adult), providing counseling to congregants, and participating in meetings and community leadership activities. Vocal demands typically increase markedly during the High Holy Days (Rosh Hashanah and Yom Kippur). A study by Hapner and Gilman (2012) indicates that for some cantors, vocal activities (speaking and singing) can exceed 40 hours per week. Cantors have varying amounts of vocal training, although most have had at least some training. Hapner and Gilman (2012) found that the cantors they surveyed had at least 3 years of vocal training, and most had more than 10 years. Notwithstanding this, 63% did not engage in daily warm-up or planned vocal rest. Over 65% of the cantors surveyed reported having a voice problem at some time in their careers.

Vocal Pacing: Special Challenges for Worship Soloists

It has been my experience that worship singers face unique challenges in that their singing lives are inextricably intertwined with their spiritual lives and worship. This can make it difficult to "unload" vocal demands if the singer feels he or she is shirking not just a professional but a *spiritual* duty, and the sense of spiritual obligation associated with job responsibilities can be very strong. This may make it hard to decline taking on additional duties or to request a decrease in vocal load or assistance with the current load. It can be very challenging for worship singers to achieve and maintain a balance of voice use that results in optimal vocal health. You may need to return to this principle time and time again as you help the singer arrive at a sustainable vocal load. Acknowledge that it may feel selfish to say "no," but remind them that they also have a responsibility to care for the gift that has been entrusted to them—the gift of singing.

Choral Singers

Choral singing is an extremely popular activity. Chorus America (2009) conservatively estimates the number of choruses in the United States at 270,000, including professional and community choruses, religious choirs, and K–12 school choruses. According to The Choral Impact Study of 2009, 32.5 million adults regularly sing in choruses in the United States. When children are included, that number jumps to 42.6 million Americans overall. Choral singing not only represents an important factor in artistic expression and enjoyment, worship, and spirituality but has been demonstrated to contribute to child and adolescent development (Brain et al., 2008; Helmrich, 2010), overall quality of life and psychological well-being (Clift & Hancox, 2010; Horn, 2013; Sandgren, 2009; Teater & Baldwin, 2014), and even as a beneficial intervention for specific disease processes (Biasutti et al., 2009; Chang, Irons, Kenny, & McElrea, 2012; Clement, Khatir, Samson, Schiaratura, & Tonini, 2012; Faunce & Kenny, 2004; Lord et al., 2010; Marchina, Norton, Schlaug, Wan, & Zipse, 2010).

Training, Singing Activities, and Vocal Pacing Considerations

Training and education can be quite variable in choral singers. Some have had extensive training and their choral singing may be part of other professional singing activities. This is most often seen in classical singers. However, as with a number of the populations discussed above, training may not be adequate or may not be aligned with performance style.

The choral demands of the singer may be associated with an academic requirement or elective, professional engagement, worship activities, community choir, or a cappella group. In singing voice rehabilitation, vocal pacing often involves short- or long-term reduction of vocal load. However, for many members of religious or community choirs, weekly rehearsals and intermittent performances may represent the full extent of singing activities. In such cases, vocal problems may develop as a result of sporadic vocal exercise and inadequate vocal conditioning as the singer vacillates between periods of prolonged and intense singing and extended periods of minimal singing. For these singers, the vocal pacing plan will likely include strategies for offloading nonsinging voice use when the choral demands increase but also establishing a regular vocal exercise and conditioning routine (i.e., increasing the amount of singing on a weekly basis) to ensure adequate vocal fitness to meet fluctuating requirements.

Ideally, the choral singer's practice sessions should include some time to work on repertoire. Often choral singers only work on their music during rehearsals. The choral rehearsal is a cognitively demanding setting, requiring the singer to simultaneously read and process the music, watch the conductor for cues and information, listen to his or her own voice as well as those of the other singers, and execute the complex coordination required to accurately sing melody, rhythm, and text, all while achieving excellent pitch accuracy and expressive interpretation. It can be very difficult to try to focus on the minutiae of improving vocal technique with such multifaceted tasks at hand. Incorporating repertoire into the home practice routine will enable the singer to deliberately focus on technically challenging portions of the choral music he or she is working on and apply skills developed through vocalizes.

Vocal Music Educators/ Choral Teachers

Vocal music educators have one of *the most* vocally demanding jobs. The reason for this is twofold: first, the extraordinary vocal demands of the typical teaching day —extending from before school to after school to nights, holidays, and weekends. Second, unlike their instrumental music or classroom teaching colleagues, vocal/choral music educators must be able to produce superior vocal quality and skill to demonstrate excellent singing to their students and must be in optimal vocal condition at all times to do so. This combination of quantitative and qualitative demands creates the perfect storm for developing a voice problem.

Although they are often not vocal performers in the same way that choral teachers are, many of the principles outlined herein are also applicable to instrumental music educators.

Teachers in general are usually generous, giving people, often wholeheartedly embodying the principle of "give until it hurts." This sense of devotion can be central to successful teaching, helping students achieve the highest performance level they are capable of. However, this same dogged commitment on the part of music educators can also lead them to put self-care on the back burner, possibly neglecting their vocal health. It is easy for them to become convinced that they can't be excellent, effective teachers without giving 110% or more.

Unfortunately, choral music educators often do not consider seeking help until they have been struggling with a voice disorder for months or even years, by which time they may have a serious injury that will require extensive rehabilitation therapy and possibly even surgery. Some even begin to consider leaving the profession they love because their voices just can't hold up anymore. However, with competent evaluation and appropriate treatment, the prognosis is usually excellent for the music educator to be able to continue his or her career, albeit with important adjustments to vocal pacing, vocal hygiene, and vocal technique for speaking and singing.

The singer may or may not want to disclose the voice injury and rehabilitation to students, parents, school administrators, or other faculty, and your recommendations on this topic must be guided by the singer's wishes and comfort level. If they are willing and comfortable doing so, sharing the experience with students can provide an important lesson in vocal health. In addition, if students are aware of the teacher's voice problem, they will likely be more than willing to help in the classroom and may serve an important role in reminding the teacher about being consistent in new vocal habits. If the teacher is willing to share information with school administrators and colleagues, they can be enlisted for support, particularly for reducing vocal demands outside the classroom, such as for lunch, recess, or after-school duty.

Training and Education

Choral music educators typically have a background in classical singing technique, but the amount of training can be inconsistent. Some may have extensive training and a high level of vocal proficiency, while others may have only had a few semesters of voice lessons in college. Assessing skill level will be an important first step in rehabilitation.

It is very common for choral music educators to consider warming up with their students to be adequate vocal exercise. However, successful rehabilitation necessitates daily individual practice during a time when the singer can focus on optimizing technical execution and can work on the exercises that have been customized for recovery. Once rehabilitation is completed, continuing regular individual warm-up time will remain an important element of ongoing vocal health.

Singing Activities and Vocal Pacing Considerations

For those teaching in primary and secondary schools, the vocal music educator's typical schedule can include 5 to 6 hours per day of choral rehearsal or classroom teaching. He or she will be lucky to have a 60-minute planning period. This schedule in and of itself exceeds that of a typical university-level choral instructor and is much more vocally rigorous than that of any other classroom teacher. In addition, they may have "extra" vocal demands during the school day such as supervising lunch in a noisy cafeteria, leading meetings, or directing students in assembly activities, among a plethora of others. And that's just the school day: the vocal music educator's schedule rarely stops at final bell. More commonly, vocal music educators engage in many more hours per week of teaching and rehearsing before and after school in activities such as directing the school musical; preparing students for All-State, Honors Choir, college auditions, or choral festivals; and teaching private lessons. They may also direct or sing in a church or community choir for another 2 to 4 hours per week. And of course, music educators have busy family and social lives. This schedule is a recipe for voice injury, and a music educator cannot sustain it full-tilt without consequences. Optimizing vocal pacing is typically a major component of singing voice rehabilitation for this population.

Use of Amplification. Use of amplification when teaching is a key factor in optimizing vocal pacing for music educators. See Chapter 14 for recommendations for voice amplification.

Voice Use in the Classroom. If possible, have the music educator video a typical rehearsal or class. Reviewing this together will reveal areas for modification. Does the arrangement of the classroom—music stand, piano, student seating—promote ideal posture and body alignment? If not, explore alternative configurations. Is the teacher expending excessive vocal energy in being a "cheerleader" for the class, shouting encouragement or providing continuous verbal feedback? Dialing back the intensity level in the classroom can create an environment in which the students are equal partners in being passionate about music and striving for excellence.

Resuming or Adding Performing Activities. As the music educator recovers and experiences improved vocal quality and stamina, he or she may wish to explore prospects for engaging in rewarding singing activities, such as singing in a church or community choir, performing in local opera or theater productions, singing in a band, or taking engagements as a concert soloist or recitalist. In all likelihood, these activities will have been abandoned or sacrificed to teaching demands or because of the voice problem. Continuing to refresh the passion for singing will be motivating and musically nourishing.

Choral Conductors

The type and context of voice use for choral conductors is similar to that of choral music educators—directing rehearsals and performances, demonstrating parts, teaching vocal technique, and so on.

Much of what was discussed in the preceding section on choral music educators will apply to this singing population, although the specific vocal demands can be quite different. Choral conductors working in a university music program may have multiple choirs as part of their academic load. Outside the academic setting, professional choir directors may conduct one or more community-based ensembles and have additional directing duties relative to symphony or opera choruses and church choirs. Many also have performing careers and additional teaching responsibilities in the classroom or private studio. Depending on the specific vocal demands, recommendations and resources from other sections may apply.

Choral conductors working in a worship setting face an additional challenge similar to that noted for worship soloists: their musical and singing lives are inextricably entwined with their spiritual lives. As for worship soloists, this factor often introduces an element of spiritual obligation associated with job responsibilities that must be sensitively considered in the rehabilitation process.

Student Singers

Student singers represent a special subset of the singing population. Although anyone who is taking voice lessons is technically a "student singer," for purposes of this section, student singers are primarily considered to be middle school through university students, whether or not they are working with a voice teacher. University students may include those enrolled in a music degree program with a voice or musical theater major or minor, college students active in extracurricular vocal activities such as musical theater productions or a cappella groups, or those taking voice lessons or choir as an elective.

As you work with student singers, it will be critical for you to obtain a clear picture of each singer not only relative to type and quantity of vocal demands, amount and stylistic appropriateness of training in singing, and the impact of both on injury and prognosis for recovery but also to informally assess the singer's maturity, level of insight and self-awareness, and motivation to recover (Harvey, 1997).

I have found that it is optimal for the student to continue voice lessons with his or her current teacher during the rehabilitation process if at all possible. The student will benefit from having additional skilled ears assessing the voice on a regular basis and from maintaining the supportive relationship with the teacher. In addition, the voice teacher can be an important advocate for the student and can reinforce rehabilitation recommendations.

Be Prepared for a Wide Range of Maturity

The period of early adolescence through early adulthood is a time of tremendous change, as young people experience dramatic physical, cognitive, and emotional growth (Andrews, 1993). The singers you work with in this age range will have achieved very different levels of emotional maturity. This can make a big difference in how much guidance and structure they need from you in order to meet their vocal health and rehabilitation goals. I have worked with 15-year-olds who demonstrated a level of maturity, discipline, and focus that exceeded that of many adults, and I have also worked with college students preparing to launch their professional singing careers who struggled mightily to make mature decisions aligned with their rehabilitation goals—especially relative to balancing singing and social priorities—and whose recovery was hindered by this struggle.

Guiding the Student Singer to Make Informed Decisions and Choices. In order for the singers you work with to reach their vocal health (and thereby vocal performance and participation) goals, you must guide them in understanding how their actions impact the goals and lead them to make decisions that will achieve the desired outcome. Presenting a list of prohibitions (particularly relative to vocal pacing) or taking the role of taskmaster or scold can undermine the effectiveness of intervention. Framing rehabilitation goals as a partnership between you and the singer and engaging the young singer's perspective with genuine attention and interest can help in establishing a relationship of trust and support, which is of critical importance in working with any singer, but especially with adolescents and young adults (Andrews, 1993). It takes skill and flexibility on the part of the singing voice rehabilitation specialist to help the singer recognize the interaction of lifestyle and vocal health and to be motivated to make healthy choices. At the same time, be aware that some singers may just not be at a level of maturity to make the necessary compromises to support recovery from injury, or may not be ready to put their singing priorities into action. We want them to achieve their rehabilitation goals, but if they are not able to optimize vocal habits in the present, our role sometimes becomes that of ensuring that they are fully informed of the ramifications their decisions may have for the future.

Training and Education

As noted above, student singers may or may not have had vocal training. Assessing training will be an important first step in the rehabilitation process.

Those who have training may be receiving instruction in classical technique and repertoire in their private voice lessons and applying this technique in school or university chorus, opera, and recital, while belting in musical theater productions or singing in a variety of CCM styles in a cappella groups, bands, in worship activities, and recreational singing. They may or may not have vocal training that specifically focuses on CCM technique and—importantly—may not have a clear understanding of the physiologic and acoustical differences between classical and CCM singing. As a result, they may be steadily advancing technical skill relative to their classical singing activities while relying on their intuition and imitation skills for the contemporary singing they are engaged in with little or no technical foundation. Or they may be trying to apply their classical technique to CCM singing, resulting in confusion and a potentially harmful somatic "argument" between inappropriate technique and the sound ideal they are trying to reproduce. In the rehabilitation process, you must carefully and thoroughly assess the amount and type of singing the student is engaged in and the degree to which training background and understanding of technique may factor into injury and recovery.

Singing Activities and Vocal Pacing Considerations

Adolescent and early adult student singers are often engaged in a great number of vocal activities that may span a wide range of types and styles of singing. They may take private voice lessons, sing in choir(s) both in and out of school, sing in musical theater or opera productions (again, in and out of school), sing in a cappella groups, and/or participate in worship singing. They typically have some vocal activities that are academic requirements (on which their academic success depends) and others that are extracurricular. In all likelihood, they are spending additional vocal time on recreational singing.

Sometimes there are family, school, or other sources of pressure on the student to be involved in various activities, and there may be a disconnect between the singer's priorities and those of peers, parents, teachers, or other adults as to which vocal activities are most important. In your role as singing voice rehabilitation specialist, your job is not to impose your opinion about what activities are most important but to elicit the priorities of the singer (considering input from adults as appropriate) and to provide education regarding the impact of various activities in supporting his or her singing goals.

Considerations for Specific Student Singer Populations

A Cappella Group Singers. A cappella singing groups are extremely popular, as evidenced not only by their legions, but as enshrined in popular culture through film and television phenomena such as *Glee, Perfect Pitch,* and *The Sing Off*. The Contemporary A Cappella Society (CASA) lists nearly 3,000 groups in its database and estimates worldwide contemporary a cappella singing groups to number in the tens of thousands (CASA, 2014). This type of singing group is certainly not limited to high school and college settings, but their proliferation in schools warrants inclusion in this section. The information and resources provided here will be applicable to anyone who participates in an a cappella group.

Unlike ensembles that students enroll in for academic credit, a cappella singing groups are typically student led and autonomous. This autonomy is an important part of the a cappella culture but lends itself to widely varying degrees of knowledge and skill relative to vocal technique and vocal health and, without adequate education, may lead to vocal excess. If group members and leaders are not sufficiently conversant in principles of vocal health, signs of vocal injury may be overlooked, and singers may not recognize the importance of seeking help for voice problems. Singers may feel pressured to go through with performances when they are sick or hoarse. If multiple members of the group ordinarily experience hoarseness or other voice changes after performances, there may be an assumption that this is a "normal" and expected part of participation instead of a dangerous manifestation of chronic voice overuse.

Vocal pacing is often a significant factor in singing voice rehabilitation for this population. A cappella groups usually rehearse two to three times per week, and rehearsals may last for 2 or 3 hours or even longer. At the college level, rehearsals are customarily augmented with extended social bonding pursuits such as weekend group retreats and numerous planning meetings. Performance schedules frequently feature extended tours during which the group visits other schools with concomitant social gatherings. These traditions contribute to a load that can be vocally burdensome and, without adaptation, may lead to vocal injury.

All of these factors combine to place the student singing in an a cappella group at high risk for vocal injury. However, students who participate in these groups often exhibit excellent leadership skills. In my experience, once armed with appropriate knowledge and information, these students do an exceptional job of incorporating good vocal habits into their traditions.

Given the collective nature of ensemble singing, the singer you are working with may be limited in how much he or she can adapt voice use and still be in the group if leadership and the rest of the group are not supportive of or receptive to recommended changes. These ensembles are often regarded on campus as elite and very competitive, and the singer may be reluctant or resistant to asking for special accommodations, fearing that doing so could jeopardize continued membership in the group. You may need to encourage the singer to effectively self-advocate. Tread carefully in making decisions about whether to intervene on the student's behalf. In autonomous, student-led organizations, your input and recommendations may not be as well received as when interacting with a voice teacher, choir conductor, or theater director. The better plan might be to empower the student with information and resources to take back to the group. The student you are working with is probably not the only one in the group experiencing vocal problems, and I have found that a cappella groups usually embrace changes that will benefit the whole group.

College Voice Performance, Music Education, and Musical Theater Majors. Students enrolled in academic vocal performance programs face intense vocal demands at a time when their voices are still developing and when their grasp and proficiency of vocal technique are in an emergent state.

In addition to weekly voice lessons, college students in academic music programs are typically required to sing in at least one vocal ensemble, usually with rigorous—sometimes daily—rehearsal schedules. Add to this daily individual practice sessions, rehearsals for opera or theater productions, coaching sessions, a job as a section leader or soloist at a church or synagogue, and recreational singing, and voice use can quickly escalate to a level that is challenging to manage.

Choral singing can represent a significant proportion of the student's vocal requirements and it can sometimes be problematic to balance choral and solo singing demands. In addition, student singers—with their emerging vocal technique—may experience confusion about the differences between solo and ensemble singing. It will be important to ascertain whether the singer notices vocal symptoms associated more with one type of singing than another.

For this population, most or all singing activities are part of their academic requirements, so adjusting vocal activities necessitates careful consideration in order to ensure academic success while promoting vocal health and recovery from vocal injury. Be prepared to advocate for the student with teachers and directors and provide recommendations as needed for adapting vocal load and activities in the short term to support recovery from injury. For example, the student might benefit from having two 30-minute lessons per week as opposed to one 60-minute lesson. If vocal quality and stamina are compromised, deferring the jury requirement to a subsequent semester may be necessary and/or the student may need accommodations in the ensemble requirement (being excused from singing for part or all of rehearsal for a period of time). Many times such accommodations can be negotiated without losing credit for the course if the student continues to attend rehearsals. In some cases of severe injury, or when surgical intervention is indicated, continuing with academic requirements may jeopardize recovery. In such cases, the student may have to cease participation in some or all academic requirements for a period of time in favor of focusing on rehabilitation therapy. This can be a difficult decision to make, as the student may not graduate on schedule as a result, but is sometimes vital for long-term vocal health and ultimate academic and professional success.

REFERENCES

Andrews, M. L. (1993). Intervention with young voice users: A clinical perspective. *Journal of Voice, 7*, 160–164.

Biasutti, E., Cavazzon, M., Di Benedetto, P., Mondolo, F., Peratoner, A., & Rugio, G. (2009). Voice and choral singing treatment: A new approach for speech and voice disorders in Parkinson's disease. *European Journal of Physical Rehabilitation Medicine, 45*(1), 13–19. Retrieved from http://www.ncbi.nlm.nih.gov/pubmed/18987565

Brain, S., Daykin, N., Evans, D., McEachran, M., Orme, J., & Salmon, D. (2008). The impact of participation in performing arts on adolescent health and behavior: A systematic review of the literature. *Journal of Health Psychology, 13*(2), 251–264. Retrieved from http://www.ncbi.nlm.nih.gov/pubmed/18375630

CASA. (2014). Retrieved March 4, 2015, from http://www.casa.org/acapedia/search/l?page=5&GroupName=&Location=&Keyword=&MusicalStyle=All&GroupComposition=All&Affiliation=&reset=Reset

Chang, A., Irons, D., Kenny, T., & McElrea, M. (2012). Singing therapy for young people with cystic fibrosis: A randomized controlled pilot study. *Music and Medicine, 10*(41). Retrieved from http://mmd.sagepub.com/content/4/3/136.abstract.

Chapline, J., Cohen, G., Firth, K., Kelly, J., Perlstein, S., & Simmens, S. (2006). The impact of professionally conducted cultural programs on the physical health, mental health, and social functioning of older adults. *The Gerontologist, 46*(6), 726–734.

Clement, S., Khatir, F., Samson, S., Schiaratura, L., & Tonini, A. (2012). Short and longer term effects of musical intervention in severe Alzheimer's disease. *Music Perception: An Interdisciplinary Journal, 29*(5), 533–541.

Chorus America. (2009). *The Chorus Impact Study*. Washington, DC. Retrieved December 5, 2015, from https://www.chorusamerica.org/advocacy-research/chorus-impact-study

Clift, S., & Hancox, G. (2010). The significance of choral singing for sustaining psychological well-being: Findings from a survey of choristers in England, Germany, and Australia. *Music and Health, 3*(1), 79–96. Retrieved from http://mpronline.net/Issues/Volume%203.1%20Special%20Issue%20%5B2010%5D/Clift%20Published%20Web%20Version.pdf

Edwards, M. (2014). I love it loud! Using audio enhancement technology. In M. Edwards (Ed.), *So you want to sing rock 'n roll* (pp. 167–191). Lanham, MD: Rowman & Littlefield.

Ellingson, T. (1987). Music and religion. In M. Eliade (Ed.), *The encyclopedia of religion* (Vol. 10, pp. 163–172). New York, NY: Macmillan. Retrieved March 28, 2015, from https://books.google.com/books?id=eIikUJpHYNQC&pg=PA268&lpg=PA268&dq=singing+in+world+religions&source=bl&ots=zzATwzZ5TO&sig=lCyO-jvJfuQVEn6Z40w9bCfcJA4&hl=en&sa=X&ei=_vj5VKbjJsS6ggSj0YNY&ved=0CDMQ6AEwAjgK#v=onepage&q=singing%20in%20world%20religions&f=false

Faunce, G., & Kenny, D. (2004). The impact of group singing on mood, coping, and perceived pain in chronic pain patients attending a multidisciplinary pain clinic. *Journal of Music Therapy, 41*(3), 241–258. Retrieved from http://www.ncbi.nlm.nih.gov/pubmed/15327342

Garnett, L. (2009). *Choral conducting and the construction of meaning: Gesture, voice, identity*. Surrey, England: Ashgate. Retrieved March 15, 2015, from https://books.google.com/books?id=LouQgvHCuZgC&pg=PA70&lpg=PA70&dq=gospel+choir+rehearsal+techniques&source=bl&ots=XBS_JKP9ml&sig=ukDbR0lNixJGeWqAR218S7qgNi8&hl=en&sa=X&ei=cfb5VIvcEIidgwTp7IC4CA&ved=0CB0Q6AEwADgK#v=onepage&q=gospel%20choir%20rehearsal%20techniques&f=false

Gellman, M., & Hartman, T. (2002). Making a joyful noise in religious ritual. *Religion for Dummies*. Retrieved January 29, 2015, from http://www.dummies.com/how-to/content/making-a-joyful-noise-in-religious-ritual.html

Hall, J. (2011). *A guide to directing a gospel choir: How to be a great gospel choir director.* Retrieved March 6, 2015, from http://choirparts.com/ebooks/A-Guide-To-Directing-a-Gospel-Choir.pdf

Hapner, E., & Gilman, M. (2012). The vocal load of Reform Jewish cantors in the USA. *Journal of Voice, 26*(2), 201–204.

Harris, H. R. (2012). In the life of the church, praise and worship leaders play a key role. *The Washington Post.* Retrieved March 6, 2015, from http://www.washingtonpost.com/local/in-the-life-of-the-church-praise-and-worship-leaders-play-a-key-role/2012/03/30/gIQAbqqKmS_story.html

Harvey, P. L. (1997). The three ages of voice: The young adult patient. *Journal of Voice, 11,* 144–152.

Helmrich, B. (2010). Window of opportunity? Adolescence, music, and algebra. *Journal of Adolescent Research, 25*(4), 557–577. Retrieved from http://jar.sagepub.com/content/25/4/557.abstract

Hopkins, V. (2015). *Rehearsal Tutorial Part 1: Introducing a new piece to your choir.* Retrieved from http://www.totalchoirresources.com/introducing-a-new-piece-to-your-choir/

Horn, S. (2013). *Imperfect harmony: Finding happiness singing with others.* Chapel Hill, NC: Algonquin Books of Chapel Hill.

Lord, V., Cave, P., Hume, V., Flude, E., Evans, A., Kelly, J., . . . Hopkinson, N. (2010). Singing teaching as a therapy for chronic respiratory disease: A randomised controlled trial and qualitative evaluation. *BMC Pulmonary Medicine, 10*(41). Retrieved from http://www.ncbi.nlm.nih.gov/pmc/articles/PMC2920262/

LoVetri, J. (2008). Editorial. Contemporary commercial music. *Journal of Voice, 22*(3), 260–262.

LoVetri, J., & Weekly, E. M. (2003). Contemporary commercial music (CCM) survey: Who's teaching what in non-classical music. *Journal of Voice, 17*(2), 207–215.

Marchina, S., Norton, A., Schlaug, G., Wan, C., & Zipse, L. (2010). From singing to speaking: Facilitating recovery from nonfluent aphasia. *Future Neurology, 5*(5), 657–665. Retrieved from http://www.ncbi.nlm.nih.gov/pmc/articles/PMC2982746/

Moss, P. (2001). *The role of the praise and worship leader: A model for preparing the singer for leadership in contemporary worship* (Doctoral dissertation submitted to the faculties of the schools of the Atlanta Theological Association). Retrieved from http://digitalcommons.auctr.edu/cgi/viewcontent.cgi?article=1081&context=dissertations

Pew Research Center. (May 2015). *America's Changing Religious Landscape.* Retrieved December 4, 2015, from http://religions.pewforum.org/reports

Robinson-Martin, T. (2009). Performance styles and musical characteristics of black gospel music. *Journal of Singing, 65*(5), 595–599.

Sandgren, M. (2009). *Evidence for strong immediate well-being effects of choral singing: With more enjoyment for women than for men.* Proceedings from ESCOM 2009: 7th Triennial Conference of European Society for the Cognitive Sciences of Music Proceedings. Jyväskylä, Finland. Retrieved from https://jyx.jyu.fi/dspace/handle/123456789/20916

Teater, B., & Baldwin, M. (2014). Singing for successful ageing: The perceived benefits of participating in the golden oldies community-arts programme. *British Journal of Social Work, 44*(1), 81–99.

Waddell, R. (2014, December 12). *Live Music's $20 billion year: Rolling Stones, One Direction, Live Nation top boxscore's year-end.* Retrieved from http://www.billboard.com/articles/business/6406028/boxscore-top-tours-2014-rolling-stones-live-nation

Weekly, E. M., & LoVetri, J. (2009). Follow-up contemporary commercial music (CCM) survey: Who's teaching what in non-classical music. *Journal of Voice, 23*(3), 367–375.

PART II

Emotional Factors

CHAPTER 8

Supporting the Singer's Emotional Needs: Working With the Psychological Impact of Voice Problems

When working with singers who have sustained a voice injury or have a voice disorder, it is essential to understand the emotional ramifications of the voice problem. The voice is central to the singer's identity and self-esteem. Singers often view their voices as an extension of themselves, as opposed to an external instrument or vehicle of expression (Eustis, 2005; Radionoff, 2004; Rosen & Sataloff, 1997). For professional singers, livelihood and income are dependent on the voice. In this case, "professional" refers not only to professional performers but to anyone who earns a living from singing, including music educators, voice teachers, choral conductors, church musicians, and so on. For others, singing is an avocation but often feels as important to them as it does to professionals. For these "avocational" singers, voice can be critical for quality of life and social interactions, especially as one becomes older. And for many, voice and singing are intrinsically connected with spiritual life and worship. Thus, having a voice problem can jeopardize income, quality of life, social connections, and support system, and can even precipitate a crisis of identity. The singer may feel lost, broken, or "defective."

Singing is an enormously vulnerable act and requires equally enormous confidence. When singers have voice injuries or voice disorders, they also acquire an injury to their confidence. This "hidden" injury must be addressed as diligently as the physical injury. It is essential that the singing voice rehabilitation specialist monitor, address, and validate the singer's feelings and reactions during the evaluation process and throughout the course of voice rehabilitation.

ESTABLISHING TRUST AND CREDIBILITY AT THE INITIAL VISIT

Upon learning that he or she has a voice injury, the singer is often flooded with emotions and questions. "Is this the end of my career? Can I ever recover from this? Did I do this to myself? Does this mean

I'm not a good singer? What will my voice teacher/director/colleagues/agent/public think? How am I going to get through the performance commitments I have? How am I going to support myself if I can't sing?" The singer feels emotionally overwhelmed and may be emotionally labile. He or she may even break down and cry upon receiving the diagnosis or at any point during the rehabilitation process when visited by such fears and questions. As a singing voice rehabilitation specialist, you must be prepared for this to happen and for what you will do when it does happen. The ability to read the singer and identify what will be most helpful is a critical skill. Some may need a shoulder to cry on and a listening ear for their fears and concerns. Others may take a no-nonsense approach and will appreciate concrete actions and clear explanations over sympathetic hand-holding. It is your job to adapt your approach based on your perception of what will best support the singer you are working with.

When addressing the questions and concerns that will inevitably arise, be honest and encouraging. What the singer needs most is to be reassured that a voice disorder or voice injury does not mean the end of a career or singing life. In many cases, simply stating that he or she can get better will provide hope and allay fears. If the singer cries or is emotional, provide reassurance that this is a normal reaction. Singers will appreciate knowing that you understand how they feel and that you recognize how important their voices are to them. This is the beginning of the bond that you will establish with each singer that will promote trust throughout the rehabilitation process.

Your honesty is equally as important as your reassurance. Be encouraging, but don't give false hope. Your enthusiasm about the prognosis must be tempered by the nature and severity of the voice disorder, and you must be guided by your knowledge and experience in explaining the injury and path to healing. Be realistic as to what the expectations should be relative to duration and degree of recovery. Emphasize that each singer's recovery is a little different, and that while there is no "crystal ball" for predicting outcome, your prognosis is based on scientific knowledge and your experience. Obviously, your credibility depends on your store of both. It takes time and practice—often over a period of years—to develop the foundation of knowledge and experience necessary to become proficient in this type of counseling, especially as it relates to being able to read the singer and to predict the outcome of the case based on the nature of the injury. Each singer provides an opportunity for you to add to that foundation. As you learn and grow, you will become more confident and accurate in prognostication, which will help you to quickly establish trust with the singers you work with.

PREPARING THE SINGER FOR THE REHABILITATION PROCESS

At the initial rehabilitation session, start by eliciting questions about the evaluation results or rehabilitation plan. When all lingering questions have been addressed, you can provide an overview of how the rehabilitation process will work. Emphasize that this process will be entirely guided by the singer's goals and is designed to facilitate achieving those goals.

Be sure that you understand what the singer's goals are in developing your treatment plan, as motivation and commitment to the process will be dependent on ensuring that your goals are aligned. This will allow you to guide expectations for results, and prepare the singer for how much time and effort will have to be expended to reach goals.

Many singers are overwhelmed by the prospect of undertaking the rehabilitation process. They may think they don't have time to undergo voice rehabilitation sessions or regular practice of vocal exercises. They may have financial concerns. They may feel the lifestyle changes you are recommending to improve vocal hygiene and vocal pacing will be impossible for them to achieve. When you encounter singers who seem resistant or overwhelmed, provide them with options and choices. For example, if they feel it will be impossible to come to sessions every week, let them know that they can still expect to make progress if they attend less frequently, although it might take more time. If they feel they won't have time to practice every day, ask them how often they think they might be able to practice, and let that be the starting point for commitment. Rather than laying out an inflexible set of rules and regulations, adapt your immediate recommendations to what you think each singer is prepared to undertake. This way, you meet them where they are and make them feel that what you are recommending is possible.

Although you must set appropriate boundaries, the singer might be reassured to know when you will be available. After you explain the nature of the injury and outline the treatment plan, let the singer know that you understand it is a lot to process, and that if questions arise after the visit, there will be time to address them in future visits or (if you are able and if you feel comfortable offering it as an option) through communication between visits.

LET'S PUT AN END TO THE BLAME GAME

One of the unique concepts in the world of singing is that of *vocal abuse*. When singers (or any other voice users, for that matter) sustain a traumatic injury to the vocal folds (nodules, polyps, cysts, hemorrhage, etc.), the etiology is often referred to as vocal abuse. This concept and terminology is not found in any other area of performing arts, in the world of athletics, or any other type of movement-related injury. Pianists and typists get tendonitis or carpal tunnel syndrome and we don't call them "hand abusers." Ballet dancers have altered foot anatomy and we don't call them "foot abusers." When a football player sustains an anterior cruciate ligament (ACL) tear, we don't call him a "knee abuser." All of these are examples of stress injuries and are regarded as an expected result of placing super-human demands on a human body. Diagnosis is made, treatment is undertaken, rehabilitation is completed, and the performer or athlete gets back into the game, all without the use of the word "abuse." Yet among singers, voice educators, and health care providers, it is very common to use this pejorative expression.

By referring to traumatic vocal injuries as vocal abuse, an element of blame is introduced into the conversation. The term suggests that singers are responsible for causing their own injuries, creating a stigma that surrounds the whole issue. The singer is viewed as being at fault, and there is an implication that if he or she only had better technique or was otherwise more accomplished, the injury wouldn't have happened. The integrity of the singer's voice is called into question, and this may persist even after the physical injury has healed. This stigma is particularly notable in the classical singing realm and is so powerful and pervasive that many singers hide their injuries, use pseudonyms when seeking medical care, and never reveal the voice problem to the public, thus perpetuating the idea that "good singers don't get voice injuries." The stigma may also make singers reluctant to seek help when they are having voice problems for fear that they will be diagnosed with the dreaded nodules, labeled as a "vocal abuser," and be forever regarded as "damaged goods."

This type of blame language is inconsistent with the expression of empathy, is counterproductive to accomplishing positive change (Behrman, 2006), and may undermine your success as a singing voice rehabilitation specialist. It creates an environment of fear and reluctance and can make it difficult to establish trust between you and the singer. A study by Gillespie and Abbott (2010) found that use of terminology such as vocal abuse and "vocal misuse" may impede self-efficacy in the context of voice care.

Furthermore, there is abundant evidence that many singers who are functioning at the peak of performance demonstrate irregularities of vocal fold edges, closure, vibration, and/or function as a part of their normal baseline (Elias, Sataloff, Rosen, Heuer, & Spiegel, 1997; Heman-Ackah, Dean, & Sataloff, 2002; Lundy et al., 1999; Sataloff & Hawkshaw, 2013). Therefore, labeling a singer as a "voice abuser" upon diagnosis of such irregularities is not only unsupportive and unproductive but also scientifically inaccurate.

Finally, vocal abuse as a clinical term presents a number of linguistic pitfalls, including circularity, nonspecificity, and ambiguity. Verdolini (1999) argues that the use of such language can have a negative impact on clinical outcomes, as it may obstruct the accuracy and clarity of clinical thinking and undermine the singer's ability to adhere to recommendations and complete rehabilitation tasks. In this case, she is referring to outcomes in a clinical setting, but the point is well taken in any context in which health care provider, therapist, or voice teacher is interacting with a singer. Verdolini (1999) further asserts that

> Vocal abuse and "misuse" are prime examples of potential sources of clinical undermining in voice therapy. . . . In lay English, the term "abuse" is deeply tied to troubling moral and health care issues, including "child abuse," "spousal abuse," and "substance abuse." Patients seeking care because of voice loss, functional deprivation, and concern over serious disease are delivered a type of inculpation along with a medical diagnosis when they are informed—often during the first clinical encounter and repeatedly thereafter—that their condition is due to an abuse. Similarly, "misuse" in our culture often implies incompetence or moral depravity ("misuse of funds"). It is difficult to conceive that the framing of patients' problems as founded in self-abuse or misuse would not undermine self-efficacy. Surely such exhortations do nothing to support or enhance it. (p. 4)

As a singing voice rehabilitation specialist, it is incumbent on you to take a leadership role in abolishing and discrediting this language. You must be diligent not only in avoiding use of the term vocal abuse when interacting with the singer but also in probing to determine whether the singer is encumbered by thoughts of self-blame. If such thoughts are present, you may need to repeatedly reassure the singer that he or she is not at fault for the voice problem.

It is also important that you endeavor to educate those you interact with as to the inappropriateness of this language. This may include voice teachers, music educators, and health care providers. This language is fairly entrenched in multiple professions, and you may encounter resistance to your appeals to eliminate it. Framing the argument in the context of athletic or other repetitive motion injuries, underlining the scientific inaccuracy of vocal abuse and the potential negative impact on rehabilitation outcome, can be a helpful way to invite more appropriate and accurate language.

MONITOR EMOTIONAL CONCERNS

Throughout the course of rehabilitation, the singer will inevitably experience ups and downs, surges of progress alternating with setbacks. At times, he or she may feel discouraged or even despairing. You may need to continuously provide reminders that such fluctuations are part of the process. In order to keep rehabilitation sessions on track, you must support the singer emotionally without letting emotional responses sidetrack the process.

There may be times when you find it necessary to devote much or all of a session to addressing the singer's emotional needs and concerns, and this is not inappropriate. It is important to read the singer and recognize when it will be beneficial to delve into and devote some time to emotional concerns. However, if it seems that every session turns into a rehashing of concerns that have been addressed again and again, it might be necessary to redirect the singer (in a supportive and compassionate manner) to ensure that you stay on track with rehabilitation goals.

If you feel the rehabilitation sessions are getting derailed by frequent emotional sidebars, you can gently guide the session back to rehabilitation goals and topics by saying something such as, "I understand that you are feeling discouraged, and this is a difficult process. Your feelings are a normal and valid response to sustaining a voice injury. Let's spend a little time working on some vocal exercises so that you can practice them between now and your next session. We can come back to these feelings whenever we need to and talk more." It can also be helpful to review the progress achieved to date. Realizing how far one has come can be enormously encouraging, even if the ultimate goal still seems to lie in the distant future.

With some singers, you may need to take a firmer hand in the redirection. Sometimes the singer may view the voice rehabilitation session as an invitation to unload all his or her problems. Discernment is required to determine when "life" issues are relevant to the voice rehabilitation process and thus worthy of addressing, and when this unloading is encumbering recovery. The following case study provides an example of discerning the relative appropriateness of addressing "life issues" as a critical factor in rehabilitation outcome.

Case Study

"Hailey" was a 37-year-old successful high school music educator with bilateral vocal fold nodules. In addition to her teaching demands, she had previously been a member of a local community chorus (which she enjoyed very much) but had to discontinue this activity due to her voice problem.

She had started voice therapy and had been extremely compliant with recommendations for improving vocal hygiene and vocal pacing. She quickly assimilated improved vocal efficiency in speaking and singing tasks in the therapy sessions, but she found it challenging to practice regularly at home. She had two young children and, when she was not teaching, devoted much of her time to caring for them and managing the household. At her fifth session, she broke down and cried, noting that she felt very discouraged and frustrated with herself for not being able to practice enough to make the progress she wanted to. She knew she should be practicing regularly, but she felt overwhelmed by the amount of work she had to do at home as well as the demands of her teaching job.

Although time management and balance of home/work life may not seem directly relevant to voice rehabilitation, she was clearly under a great deal of stress, and this was interfering in her ability to achieve her voice goals. She was motivated and committed to her voice recovery, but the voice practice was becoming just another chore in her already too busy life.

In this case, simply reiterating the importance of practicing exercises may have been counterproductive and may have made her feel even more discouraged. We discussed the importance of self-care in general. It became clear that what was frustrating her was the fact that she felt she never had time for herself. We talked about the things she found relaxing and rejuvenating. We set a goal for her to allow herself 15 to 20 minutes per day to devote to something she enjoyed, such as scrapbooking or taking a relaxing bath. At first she thought this would be impossible, since she always arrived at the end of the day with chores left to do. However, she agreed to try it for the next week.

At her next session, she arrived beaming. "I did it!" she said. She reported that initially, she found it difficult. She even had to lock the bathroom door to keep her family from intruding on her brief restoring bath, but they quickly understood that she needed this quiet time for herself and respected and supported it. "I feel like a new person," she said.

By allowing herself this little bit of stress-relieving time, she demonstrated to herself that it was possible to carve out time from her busy day to do things that were important to *her*. In the following week, she applied the same strategy to practicing vocal exercises for 15 minutes per day. She began to make progress more quickly, which she found very rewarding. The better her voice got, the more encouraged she felt and the more time she found she was able to devote to her recovery.

This is an example of how the singer's frustration about *life* issues was affecting her ability to make progress in voice rehabilitation. By allowing space in the rehabilitation context to express and explore this frustration, she was able to experience a breakthrough in self-care that ultimately helped her meet her voice goals.

Had she not experienced this breakthrough so quickly, or had she continued to demonstrate emotional breakdowns on a regular basis in rehabilitation sessions, it would have been important to consider referral to resources that would help her manage stress and her emotional response to her voice injury more directly, as we will discuss below.

MAKE APPROPRIATE REFERRALS WHEN NECESSARY

Sometimes the singer's emotional struggle relative to the voice problem may be encumbering recovery so much that including a mental health professional on the voice rehabilitation team is indicated. The singer may have significant problems in his or her personal life related to work, family, relationships, self-esteem, or other difficulties that are impeding the ability to make progress in voice rehabilitation and/or causing general malaise. Knowing when the problem is beyond your scope of practice and when to refer to another professional is essential. At times, the line can be blurry. It is often best to err on the side of caution by gently introducing the possibility of seeking additional care. You might say something like, "Sometimes it can be really helpful to have someone to talk to during a difficult time. Can I help you find resources?" It doesn't have to be presented as a "mental health problem" but can be framed as a means of achieving support and assistance during challenging times.

You will be best equipped to help the singer if you educate yourself regarding local mental health resources and professionals. You may query local or national professional organizations such as the American Psychological Association (http://www.apa.org/) to locate mental health professionals who specialize in treating performers. This may include psychiatrists, psychologists, and/or social workers (Davis, 2004). Some singers may find it particularly helpful to include trusted clergy or religious leaders as part of their mental health team. Stress reduction programs may be beneficial as well, such as Mindfulness-Based Stress Reduction (Edman, Kondrad, & Rakel, 2011).

It is important to realize that some medications—many of which are commonly prescribed or recommended by otolaryngologists—can have significant psychiatric side effects (Levy, Abaza, Hawkshaw, & Sataloff, 2001). Although the singing voice rehabilitation specialist should never make recommendations to singers regarding changing medications, he or she can recommend that the singer have a discussion with the prescribing doctor about medications. Being well-informed about how medications may be affecting any aspect of the singer's recovery is an important part of advocating for and supporting singers' health.

CREATING A SAFE ENVIRONMENT FOR HEALING

Once the rehabilitation process is under way, there are further considerations for the singer's emotional needs that should guide you in structuring the rehabilitation sessions and in interacting with the singer.

The singer will likely be in an emotionally fragile state and may be reactive to vocal symptoms such as loss of pitch and dynamic range, strain or pain when singing, loss of vocal stamina, and—often most disturbing—compromised vocal quality. As a result, the singer may feel very nervous and self-conscious about singing or even speaking in front of you. He or she may feel "in the spotlight" and may expect criticism and a negative reaction from you. It is vital that the singer immediately feels that he or she is ensconced in an environment that is safe, nonjudgmental, supportive, and encouraging. As we discussed in Chapter 6, creating such an environment depends largely on the language you use in rehabilitation sessions and the manner in which you interact with the singer. You convey feedback not only verbally but also by facial expression and body language, and you must be mindful at all times of what you are communicating via all of these pathways.

You can help this process by immediately establishing that the singer is a partner in rehabilitation: that rehabilitation is something you will *do* together versus something that will *happen to* him or her. One of the ways in which I try to achieve this is by minimizing the medical atmosphere as much as possible. For example, although I wear the usual clinical white lab coat when collaborating with my physician colleagues during evaluations, I take it off for therapy sessions in an attempt to remove a layer of clinical distance between myself and my singer patients.

We will revisit strategies for addressing the singer's emotional needs and creating a supportive rehabilitation environment throughout the book, as well as supporting the singer in the return to performing.

REFERENCES

Behrman, A. (2006). Facilitating behavioral change in voice therapy: The relevance of motivational interviewing. *American Journal of Speech Language Pathology, 15*(3), 215–225.

Davis, J. (2004). How to find a therapist. *WebMD .com*. Retrieved April 4, 2014, from http://www.webmd.com/anxiety-panic/guide/how-to-find-therapist

Edman, J., Kondrad, L. & Rakel, B. (2011). The use of nutrition and integrative medicine or complementary and alternative medicine (CAM) for singers, Part 1. *Journal of Singing, 68*(2), 165–173.

Elias, M., Sataloff, R. T., Rosen, D. C., Heuer, R. J., & Spiegel, J. R. (1997). Normal strobovideolaryngoscopy: Variability in healthy singers. *Journal of Voice, 11*(1), 104–107.

Eustis, L. (2005). *The singer's ego*. Chicago, IL: GIA.

Gillespie, A. I., & Abbott, K. V. (2010). The influence of clinical terminology on self-efficacy for voice. *Logopedics Phoniatrics Vocology, 35*(3), 91–99.

Heman-Ackah, Y., Dean, C., & Sataloff, R. T. (2002). Strobovideolaryngoscopy: Findings in singing teachers. *Journal of Voice, 16*(1), 81–86.

Levy, S., Abaza, M., Hawkshaw, M., & Sataloff, R. (2001). Common otolaryngologic medications: Psychiatric side effects. *Journal of Singing, 57*(5), 35–40.

Lundy, D. S., Casiano, R. R., Sullivan, M. S., Roy, S., Xue, J. W., & Evans, M. M. (1999). Incidence of abnormal laryngeal findings in asymptomatic singing students. *Otolaryngology–Head and Neck Surgery, 121*(1), 69–77.

Radionoff, S. (2004). Preparing the singing voice specialist revisited. *Journal of Voice, 18*, 513–521.

Rosen, D. C., & Sataloff, R. T. (1997). *Psychological aspects of voice disorders*. San Diego, CA: Singular.

Sataloff, R. T., & Hawkshaw, M. J. (2013). Singers: What is normal? *Journal of Singing, 69*(3), 301–303.

Verdolini, K. (1999). Critical analysis of common terminology in voice therapy: A position paper. *Phonoscope, 2*(1), 1–8.

PART III

Vocal Coordination and Conditioning

CHAPTER 9

Shaping Voice

As noted in Chapter 1, shaping voice is perhaps the most important critical skill for the singing voice rehabilitation specialist and forms the foundation of the vocal coordination and conditioning component of singing voice rehabilitation. The process of shaping voice is highly interactive. As you listen to the singer, you should be able to analyze the sound he or she is producing and rapidly assess whether or not vocal production is safe, healthy, and efficient and whether it results in a vocal quality that is desirable and appropriate for the singer's chosen style. If the singer is not meeting the target (whether due to injury or function), you must be able to quickly determine where the problem lies, why it is occurring, and how you will collaborate with the singer to lead him or her to adapt and adjust various aspects of coordination in a way that positively impacts the output and incrementally moves the singer toward the sound ideal. You will do this by using various forms of feedback, education, instruction, demonstration, or modeling, all while constantly assessing which methods are best suited to the particular singer you are working with and adjusting your interactions accordingly.

Shaping voice will require you to bring all your artistic skill and scientific knowledge to bear. By now, your studies should have prepared you to be thoroughly conversant with principles of the anatomy, physiology, and acoustics of singing. An in-depth exposition of pedagogic skills relative to the mechanics of singing for respiration, phonation, resonance, and alignment necessary for effective shaping of voice is beyond the scope of this text. If your knowledge and understanding of these topics is at all shaky, or if you are not well acquainted with the concepts presented here, I strongly recommend that you go back to the basics so that you are well prepared for the task of shaping voice and designing an exercise regimen. This is of utmost importance when working with singers who have a voice injury or disorder.

WHAT IS SHAPING VOICE?

The conditioning paradigm of "shaping" was first introduced by B. F. Skinner. The underlying principle of shaping is to reinforce successive approximations of a desired behavior until the target behavior has been achieved. Although initially utilized in scientific experimentation with animals using rewards such as food for reinforcement, shaping can be applied to virtually any training paradigm. In the case of singing voice rehabilitation, what is being shaped is subtle change in movement, position, coordination, sensation, awareness, or thought processes resulting in changes to vocal sound through optimizing the function of individual subsystems of voicing and their interaction. The reinforcement is often the improved singing experience itself. The singer may observe that the voice sounds better or may perceive improvement via kinesthetic feedback such as greater ease of phonation or absence of pain or discomfort during phonation. This favorable experience can in and of itself serve as an incentive to repeat the behavior that led to the change. In order to grasp how the singer gradually acquires and perfects new skills, it is necessary to understand the basics of motor learning.

MOTOR LEARNING

Schmidt and Lee (2014) define motor learning as "a set of processes associated with practice or experience leading to relatively permanent gains in the capability for skilled performance." They also point out that learning is inferred rather than directly observed: We infer that learning has taken place based on the improvement in performance that we observe (Schmidt & Lee, 2010).

Motor learning is distinguished from *motor performance*, which is how well the learner succeeds on any given attempt at execution of a learned task. For example, a singer may have diligently learned, practiced, and prepared a song and sung it perfectly multiple times in the practice room or studio. However, when it is time for this particular singer to perform the song in front of an audience—say for an end-of-semester graded jury or important professional audition—he or she does not sing nearly as well. The motor learning may indeed have occurred, but the motor performance was thrown off by circumstances that undermined the execution of that specific attempt. Motor performance can be affected by a number of internal or external factors (room acoustics, distraction, fatigue, anxiety, etc.) and does not necessarily reveal whether or not motor learning has taken place.

Motor learning has three stages: the verbal/cognitive stage, the motor learning stage, and the automatic stage (Schmidt & Wrisbreg, 2008), also referred to as the cognitive, associative, and autonomous stages (Fitts & Posner, 1967). Relative to singing voice rehabilitation, the *verbal/cognitive stage* is when the singer is "getting the hang of" a new skill. During this stage, the singer has to devote significant attention to executing the task, the error rate is high, and the singer is highly reliant on extrinsic feedback (e.g., your cueing and instruction) to ascertain whether he or she is on the right track. This is the stage during which you will see and reinforce successive approximations the most, as the skill will be fairly error prone and perfection is not expected. During the *motor learning stage*, the skill has basically been learned, and the singer is refining the movement pattern. At this stage, the singer will demonstrate increased independence in self-assessment and self-correction and will be less reliant on your cues and feedback. Keep in mind that this stage can go on for years—well beyond the span of the rehabilitation process. Even though the learner becomes quite proficient in this stage, tiny adjustments can still take place that make the execution more and more accurate and reliable. In the *automatic stage*, the singer is able to execute the task with very little active processing. The movement has become fast and automatic.

Motor learning of *inefficient* patterns is very common and may be at the automatic stage by the time you begin to work with the singer. An example is maladaptive muscle tension (in the neck, jaw, tongue, etc.) that develops as a compensation for an underlying injury or loss of function. In such cases, the inefficient pattern will have to be unlearned and replaced with more efficient patterns. This can take time, and it is important to let the singer know that the voice may fluctuate a lot during this process until the new patterning is solidified.

Demonstration and Modeling

Learning through demonstration and modeling is an example of observational learning, in which the learner gains information by watching (or, in the case of singing, watching and listening to) another. According to Schmidt and Lee (2014), this can be a powerful and beneficial tool but must be utilized in combination with appropriate feedback and cueing. Overreliance on modeling can undermine long-term learning.

Feedback and Cueing

Feedback is information the learner receives about a specific execution and outcome of a task. Feedback is generally considered to be related to information the learner receives during or after the movement and may be motivational, informational, or attention focusing (Schmidt & Lee, 2014). Feedback may or may not include information about errors for the learner to apply to subsequent attempts to make them more successful (Schmidt & Lee, 2014).

Intrinsic Feedback

Intrinsic feedback arises as a natural consequence of executing the task and is available to learners through information they can observe and perceive directly. For singers, this might include how the voice sounds, the sensations they experience in the body while singing, perception of relative ease or effort, or kinesthetic awareness of body position and movements. Intrinsic feedback may also be a function of tactile information such as vibration or body movement (e.g., putting the hands on the face to feel for vibration or on the abdomen to feel for respiratory movement). Visual information such as observation of body position or watching movements in the mirror are also forms of intrinsic feedback.

Extrinsic Feedback

Extrinsic (or augmented) feedback is information that is fed to the learner from an outside source (such as an instructor) and is a feedback layer that occurs over and above the intrinsic feedback the learner is already receiving (Schmidt & Lee, 2014). Extrinsic feedback is a supplement to intrinsic feedback, and the frequency and nature of this augmented feedback is under the control of the instructor. In the case of singing voice rehabilitation, extrinsic feedback is the verbal or nonverbal information you provide to let the singer know how he or she is doing. Acoustic feedback using spectrograms and/or power spectra or physiologic feedback using equipment such as electroglottography to monitor phase closure can also be useful for some singers (Miller, 2008). Miller's Voce Vista is a program that provides this type of feedback with minimal equipment requirements.

The feedback or cueing you provide to the singer may fall into two categories: knowledge of performance (KP) or knowledge of results (KR) (Schmidt & Lee, 2014). Knowledge of performance tells the learner something about kinematics (e.g., "I saw your abdomen expand when you inhaled just then" or "your lips were rounded rather than retracted there"). Knowledge of results (KR) tells the learner how successful the execution was relative to an environmental goal (e.g., "you sang the wrong note" or "you missed the entrance"). Receiving a score on a performance (such as a test) is also a form of KR feedback. KR tells the singer how close he or she came to the target but provides no qualitative feedback. According to LeBorgne and Rosenberg (2014), KR is only helpful if the singer has a reference for what the target is. Both forms of feedback can be beneficial, but what is most important for learning to take place is the precision of the feedback: how accurately the feedback you provide describes the outcome (Schmidt & Lee, 2014).

When we are speaking or singing, we hear our own voices both through external air and bone conduction (from the outside) but also through internal bone conduction (from the inside). For this reason, our voices sound different to ourselves than to others. We cannot hear our instruments accurately in the same way that guitar or flute players can hear theirs. This phenomenon can make the singer more dependent on sensation than sound for intrinsic feedback, and he or she may need extrinsic feedback from the instructor to develop sensory references to support the intrinsic aural feedback that promotes accurate self-assessment. Recording oneself singing is also a helpful way to facilitate development of reference sensations associated with particular vocal sounds or productions.

Effects of Feedback on Learning and Performance

Research indicates that attention to the outcome of a task is more beneficial in learning than attention to the mechanics of a task (LeBorgne & Rosenberg, 2014; Titze & Verdolini Abbott, 2012), and executing and experiencing movements is more powerful for learning than verbal instruction on mechanics (Wulf & Weigelt, 1997; Yiu, Verdolini, & Chow, 2005). When working with singers, questions such as "How did that feel?" or "How did that sound?" may promote learning better than "What did you do?" Singers certainly can benefit from learning about the anatomy, physiology, and acoustics of singing. However, although this declarative knowledge can support motor learning, it does not necessarily translate into developing the procedural knowledge specifically required for motor learning to take place.

In my experience, some singers (especially those who are highly analytical) do benefit from feedback regarding the mechanics of singing. I suspect that in these cases, the singer is using the mechanical information as an added layer of interpretation within their intrinsic sensory feedback. However, it is important for the singer to avoid becoming tied up in knots by thinking about the movements rather than doing them.

Interestingly, a 1990 study by Winstein and Schmidt found that trials without feedback can also produce learning, suggesting that it may be beneficial to sometimes just let the singer experiment, which I have certainly found to be true.

Although external focus is thought to have more long-term benefit to learning than focus on coordination, attention to coordination may be beneficial in the early stages of learning. When this is the case, it is better to encourage the learner to think about coordination before or after, but not during execution of a task (Singer, 1985). In fact, it has been established that, in general, feedback that occurs concurrently with task performance undermines learning (Schmidt & Wulf, 1997). Providing feedback at the same time that the singer is singing may appear to be immediately helpful, but it can impede learning in the long term because it fosters dependence and hampers carryover (plus it requires the singer to focus on what you're saying rather than processing the experience). It is better to wait until the singer finishes before providing verbal feedback. Briefly delaying the feedback can afford the singer added time to more fully process the sensory experience.

Physical guidance (for example, manually guiding the singer's body position) tends to be helpful in the short term but will likely not generalize (Schmidt & Lee, 2014). This doesn't mean you should never use this technique, only that it should be used judiciously, and you should move as quickly as possible to focusing on the outcome ("How does that alignment feel?").

Fading feedback as soon as possible is beneficial to learning. For this reason, it will be best to provide more frequent feedback in the early stages and gradually reduce the frequency as the skill develops to prevent dependency (Winstein & Schmidt, 1990). Switching from extrinsic to intrinsic feedback as soon as possible also fosters independence. This is the mechanism through which accurate self-assessment increases, which will make home practice more successful.

Titze and Verdolini Abbott (2012) suggest that the mental imagery that has long been a mainstay of teaching voice may actually undermine learning by favoring declarative rather than motor learning. On the other hand, use of imagery may provide a beneficial external focus for the singer that prevents undesirable over-analysis of singing mechanics.

Summary of Feedback and Singing Voice Rehabilitation

- In the early stage of learning (verbal/cognitive), modeling, cueing, and extrinsic feedback can facilitate fast acquisition of skill and promote sensory reference.
- Allow time for self-assessment and processing on the part of the singer before providing information. Avoid giving feedback while the singer is singing.
- Focus on outcome more than on mechanics when providing feedback.
- Feedback that is either too frequent or too infrequent can hinder learning. Provide adequate feedback to support learning, but fade frequency of feedback as soon as possible.
- Consider allowing the singer to experiment and experience for a time without providing extrinsic feedback.

- Move the singer to independence in self-assessment and reliance on intrinsic feedback quickly for successful home practice and automaticity. Record the singer (audio and/or video) and use playback of the recording to develop shared references and increase accuracy of intrinsic aural and sensory feedback.

Practice and Learning

In the singing voice rehabilitation session, you will be illustrating to the singer how to practice. Blocked practice (performing the same task multiple times) helps the learner to quickly acquire a sensory reference. This type of practice can be beneficial when first learning a task. For example, working on respiratory coordination in isolation before trying to coordinate respiration with phonation and resonance. In random practice, the learner practices multiple skills at the same time (e.g., resonance, breath support, register transition all in the same task). Random practice usually results in increased short-term errors but is beneficial for long-term learning (Shea & Morgan, 1979).

I have found that negative practice —that is, deliberately executing a task with the undesirable coordination pattern—can be beneficial, if used judiciously. This technique helps to establish a reference sensation for the behavior one wants to "undo," which can help the singer to realize when he or she is slipping into an old pattern.

For in-depth information on motor learning, see Schmidt and Lee (2010, 2014) and Schmidt and Wrisberg (2008). For application of motor learning to the teaching of singing, see LeBorgne and Rosenberg (2014, Chap. 16).

VOCAL COORDINATION AND CONDITIONING: INTERACTION OF SYSTEMS

The application of motor learning in shaping voice will certainly involve optimizing mechanical coordination of the voicing subsystems (respiration, phonation, resonance) but also optimizing the interaction of these systems with each other and with the entire body. This necessitates a thorough understanding of the principles of voice *habilitation* relative to the mechanics and acoustics of singing. As I have already stated, a prerequisite for applying the information provided in this book is that you already possess this understanding and that you are experienced in using it relative to voice habilitation. Therefore, our discussion here will be limited to a few key features of the interaction of these subsystems that are especially important in shaping voice for singing voice rehabilitation.

Interaction of Respiration and Phonation

Vocal fold vibration is powered by air from the lungs in accordance with Bernoulli's law. The activation of the muscles of respiration—both inspiratory and expiratory—is responsible for controlling pulmonary pressures. The vocal folds in turn aid in pacing the elastic recoil pressure of the expanded lungs so that phonation can be sustained for extended periods of time. If the air is released passively, phonation will become weaker as lung volume decreases. To sustain phonation consistently, the singer must deliberately mete out the airflow through coordination of respiratory action (antagonistic activation of the muscles of inspiration and expiration) using the glottal valve to slow down the release of the air, resulting in what is referred to as "appoggio" or "leaning against the breath." Thus, *appoggio* describes the interaction of vocal fold valving and respiration. Adducting vocal folds too firmly and activating lung pressure at a high level will result in a long closed phase of vibration, "clapping" motion of the vocal folds, strong mechanical stress on the vocal folds, and pressed vocal quality. Conversely, if the vocal folds are not adequately adducted, there will be inadequate resistance to the airflow. Vocal quality will be breathy, and the lungs will be emptied relatively quickly, shortening the duration of phonation the singer is able to sustain. Thus, the singer must exactly balance the interaction of pulmonary forces with glottal valving. This interaction is further influenced "up the phonatory chain" by the interaction of vocal fold vibration with the vocal tract. If the singer can optimize vocal fold vibration with the aid of the vocal tract, the vocal folds will more efficiently valve the airflow, facilitating breath support. We will explore how this favorable interaction of vocal fold vibration and the vocal tract can be accomplished in the next section.

Changing the length and stiffness of the vocal folds through the interaction of the thyroarytenoid and cricothyroid muscles not only influences frequency of vibration (varying the pitch) but also impacts the interaction of airflow and glottal valving by varying the manner in which vocal fold tension is achieved. When the vocal folds are stretched longer and thinner, the strategy for maintaining vocal fold tension must change to maintain resistance to the airflow. At relatively low pitches, vocal fold tension is controlled by the thyroarytenoid muscle. As pitch increases, the vocal ligament plays a greater role in maintaining vocal fold tension (Titze, 2000; Titze & Verdolini Abbott, 2012).

Epigastric Movement in Singing

The epigastric region (located between the xiphoid process and the lower border of the ribs) is part of the area that expands on inhalation during abdominal breathing. When both the diaphragm and rectus abdominus muscles are contracted on exhalation, outward bulging of the upper abdominal wall in the epigastric area is produced. This action occurs naturally during laughing and coughing and can facilitate strong adduction of the vocal folds. Although constant activation of this gesture would likely produce excessive subglottic pressure and forceful collision of the vocal folds, used gently and judiciously, it may facilitate the strong thyroarytenoid (TA) activation needed for loud singing in general, for belting, and also for "safe" yelling. The gesture can be elicited by having the singer explore abdominal movements in the epigastric region while producing phonemes such as /k, t, p, ʃ, tʃ/. The engagement of the epigastric area should be palpable but not clenched or tight. Lisa Popeil (1996) refers to this gesture as using "the magic spot" and endorses it as a component of her pedagogy of belting.

Onsets

The onset of phonation is determined by the manner in which the closure of the vocal folds interacts with breath acceleration. This can be accomplished in a number of different ways. In a glottal onset, vocal fold closure is initiated prior to breath flow, subglottic pressure builds to a high level, and the vocal folds "pop" open. Although chronic or consistent use of this manner of onset has vocal health implications associated with the ensuing forceful collision of the vocal folds, glottal onset is not universally "bad" (in fact, the glottal stroke is phonemic in languages such as German and Hawaiian). The glottal onset can also be useful for expressive purposes.

If breath flow is initiated prior to vocal fold adduction, the result is an aspirate onset, which has a slightly breathy quality. This can be elicited by releasing the breath on /h/ prior to phonation.

Either type of onset can be used as a correction for excessive use of the other. Much of the time, the objective is to strike a balance somewhere in between the extremes, but potentially any of these onsets can be functional in singing, depending largely on style and expressive objective.

Interaction of Vocal Fold Vibration and the Vocal Tract

The vocal tract is the tube (or series of tubes) formed by the structures between the vocal folds and the point where the sound leaves the body (lips or nose). The vocal tract thus encompasses the epilarynx (the area immediately superior to the vocal folds, including the ventricle and laryngeal vestibule), the pharynx, the mouth, and (if the velopharyngeal port is open) the nose. The movements of these structures, along with the articulators (velum, tongue, lips, jaw), change the configuration of the series of tubes.

Formants

The resonating frequencies of the vocal tract are called formants, and they change depending on the vocal tract's configuration. The vocal tract has many formants, but for purposes of singing, we are primarily interested in the first five. The frequencies of the first and second formants (F1 and F2) determine what the vowel is. Formants 3 to 5 form the singer's formant cluster (more on that in the next chapter).

In singing, the vowel can be modified quite a bit before there is an external perception that the vowel has changed. See Table 9–1 for a summary of how F1 and F2 can be manipulated to modify the vowel.

The degree to which the vowel is closed or open influences F1. Closed vowels have a lower F1, while open vowels have a higher F1. F2 is higher for front vowels and lower for back vowels (Figure 9–1).

The way in which we modify vowels (i.e., by movement of the lips, tongue, and adjustments in laryngeal height) either enhances or inhibits the sound. This tweaking of vowel color associated with adjustments in F1 and F2 (sometimes referred to as "formant tuning" or "vowel tuning") is a big part of how singers can learn to optimize resonance.

Vocal Tract Inertance

If the vocal folds and vocal tract have comparable impedance, they can interact in such a way that each facilitates the function of the other. Thus, their interaction is nonlinear. See Titze (2000) and Titze and Verdolini Abbott (2012) for in-depth descriptions of the complex phenomenon of vocal production relative to impedance, reactance, inertance, and compliance. To summarize, impedance is a lack of

Table 9–1. *F1 and F2 are Adjusted by Degree of Lip Rounding, Larynx Height, and Tongue Position (Miller, 2008)*

Degree of lip rounding	Increasing lip rounding lowers all formant frequencies, but especially F2 Lip retraction raises all formant frequencies
Laryngeal height	Lower larynx results in lower formant frequencies, but especially F1 Raising the larynx raises formant frequencies
Tongue position	Moving the tongue constriction forward raises F2 and lowers F1 Moving tongue constriction backward lowers F2 and raises F1

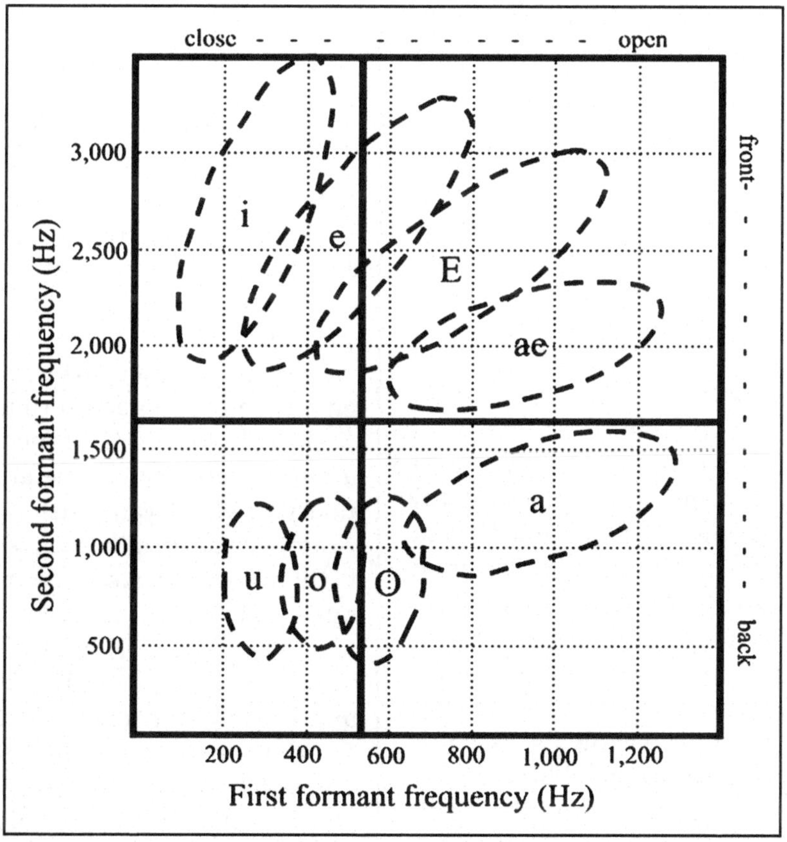

Figure 9–1. *Vowel chart illustrating 1st and 2nd formant ranges (F1 and F2) for various vowels. Reproduced with permission from Inside View Press. Miller, D. (2008).* Resonance in Singing. *Princeton, NJ: Inside View Press.*

response to a stimulus. In the vocal tract, impedance is the ratio of the oscillatory acoustic pressure and the oscillatory airflow of the column of air at the entrance to the vocal tract (glottis). Reactive impedance refers to the timing of the response. In inertive reactance, flow and pressure are out of phase, with flow being delayed relative to pressure (pressure peaks before flow). In compliant reactance, flow and pressure are also out of phase but with an advance response, so that flow peaks before pressure. Inertive reactance of the vocal tract helps the vocal folds vibrate more easily. The result is known as resonant voice. Compliant reactance actually makes it more difficult for the vocal folds to vibrate and undermines resonant voice (Titze & Verdolini Abbott, 2012).

Obviously, vocal tract inertance is desirable to optimize vocal production. When vocal tract inertance is achieved, formant frequencies of the vocal tract can boost the fundamental frequency and harmonics generated by the vocal folds, resulting in increased acoustic output with minimal effort. The ways in which vocal tract inertance can be altered include modifying the length of the vocal tract, modifying the shape of the vocal tract, and narrowing the epilaryngeal tube. The length of the vocal tract can be altered by changing laryngeal height and the relative positions of the jaw, lips, and tongue. The shape of the vocal tract can be altered by lip position and degree of pharyngeal widening or narrowing. According to Titze and Verdolini Abbott (2012), narrowing of the epilaryngeal tube is primarily accomplished indirectly through adjustments the singer makes to perceptually achieve a "ringing" quality. Use of "twang" resonance is one way to narrow the epilarynx tube and pharynx, characteristic of belting (Sundberg & Thalen, 2010). Semi-occluded vocal tract sounds (lip/tongue/labio-lingual trills, straw phonation, nasal consonants, etc.) also facilitate vocal tract inertance. This is particularly true for phonation with a small-diameter straw (Titze & Laukkanen, 2007). We will explore this further in Chapter 11.

The exact nature of the modifications of the vocal tract vary depending on the resonance strategy for a particular vocal sound. There are significant ways in which the strategies differ for classical singing and belting, which we discuss in the next chapter.

"Twang"

Although sometimes referred to as a "nasal" quality, twang may or may not actually feature nasal air emission. Klimek (2013) describes twang as a bright, piercing sound that has the quality of a cackling witch or schoolyard "nyae nyae" taunt. Acoustically, twang is characterized by strong energy in the singer's formant cluster (2–4 kHz). Twang resonance results in a narrow epilarynx tube and narrow pharynx, which can assist in raising F1 to achieve the bright, brassy quality of belting without excessive mechanical stress on the vocal folds (Sundberg & Thalen, 2010). Klimek (2013) provides a tutorial on eliciting twang and applications for voice rehabilitation. In addition to the school yard taunt and witch's cackle, she suggests using "baaah" (like a sheep), "neigh" (like a horse), "MBeep-beep" (as in the cartoon Road-Runner), or the "nyuk-nyuk-nyuk" of the Three Stooges as references for twang quality.

Registers: Interaction of Airflow, Glottal Configuration, and Vocal Tract

The topic of registers can be a thorny one, in part due to terminology and conceptions that emerged centuries ago in classical singing that have persisted into the modern age of voice science. The topic is further complicated by differences in how register terminology is used in speech-language pathology and singing. Furthermore, the degree to which registers are understood and the manner in which they are described and labeled within the realm of voice performance and pedagogy vary greatly, which can make it even more challenging to grasp what vocal registers are really all about.

Registers may be conceptualized as perceptually distinct segments of the span of vocal range. In speech pathology, these distinct segments are referred to as *pulse* (or fry), *modal* (or speech register), and *loft* (or falsetto). In singing, the segments are broadly labeled *chest voice* or *head voice*. These two registers may be combined or *mixed* in various ways. Singing language relative to this concept of mixing may include *chest mix, head mix,* or *upper extension*. In classical singing, a transition between registers is referred to as a *passaggio* (meaning "bridge"), and the singer may use "covering" to achieve smooth navigation of transitions, sometimes referred to as *turning over*.

Comprehensive overview of the historical use of register terminology and associated definitions is beyond the scope and intention of this book. Instead, we will briefly explore the physiologic and acoustical underpinnings of what is currently understood about registers.

Physiology of Registers

If we move away from traditional singing language for a moment, we can conceive vocal registers as being a function of vocal fold adduction, phase closure, lung pressure, and source-filter interaction.

The TA and cricothyroid (CT) muscles are the key players in controlling vocal fold adduction. When TA is predominantly activated, the vocal folds become shorter and fatter. The vertical dimension of the vocal folds is thick and relatively squared up. If TA adduction is decreased and CT is allowed to become more active, the vocal folds become longer and thinner, the vertical dimension becomes thinner, and there is less contact between the vocal fold edges (McCoy, 2004 and 2014; Titze, 2000). The degree of adduction influences phase closure, with greater adduction resulting in a longer closed phase, and decreased adduction a shorter closed phase. The TA-dominant/thicker edge/long closed-phase configuration is characteristic of what has traditionally been called "chest voice." The CT-dominant/thinner edge/short closed-phase configuration is associated with falsetto. "Mixing" involves gradually increasing or decreasing TA and CT interaction so that the degree of adduction and phase closure falls somewhere between the extremes (McCoy, 2014).

The strategy for controlling vocal fold tension varies depending on register. When TA is used to control vocal fold tension, the vocal fold cover is relatively lax and the body of the vocal fold is fully involved in vocal fold vibration. As CT activation increases, the vocal folds are stretched and stiffened, the vocal ligament takes over control of tension, and the epithelium and superficial lamina propria are lax (Titze & Verdolini Abbott, 2012). Thus, the smoothness or abruptness of a register change results in part from the degree to which TA and ligament alternate to bear the tension (Titze & Verdolini Abbott, 2012). Yodeling is an example of a highly controlled, abrupt alternation of tension control between TA and vocal ligament. In other forms of singing, the "passing off" of tension control and intrinsic laryngeal muscle activation occurs in a more gradual manner.

The way in which vocal fold tension and degree of adduction interact with lung pressure is also part of determining register, with greater adduction being associated with higher lung pressure and vice versa. Air pressure changes can destabilize register. This interaction is illustrated in *messa di voce,* in which the singer spans the full dynamic range in a crescendo and decrescendo on a single note. To achieve a consistent tone quality and avoid abrupt register changes or phonation breaks, the singer must slightly abduct during the crescendo and slightly adduct during the decrescendo (Titze & Verdolini Abbott, 2012).

The interaction of source-filter also influences register. If the singer does not achieve a favorable interaction between the fundamental frequency and harmonics (source phenomena) and the resonating frequencies of the vocal tract, register can become destabilized (Titze & Worley, 2009). In fact, register "breaks" often result from a failure to optimize this interaction. For example, the resonance strategy for belting is to use the first formant to reinforce the second harmonic (more on this resonance strategy in the next chapter). This means that as the fundamental increases, F1 must increase with it. If the singer doesn't modify the vocal tract to raise F1, the voice may suddenly "flip" into head or falsetto register.

Vocal fry or pulse register is characterized by low pitch (below 70 Hz), brief interruptions in acoustic energy within a vibration cycle, low to moderate TA activation, and vocal folds that are short and very lax (Titze & Verdolini Abbott, 2012). *Creaky voice* has a similar adduction to vocal fry but is characterized by an irregular vibration pattern and can be accomplished on any pitch. The highest of all registers is called whistle or flageolet. This is the kind of extremely high-pitched sound often associated with female singers like Mariah Carey. In whistle register, the vocal folds are extremely stretched and thin and do not make contact, although they continue to oscillate (McCoy, 2004). Titze (2000) speculates that whistle register may be created with air turbulence in the glottis in the absence of significant vocal fold vibration.

For detailed explanation of mechanics of vocal registers, see Titze (2000); relative to formant tuning, see Titze and Verdolini Abbott (2012), Miller (2008), and McCoy (2004, 2014). For strategies on teaching registers, particularly mixing and the difference between classical and belt singing, see Edwards (2014, Chap. 4).

Body Alignment

The larynx is freely suspended in the neck by the extrinsic laryngeal muscles and other connective tissue—it does not articulate with the skeleton. This is what allows the mobility necessary for swallowing, breathing, and phonation. The alignment of the body can tremendously influence vocal health and function. The subsystems of voicing—respiration, phonation, and resonance—interact with each other but also function in relation to the alignment of the body. For example, if the rib cage is collapsed in a "slouching" posture, the ribs will not be able to fully expand and the abdomen will be limited in its excursion, making it nearly impossible to achieve optimal coordination of respiration to support phonation. Relative positioning of the entire body—from the toes to the crown of the head—can be manipulated to enhance or hinder phonation. Optimizing this positioning can be an important component of singing voice rehabilitation.

Voice teachers sometimes endorse a "military" posture, with the chest held high and shoulder blades squeezed together. This is similar to "plumb line" posture, in which one stands in such a way that an imaginary line could be drawn "from the top of the head, through the external meatus of the ear, the acromion of the shoulder, the highest point of the pelvis, and the front of the ankle" (Gilman, 2014, p. 17). Gilman reports that the historical basis for this recommendation was in fact to achieve optimal alignment for carrying military equipment, a task not typically required in singing. Fortunately, there are abundant resources for achieving alignment that is much more favorable for singing. Among those are the Alexander Technique and the Feldenkrais Method. Both focus on postural efficiency, stability, and coordination and have a basis in the principles of motor learning previously discussed. Training in techniques such as these can be enormously beneficial in voice habilitation and rehabilitation. To learn more about these techniques, see www.alexandertechnique.com and http://www.feldenkrais.com. For further information on alignment and voice, see Schneider, Dennehy, and Saxon (1997). For detailed strategies and exercises to optimize physical alignment for singing, see Gilman (2014).

In the following chapters, we explore the ways in which principles of motor learning and the interaction of phonation subsystems have a direct application for optimizing vocal coordination and conditioning in singing voice rehabilitation.

REFERENCES

Edwards, M. (2014). *So you want to sing rock 'n' roll.* Lanham, MD: Rowman & Littlefield.

Fitts, P. M., & Posner, M. I. (1967). *Human performance.* Belmont, CA: Brooks/Cole.

Gilman, M. (2014). *Body and voice: Somatic re-education.* San Diego, CA: Plural

Klimek, M. M. (2013). Using twang. In A. Behrman & J. Haskell (Eds.), *Exercises for voice therapy* (2nd ed.). San Diego, CA: Plural.

LeBorgne, W. D., & Rosenberg, M. (2014). *The vocal athlete.* San Diego, CA: Plural.

Miller, D. G. (2008). *Resonance in singing.* Princeton, NJ: Inside View Press.

McCoy, S. (2004). *Your voice: An inside view.* Princeton, NJ: Inside View Press.

McCoy, S. (2014). Singing music theatre and voice science. In M. Edwards (Ed.), *So you want to sing rock 'n' roll* (pp. 41–52). Lanham, MD: Rowman & Littlefield.

Popeil, L. (1996). *The total singer* (DVD). Los Angeles, CA: Voiceworks Method.

Schmidt, R. A., & Lee, T. D. (2010). *Motor control and learning: A behavioral emphasis* (5th ed.). Champaign, IL: Human Kinetics.

Schmidt, R. A., & Lee, T. D. (2014). *Motor learning and performance: From principles to application* (5th ed.). Champaign, IL: Human Kinetics.

Schmidt, R., & Wrisbreg, C. (2008). *Motor learning and performance: A situation-based learning approach* (4th ed.). Champaign, IL: Human Kinetics.

Schmidt, R. A., & Wulf, G. (1997). Continuous concurrent feedback degrades skill learning: Implication for training and simulation. *Human Factors: The Journal of the Human Factors and Ergonomics Society, 39*(4), 509–525.

Schneider, C., Dennehy, C. A., & Saxon, K. G. (1997). Exercise physiology principles applied to vocal performance: The improvement of postural alignment. *Journal of Voice, 11*(3), 332–337.

Shea, J. B., & Morgan, R. L. (1979). Contextual interference effects on the acquisition, retention and transfer of a motor skill. *Journal of Experimental Psychology: Human Learning and Memory, 5*, 179–187.

Singer, R. N. (1985). Sport performance: A five-step mental approach. *Journal of Physical Education and Recreation, 57*, 82–84.

Sundberg, J., & Thalen, M. (2010). What is twang? *Journal of Voice, 24*(6), 654–660.

Titze, I. R. (2000). *Principles of voice production* (2nd printing). Iowa City, IA: National Center for Voice and Speech.

Titze, I. R., & Laukkanen, A. M. (2007). Can vocal economy in phonation be increased with an artificially lengthened vocal tract? A computer modeling study. *Logopedics Phoniatrics Vocology, 32*, 147–156.

Titze, I. R., & Verdolini Abbott, K. (2012). *Vocology: The science and practice of voice habilitation.* Salt Lake City, UT: National Center for Voice and Speech.

Titze, I. R., & Worley, A. (2009). Modeling source-filter interaction in belting and high-pitched operatic male singing. *Journal of the Acoustical Society of America, 126*(3), 1530–1540.

Winstein, C. J., & Schmidt, R. A. (1990). Reduced frequency of knowledge of results enhances motor skill learning. *Journal of Experimental Psychology: Learning, Memory and Cognition, 16*, 677–691.

Wulf, G., & Weigelt, C. (1997). Instructions about physical principals in learning a complex motor skill: To tell or not to tell. *Research Quarterly for Exercise and Sport, 68*, 362–367.

Yiu, E., Verdolini, K., & Chow, L. (2005). Electromyographic study of motor learning for a voice production task. *Journal of Speech, Language, and Hearing Research, 48*, 1254–1268.

CHAPTER 10

Stylistic Considerations in Singing Voice Rehabilitation: Classical and Contemporary Commercial Music (CCM) Singing

Singing is the oldest music, and the styles and genres of singing in the world are myriad. In your work as a singing voice rehabilitation specialist, you will encounter a lot of them. This includes a wide range of Western singing styles, but possibly those from a diverse spectrum of world musics as well. In all likelihood, most of the singers you work with will fall into Western classical, musical theater and contemporary styles. Although you do not necessarily have to possess a deep knowledge of the minutiae of stylisms and traditions for every single genre, you will need to have a clear understanding of the underlying mechanics (at least for the most common styles) so that you can guide the singer on an appropriate technical path and design exercises that are consistent with the physiology and acoustics of the chosen style. One size definitely does not fit all when it comes to singing voice rehabilitation.

HISTORICAL CLASSICAL SINGING BIAS IN VOICE PEDAGOGY

There is unfortunately a long history of classical singing bias in Western voice pedagogy, as I witnessed in my own training. From the time I was in high school right through my master's in voice, I learned from multiple sources that "belting is bad," "belting will give you vocal nodules," and "if you can sing with classical technique, you can sing anything." These views were widely held and persisted well into the 20th century, as evidenced by a 1990 literature review and survey of "individuals whom we consider knowledgeable in this area" by Miles and Hollien, 1990, pp. 67–68). "To belt 'is to use the vocal instrument in a pathological fashion'" was among the reported comments. Fortunately, we now know that none of this is true. It is certainly possible to belt with excellent technique, making this type of singing no more dangerous than classical singing. Phyland, Oates, and Greenwood (1999) reported no difference in experience of vocal impairment, disability, or handicap between groups of opera, musical theater, and contemporary singers. Furthermore, there have been numerous studies demonstrating the physiologic and acoustic differences between classical singing and belting, which conclude that the techniques are not interchangeable and thus require distinct pedagogical approaches. A number of these studies are cited in this chapter and elsewhere in this book.

Classical singers almost universally have extensive training over a period of many years before beginning their professional singing careers. Singers in contemporary styles may have little or no training, yet may have performance schedules that are even more demanding than classical singers. Contemporary commercial music (CCM) singers often develop their technique through imitation and intuition with minimal training and with remarkable results. Just imagine what would happen if someone tried to become a professional opera singer by imitation and intuition, with no training, engaging in multiple performances per week, trying to project over an orchestra without amplification. It's hard to conceive that the singer in that scenario would *not* end up with a voice injury! Thus, risk of injury may be a function of vocal load combined with inadequate training rather than an inherent stylistic factor. In your work as a singing voice rehabilitation specialist, you can do a lot to dispel misguided beliefs about the relative "safety" of different kinds of singing.

WESTERN CLASSICAL SINGING

Western classical singing emerged centuries ago. Thus, there is a long tradition of voice pedagogy associated with this vocal style and technique. The teaching of classical singing became more systematized in the 18th and 19th centuries with the emergence of "Bel Canto" ("Beautiful Singing"). Genres of classical singing include opera, choral, concert, and art song. Although there are stylistic differences between these genres, they are fairly subtle, and vocal technique is relatively consistent throughout.

Some of the vocal characteristics associated with classical singing include a "ringing" resonance, clarity of tone and evenness of quality throughout the range, imperceptible register transitions, legato, and agility (Ekholm, Papagiannis, & Chagnon, 1998). Vocal timbre in classical singing is characterized by both "roundness and brightness" (Green, 2014). Vowels are expected to be "pure" (e.g., avoiding diphthongs or "chewing" vowels). Classical singers are expected to demonstrate a high level of dynamic control, and vibrato is used consistently (although the latter is less characteristic in some choral singing). Ornamentation in classical singing is fairly circumscribed and improvisation is minimal (at least in this day and age). Transitions between notes are expected to occur smoothly and without aspiration, and onsets are also expected to be smooth.

Physiologic and Acoustical Characteristics of Classical Singing

Western classical singing emerged long before microphones and electronic amplification, and many of the sound characteristics and technical strategies associated with classical singing developed to allow the singer to project in a large performances space with no amplification. Skillful projection is further necessitated by the fact that classical singers often perform with a range of instrumental and vocal ensembles. Thus, a single voice must be able to project over 60 to 80 instruments and chorus.

Singer's Formant Cluster

This projection is largely achieved via the singer's formant cluster (third, fourth, and fifth formants of the vocal tract), which has acoustic energy in the range of 2,500 to 3,500 Hz. Most of the orchestral sound energy is below 500 Hz. Accessing the singer's formant cluster gives the voice a "ringing" quality and enables the singer to be heard above the orchestra (Sundberg, 1977). According to Titze and Verdolini Abbott (2012), one of the ways the classical singer accesses the singer's formant cluster is by narrowing the epilarynx tube (the space just above the vocal folds, including the ventricular space and laryngeal vestibule), which is primarily accomplished indirectly through adjustments the singer makes to perceptually achieve the aforementioned "ringing" quality.

Resonator Shape

The resonator shape in classical singing is characterized by a relatively low laryngeal position, wide pharyx, and rounded lips. The wide pharynx is accomplished in part by raising the soft palate and creating a "yawning" posture. Titze and Verdolini Abbott (2012) refer to this resonator shape as an "inverted megaphone" (e.g., wide in the back and narrow in the front), which has the benefit of creating vocal tract inertance over a frequency range of 500 to 1,500 Hz (see Chapter 9 regarding vocal tract inertance). This wide inertance range enables the singer to capitalize on the interaction of source and filter such that the second, third, and fourth harmonics of the source can be reinforced by F2, while the fundamental frequency is reinforced by F1 (Titze & Verdolini Abbott, 2012). Thus, the singer has a number of options for achieving an acoustic "boost" throughout the range. Titze and Worley (2009) posit that the relatively low F1 in classical singing helps the singer move through the range smoothly without the instabilities (breaks) that occur when a harmonic passes through a formant. This explains why closed vowels (which have lower F1) are typically facilitating in classical singing, while open vowels that have a higher F1 (such as /a/) tend to present greater challenges in achieving a stable tone. Throughout the range, the singer can make adjustments in vowel color to realize optimal resonance, quality, and projection.

Registers

The classical singer is expected to have a seamless vocal quality throughout the range, with no perceptible transition. Classical singers do have to work to balance TA/CT engagement, but in a way that is consistent with the resonance strategies described above. For men, this means developing TA-dominant registration ("chest voice") into the range where the male voice naturally transitions to falsetto. For women, this often means minimizing TA-dominant registration so that head voice quality is carried into the lower range, sometimes even into the speaking range. When singing in TA dominant registration—male or female—the tone quality and timbre match the rest of the range and are decidedly not speech-like.

Breath Support

There are various pedagogical schools relative to breath support (or breath management) in classical singing, but most advocate *appoggio*, or the balanced activation of the musculature of inhalation *and* exhalation to control airflow during phonation. Classical singing often requires long phrases and very controlled release of air. Subglottic pressure is achieved by a combination of glottal adduction and abdominal compression, and there is a balance of breath pressure and breath flow.

Implications for Singing Voice Rehabilitation

Understanding the resonance strategy described above is crucial for optimizing vocal coordination and conditioning and designing appropriate rehabilitation exercises for the classical singer. For example, tongue tension may elevate the larynx, resulting in a suboptimal resonator shape that undermines source-filter interaction, increasing phonatory effort. In this case, you will need to employ strategies to unload the tongue tension and achieve a lower larynx position, such as instructing the singer to maintain the laryngeal posture that naturally occurs when yawning. As lip rounding is a critical element of the "inverted megaphone" resonator shape, vowels that have lip retraction (such as /i/) may need to be modified by rounding the lips. Vowel choices and modification should be guided by the principles outlined above.

CONTEMPORARY COMMERCIAL SINGING STYLES

Contemporary singing styles include pop, rock, jazz, blues, country, bluegrass, gospel, R&B, folk, and many more. Historically, there have been few options for vocal training in these styles and genres. Singers have learned mainly by imitation and intuition. When CCM singers do seek training, it is not unusual for them find themselves under the tutelage of a classical voice teacher who teaches them a technique that has very little to do with their style. They may come away from the experience feeling vocally confused. As we will discuss below, the physiologic and acoustic characteristics of CCM singing are in many ways opposite those of classical singing. Trying to impose classical technique onto CCM styles can result in a potentially harmful somatic "argument" between inappropriate technique and the sound ideal the singer is trying to reproduce. It's kind of like putting ballet pointe shoes on a student who wants to learn tap dancing.

Fortunately, the last several decades have yielded a surge in research and pedagogical development that has significantly increased our understanding of the difference between classical and contemporary singing styles, and pioneers in CCM pedagogy have helped us understand how to teach CCM singing. Classical voice teachers still outnumber those with expertise in teaching vocal technique for CCM singing, and academic music programs are still largely classically oriented, but the tide has turned, and all signs indicate that in the next decades, we will see increasing opportunities for training CCM singers to sing in a safe, healthy, and systematic way.

Characteristics of CCM Singing

Unlike classical singing, which has fairly circumscribed parameters for sound quality and performance practices, CCM singing features a wide range of acceptable sounds. Although there may be stylistic expectations within genres, the overall array of vocal options spans the gamut from wispy and breathy, to bright and brassy, to growling and gravelly, to shouting and screaming, and virtually anything in between. Since most CCM singers perform with amplification, the singer may employ quieter tones and still be heard, and may use the sound system to enhance desired vocal qualities. The audience expects individualized, unique characteristics that create a "vocal signature" that is distinct and recognizable.

The singer doesn't necessarily have to execute register transitions smoothly—abrupt transitions are acceptable and at times even desirable. Transitions from one note to the next can be smooth or choppy. The consistency with which vibrato is used is more variable than in classical singing. Vibrato is often used more as an ornament or expressive device. It is acceptable for the singer to breathe in the middle of a phrase or even in the middle of a word, something that would be anathema to the classical singer. Most CCM styles have a speech-like vocal quality that is distinct from classical singing. The diction is typically in the vernacular of the singer (or, at least, of the genre).

Physiologic and Acoustic Characteristics of Belting

Many CCM singing styles employ belting, which is a vocal technique characterized by bright, brassy, piercing vocal timbre, relatively high intensity, and a speech-like quality. Vibrato is minimally employed (usually at the end of the phrase). Belting can be found in rock, pop, jazz, blues, gospel, R&B, country, bluegrass, folk, and other CCM genres, as well as in musical theater singing.

Resonator Shape

Belting is characterized by a resonator shape that in many ways is opposite that of classical singing. The lips are retracted and the pharynx is somewhat narrowed, yielding a resonator that is narrow in back and wide in front. Titze and Verdolini Abbott (2012) describe this as a "megaphone" shape, in contrast to the "inverted megaphone" of classical singing. The larynx is slightly elevated (as opposed to the lowered larynx of classical singing). This resonator shape raises the first formant (F1) to about 1,000 Hz in males and 1,200 Hz in females, which is facilitated by vowels with a high F1 such as /æ/ or /a/. Keeping F1 relatively high enables the singer to use F1 to reinforce the second harmonic of the fundamental (H2). H2 approaches but does not cross F1 (Titze & Verdolini Abbott, 2012; Titze, Worley, & Story, 2011).

The effect of this strong energy in H2 is that the listener perceives most of the acoustic energy an octave above the pitch that the singer is singing. So for a female belter singing C5, we get the same thrill we do when we hear a soprano sing a high C (C6). "Twang" resonance (see Chapter 9 for review) results in a narrow epilarynx tube and narrow pharynx, which can further assist in raising F1 to achieve the bright, brassy quality of belting without excessive mechanical stress on the vocal folds (Sundberg & Thalen, 2010).

Registers

In belting, a relatively high amount of TA adduction is desirable to keep a good amount of H2 energy in the source (i.e., at the vocal folds). Thus, there is a physiologic and acoustic rationale for employing a TA-dominant register relatively high into the singing range—up to about E5 for women and C5 for men (Titze & Verdolini Abbott, 2012; Titze et al., 2011). The degree of TA activation will be adjusted depending on range (e.g., less for higher notes and more for lower notes). The register "mix" for belting typically has TA in the driver's seat, collaborating with CT for optimal balance. This doesn't mean that *chest voice* is synonymous with *belting*, though. Belting is about the whole physiologic and acoustic package: strong TA adduction *plus* H2 reinforced by F1 (Titze & Worley, 2009; Titze et al., 2011), allowing the singer to use source-filter interaction rather than laryngeal effort to achieve the desired sound. This is the key to safe and healthy belting.

Breath Support

Because of the relatively strong TA activation, which yields a long closed phase of vibration, subglottic pressure is achieved more through vocal fold adduction than with abdominal pressure. In fact, excessive abdominal compression is contraindicated, as it may increase mechanical stress on the vocal folds. The amount of abdominal compression utilized for classical singing is often too much for belting, and thus the inhalation posture may be more static during phonation in belting. For musical theater singers who are also dancers, maximal abdominal expansion is visually undesirable, and thus the thoracic component of inhalation may be utilized more than in classical singing. See Chapter 9 for discussion of epigastric gesture, which may also be facilitating in belting.

Extended Vocal Techniques

Many CCM genres employ extended vocal techniques such as deliberately breathy tone, growls, screams, squeals, shouts, and other distorted sounds. Some of these sounds are achieved with a degree of pharyngeal constriction and laryngeal compression that can potentially be phonotraumatic. However, they are key elements of certain styles of singing and the goal should be to help the singer achieve them in the safest way possible rather than trying to eliminate them. We will discuss this further below.

Registers in Extended Techniques

Lest you have the idea that CCM singing is all about TA-dominant registration, we will discuss a few examples of CT dominant register (head voice) in CCM singing. Falsetto is commonly employed in many CCM styles. This is the natural "loft" register for male voices, however, women achieve a similar quality by using very thin vocal fold edges (with a relative disengagement of TA) and long open phase of vibration, resulting in a breathy or "wispy" quality. Utilizing a CT-dominant mix, high larynx, and lip retraction with increased vocal fold adduction (and associated increased subglottic pressure), the singer can extend a bright, piercing quality beyond the range limitations of belting. This can be used to achieve a "squealing" quality characteristic of a lot of rock singing (as in the climax of Aerosmith's "Dream

On," as noted by Edwards, 2014). In the male voice, this is sometimes referred to as "reinforced falsetto."

Deliberate register "breaks" (e.g., abrupt transition from TA dominant to CT dominant as in yodeling) is also a common stylism in CCM singing.

Implications for Singing Voice Rehabilitation

Singing voice rehabilitation for CCM singers must be customized to meet the individual stylistic characteristics of the singer. Technical instruction on vocal coordination and vocal exercise design should be based on the physiologic characteristics associated with the style or genre. For example, if you are working with a belter, cuing the singer to widen the throat and lower the larynx will undermine the resonator shape and resonance strategy of belting and may result in exacerbating muscle tension and laryngeal strain. Raising the chin a bit will be helpful in elevating the larynx, a strategy that would be contraindicated for the low-larynx posture of classical singing. Vocalizing on vowels that have a low first formant frequency (such as /i/ or /u/) will limit the range in which the interaction of F1 and H2 described above is possible. High F1 vowels such as /æ/ or /a/ will be better vowel choices for belting, as noted above. See Chapters 11 and 12 for more details about designing exercises for specific singing styles.

Regarding vocal effects or distortions (growls, screams, shouts), I usually advise the singer that such sounds can be vocally "expensive" and encourage them to be judicious in employing them. What do I mean by judicious? If the sound is intended to be emotionally evocative, it will be more meaningful and effective if it is only used at the point(s) in the song that meet that criterion, rather than being peppered throughout the song. This makes the distorted sound a sort of expressive device that carries an interpretive intention. A growling or distorted quality can also be simulated by employing vocal fry or "creaky" voice (as described in Chapter 9), especially when using a sound system. If you work a lot with singers who employ this type of vocal effect, consider advancing your training with a reputable pedagogue to learn how you can teach them effectively. Melissa Cross (MelissaCross.com) has achieved excellent results in teaching "safe screaming." See Edwards (2014) for a tutorial on teaching extended vocal techniques and distorted vocal sounds.

The "Vocal Signature"

The voices of many iconic singers have characteristics we might consider dysphonic—raspy, rough, or gravelly. Some historic singers who fit this description include Louis Armstrong and Joe Cocker. You may work with singers who have a "vocal signature" that is similarly dysphonic. If they have come to you for help, they are likely having trouble meeting their singing demands. Their vocal quality may well be associated with a vocal pathology, but if it is part of what sets them apart and makes them successful singers, eliminating the dysphonia entirely is not the rehabilitation goal. Rather, the goal is to help them produce the sound that is uniquely theirs with the best possible coordination and efficiency and to ensure that all other contributing factors are adequately addressed (vocal hygiene, medical factors, vocal pacing, etc.) so that they are able to continue performing.

MUSICAL THEATER SINGING

Stylistically and technically, musical theater singers have the most challenging singing job. The professional expectation is that singers in this genre not only will be accomplished in "legit" singing (necessitating a classical foundation) but must also be skillful belters. Furthermore, the spectrum of styles featured in Broadway musicals requires the singer to be capable of singing convincingly across genres, including pop, rock, country, gospel, R&B, and many more (Green, Freeman, Edwards, & Meyer, 2014). Some musicals not only require the singer to nail the style but also to pull off vocal impersonations of singers well known to the audience (as in *Motown* and *Jersey Boys*).

Implications for Singing Voice Rehabilitation

The musical theater singer has to be a vocal acrobat, and singing voice rehabilitation with this type of singer will likely involve working across techniques to ensure healthy coordination in all relevant styles. The singer's training may not have addressed the full span of the required singing skills, which means you may need to incorporate voice habilitation in one or another style to ensure recovery and long-term vocal health. The exercise regimen will need to be appropriately comprehensive as well.

A WORD ABOUT WORLD MUSICS

An in-depth exploration of singing styles across the world is certainly beyond the scope of this text, but the topic warrants at least a brief mention, as you are likely to encounter singers who come from singing traditions that are unfamiliar to you. When this happens, it is incumbent on you to find out as much as you can about the style and genre. Ask the singer to give you a list of iconic artists of the genre, and watch and listen to recordings so that you can glean as much as possible about the technical characteristics of the style. Use this knowledge to guide the singer to optimal coordination and conditioning and for designing exercises. For example, if the genre employs scales that differ from those in Western music, use them to design your exercises. Are there speech sounds that are particularly characteristic of the language and the genre? If so, incorporate them into the exercise as well. The important thing is to adapt the rehabilitation design to the singer, not vice versa. Remember that one of the differences between voice lessons and voice rehabilitation is that you do not necessarily need to teach the singer the *style*; you just need to use your knowledge of the acoustic and physiologic basis of the target sound to help him or her achieve healthy and efficient *coordination*. You can always refer to an appropriate expert in the style for pedagogy follow-up if needed once the injury has resolved.

REFERENCES

Edwards, M. (Ed). (2014). *So you want to sing rock 'n' roll.* Lanham, MD: Rowman & Littlefield.

Ekholm, R., Papagiannis, G., & Chagnon, F. (1998). Relating objective measurements to expert evaluation of voice quality in Western classical singing: Critical perceptual parameters. *Journal of Voice, 12*(2), 182–196.

Green, K. (2014). Classical training and Bel Canto. In M. Edwards (Ed.), *So you want to sing rock 'n' roll* (pp. 239–243). Lanham, MD: Rowman & Littlefield.

Green, K., Freeman, W., Edwards, M., & Meyer, D. (2014). Trends in musical theater voice: An analysis of audition requirements for singers. *Journal of Voice, 28*(3), 324–327.

LeBorgne, W. D., & Rosenberg, M. (2014). *The vocal athlete.* San Diego, CA: Plural.

Miles, B., & Hollien, H. (1990). Whither belting? *Journal of Voice, 4*(1), 64–70.

Phyland, D. J., Oates, J., & Greenwood, K. M. (1999). Self-reported voice problems among three groups of professional singers. *Journal of Voice, 13*(4), 602–611.

Sundberg, J. (1977). The acoustics of the singing voice. *Scientific American, 236*, 82–91.

Sundberg, J., & Thalen, M. (2010). What is twang? *Journal of Voice, 24*(6), 654–660.

Titze, I. R., & Verdolini Abbott, K. (2012). *Vocology: The science and practice of voice habilitation.* Salt Lake City, UT: National Center for Voice and Speech.

Titze, I. R., & Worley, A. (2009). Modeling source-filter interaction in belting and high-pitched operatic male singing. *Journal of the Acoustical Society of America, 126*(3), 1530–1540.

Titze, I. R., Worley, A. S., & Story, B. H. (2011). Source-filter interaction in female operatic singing and theater belting. *Journal of Singing, 76*(5), 561–572.

CHAPTER 11

Designing Vocal Exercises for Singing Voice Rehabilitation

Much of your work with singers will involve designing an appropriate vocal exercise regimen. In selecting exercises, you should have a clear rationale for how each exercise will address the underlying voice problem based on your knowledge of the anatomy, physiology, and acoustics of singing. The exercises also must be consistent with the singer's training background and style of singing. This vocal exercise regimen will form the foundation for the improvement in vocal coordination and conditioning that is necessary for singing voice rehabilitation.

EXERCISE PHYSIOLOGY AND VOICE

Although exercise physiology is not nearly as well studied relative to voice as it is for fitness and sports, there is a firm basis for application of general principles for singing, and exercise physiology concepts and principles have a direct bearing on the design of an effective and appropriate rehabilitation protocol. For an excellent overview of fundamentals of exercise physiology and application to singing as well as review of relevant research, see LeBorgne and Rosenberg (2014, Chap. 15) and Titze and Verdolini Abbott (2012, Chap. 6).

It is of critical importance for both you and the singers you work with to understand the difference between "warming up" the voice and engaging in vocal exercise that will advance vocal technique and support recovery from injury. Vocal "warm-ups" are relatively simple exercises that increase blood flow to muscles, increase muscle temperature, and increase flexibility and range of motion of muscles and joints gently and easily (LeBorgne & Rosenberg, 2014). The goal of the vocal warm-up is to prepare the body-instrument to work, which can usually be accomplished in 5 to 10 minutes. However, the warm-up does not necessarily address development of technique and skill. This type of work is accomplished through a regimen of exercises that target specific rehabilitation objectives and technical goals, and may range from 15 to 45 minutes in duration. For the singer, the performance improvement achieved in vocal exercises must also be realized in the context of the music typically performed, and this often requires the guidance of the singing voice rehabilitation specialist. Thus, addressing vocal coordination and conditioning in singing voice rehabilitation encompasses both vocal exercises and work on repertoire, always bearing in mind the line between *rehabilitation* and *habilitation*, as discussed in Chapter 6.

As in physical fitness, the objective in vocal exercise is to train muscles in a manner that promotes changes in muscle fiber as well as neural and metabolic changes. These adaptations will yield increased function as the entire vocal mechanism adapts to the new demands (LeBorgne & Rosenberg, 2014). Keep in mind that all subsystems of voice—respiration, phonation, resonance—involve skeletal muscle, as do the muscles involved in alignment, articulation, and many necessary movements of singing—thus, all will be responsive to physical training. A minimum of 3 days of training per week is recommended for successful outcome (Saxon & Schneider, 1995).

The underlying principles of exercise training may be considered to include intensity, frequency, overload, specificity, and reversibility (LeBorgne & Rosenberg, 2014; Titze & Verdolini Abbott, 2012). *Intensity* and *frequency* are self-explanatory concepts. *Overload* refers to exceeding the current ability of the muscle, *specificity* to targeting a specific muscle or group of muscles, and *reversibility* to the fact that muscles will "detrain" if the exercise regimen is stopped or suspended. Titze and Verdolini Abbott (2012, p. 192) explore additional terminology related to exercise, including *individuality*, "the degree to which a particular individual's response to a specific load or training program is largely unpredictable," a strong argument for tailoring the exercise regimen to each singer individually.

These principles translate fluidly to voice habilitation, but in the context of rehabilitation, the balance of healing and strengthening must be carefully weighed. Frequency and intensity of exercise must be calibrated to a level that does not promote excessive fatigue or maladaptive compensatory effort. However, the recommendation of a minimum of 3 days of training per week endorses regular practice of exercises and provides an argument against prolonged periods of complete vocal rest or elimination of singing. The principle of *overload* may need to be applied conservatively in cases of phonotrauma depending on severity of injury but is appropriate for cases of hypofunction, such as with vocal fold atrophy or paresis. LeBorgne and Rosenberg (2014) recommend alternation of muscle groups when overloading muscle to promote strength and endurance. This practice will promote healing while minimizing risk of reinjury or worsening of existing injury. *Specificity* pertains to developing rehabilitation exercises that are style specific but may also apply to training muscles and muscle groups that are relatively weak to promote adaptive compensation, especially in cases where the singer has become overly reliant on maladaptive effort, or "pushing," to the detriment of balanced effort. *Reversibility* provides an argument for regular practice of appropriate duration, for achieving tolerable balance of voice use and voice rest, and against blanket recommendations of "no singing" or prolonged complete voice rest.

Vocal Cool-Down

Although most trained singers are at least familiar with the concept of warming up the voice and many engage in a regular warm-up routine, cooling down the voice is generally less familiar and less often applied. Most athletes engage in some sort of cool-down following intense physical activity. Although there has been limited research on the subject relative to singing, it seems plausible that at least a brief period of structured vocal recovery following intense voice use could be beneficial, especially considering the parallels that have been drawn and demonstrated relative to other aspects of exercise physiology. Examples of vocal cool-downs will be provided in the case studies in Chapter 12.

WHEN TO START SINGING EXERCISES

For singers who have a voice problem, singing is usually their top priority when they arrive at the first rehabilitation session. For this reason, I try to get at least some singing in at the very first session. I have found this practice to be very effective for bestowing credibility to the rehabilitation process, as well as promoting the bond of trust that is so important for successful outcome. Digging into the singing right away shows the singer that you not only recognize the urgency, but you agree that singing is the prime order of business. This doesn't mean that you completely ignore the other important elements of recovery in the first session. A quick review of the overall plan, possibly using a visual organization aid as described in Chapter 6, will help the singer to see the big picture and underscores the multifactorial nature of the rehabilitation process.

There will likely be situations in which you will not be able to get much singing into the first session. If the singer has a lot of questions about the injury or rehabilitation process, is struggling with anxiety or other strong emotions

When I first began working as a singing voice rehabilitation specialist, I felt I needed to do a lot of ground work with the singer before starting to work on singing exercises. I had just completed my speech-language pathology master's degree after 18 years of teaching voice and performing professionally. I wanted to teach my patients about vocal anatomy, and I spent a lot of time going over vocal hygiene goals and thoroughly reviewing voice use and vocal pacing. Often the singer's speaking voice was more dysphonic than the singing voice, and I felt I needed to address that domain before proceeding to singing. Sometimes I wouldn't get to singing until the second or third session. As a freshly minted SLP, my approach was all in the interest of following the rehabilitation plan I had developed and sticking to that plan in a linear fashion. Most of my patients made very good progress, which I attribute to their commitment and motivation much more than my misguided pursuit of order. Gradually, I started to notice that the singers seemed to be anxiously tolerating our work on the other rehabilitation elements while eagerly awaiting the singing work. I went back to my voice teacher "roots" and began to shift my rehabilitation procedure so that singing occurred earlier in the process—in the first session if possible—even if it meant putting in-depth work on other aspects of recovery on the back burner in the short term. The more I did this, the more quickly the singer's "buy-in" to rehabilitation appeared to emerge. For those of you on a dual-training path, the lesson here is to keep both your clinical and pedagogical hats firmly in place at all times.

surrounding the voice problem, or if your judgment leads you to believe that another component of the process should take priority, it's perfectly reasonable to defer singing for a bit.

You may need to explicitly convey to the singer that the rehabilitation exercises constitute singing. I was once surprised to hear a postsurgery singer I was working with ask, after weeks of therapy during which we had developed a complex and thorough vocal exercise regimen that he was executing on a daily basis, "When are we going to start singing?" Many times singers feel the work they are doing doesn't "count" if they are not back to their preinjury performance schedule. Let them know that the exercise regimen will be a lifelong component of their singing activities, and give them regular updates on the prognosis for returning to performing.

VOCAL EXERCISE BY DESIGN

The Singing Voice Rehabilitation Specialist as Master Chef

Imagine that in your pantry you have flour, salt, sugar, baking powder, olive oil, rice, potatoes, canned tomatoes, a few kinds of pasta, garlic, and some dried beans. In the refrigerator, you have butter, milk, eggs, cheese, a fresh whole chicken, lemons, strawberries, onions, carrots, squash, salad greens, and peppers. You have fresh herbs like basil, thyme, oregano and rosemary, and a loaded spice rack. Just imagine all the different things you could make with these ingredients! You could make a pound cake with strawberries, for example, or an herb-roasted chicken with rosemary potatoes and baked squash. You could make a fresh salad with lemon dressing, or a shepherd's pie, or pasta with a hearty tomato sauce.

A few key principles apply if you want to create a delicious and successful meal: (1) You can't just dump all the ingredients in together indiscriminately and expect something wonderful to emerge; (2) you have to know the properties of the ingredients and how they will combine with other ingredients; (3) you have to measure carefully and periodically taste to make sure the flavor is right; and (4) you have to customize the dish so that it is suitable for a given occasion (e.g., don't make a dessert when a main dish is called for). Some ingredients—like salt—will be used for all the recipes. Other ingredients will be used differently in one recipe versus another. Sometimes you may not have the ingredients you need, in which case you have to go shopping.

Customizing an exercise regimen for a particular singer can be a lot like making a great meal: It works best when you have lots of ingredients to choose from, can choose the right ingredients depending on what the occasion calls for, know how to use and combine the ingredients, and know when and where to shop.

My goal in this chapter is to provide you with a few basic resources (ingredients) and to explore the properties of these elements so that you will be able to tailor the vocal exercise regimen depending on the singer's injury or disorder, singing style, technical skill, learning style, and singing goals. What you won't find here is a one-size-fits-all or cookie-cutter approach to developing an exercise program, nor will you find an exhaustive catalogue of every possible exercise in every possible permutation—that's where the shopping comes in. There are numerous excellent resources—some of which will be mentioned herein—for specific exercises and their possible application for healing voices. Observing or discussing cases with colleagues and/or attending master classes, conferences, and workshops will provide additional opportunities to "shop." Ideally, you will be shopping at these "stores" for your entire career, ever increasing the provisions in your vocal exercise pantry and your collection of recipes. Our focus here will be on inspecting the underlying principles and assembling the building blocks which will guide you in selecting the most suitable recipe for each and every singer you work with.

Don't Throw the Baby Out With the Bathwater

If the singer has a regular warm-up routine, have him or her demonstrate it for you. This is a great way to get singing into the very first session and has advantages beyond the "buy-in." Observing the singer executing the warm-up provides you with another layer of assessment to augment your initial singing voice evaluation, to determine if there has been any change since that initial evaluation and to make an estimation of what principles of singing the singer is already acquainted with. If the singer is taking or has taken singing lessons, the warm-up routine he or she is currently using likely already includes some appropriate exercises (such as pitch glides, semi-occluded vocal tract exercises, etc.) that you may immediately incorporate into your exercise design. Let them know this by saying something like, "There are a lot of [or some] great exercises here that we're going to keep in your routine." This can be very encouraging and validating to singers, making them feel they are on the right track. If they have a warm-up routine and it gets tossed out completely in favor of starting from scratch, the singer may be left with the feeling that there is something "wrong" with what he or she has been doing up to this point.

If the singer is presently working with a teacher and the current warm-up routine has useful components, you can dovetail your exercise design with the current routine so that the singer doesn't feel the voice lesson exercises and rehabilitation exercises constitute separate practices. Be sure to evaluate the routine for acceleration of intensity. Adjustments may be needed to ensure a lower intensity or more gradual warm-up, especially if the injury is significantly affecting technique.

Conversely, if the singer has a well-established warm-up regimen that he or she appears to execute in a manner that exhibits entrenched maladaptive compensatory behaviors, it can be helpful to make a fresh start to avoid reinforcing the muscle memory associated with those well-known exercises.

If the singer doesn't have a regular exercise regimen, the first session is a good time to get started, even if you are only able to cover a few simple exercises or teach basic respiratory mechanics or principles of resonant voice. At the very least, send the singer out the door practicing abdominal breathing. This makes the process kinesthetic and somatic from the start.

A Word About Prerecorded Vocal Exercise Programs

Sometimes singers will come to you with a warm-up routine they have obtained by purchasing a CD or DVD voice training program, or from downloaded apps. Although some of these programs include excellent teaching and materials, some do not. Often, the exercises are quite elaborate and way beyond the skill level of the singer using them. Sometimes the exercises are not style or range appropriate, and even though the instructor usually says something along the lines of, "Come in at the pitch that feels comfortable to you and drop out when it gets too high," I have observed singers working way out of their controllable range when singing along with such a recording. In my opinion, the greatest obstacle in using prerecorded voice training or vocal exercise programs is that the singer is usually just drilling through the exercises and gets no immediate instructional feedback (e.g., there is no shaping of voice going on). The singer may become very skilled at following the recording, but I question whether technique is developing optimally.

Having said that, if a singer comes to you who has worked on one of these programs, it is clear that he or she is hungry to learn how to sing better and has already demonstrated the ability to engage in regular practice. Prognostically, this is great news—this singer will likely have a very good outcome in rehabilitation. Adding personalized feedback, education, and voice shaping to the discipline and motivation they bring to the table will likely result in steady or even rapid improvements in vocal coordination and conditioning. Again, be careful not to give the singer the impression that the work he or she has done with the recorded program is "wrong" or "bad." Determine whether any of the exercises are appropriate for rehabilitation or can be modified to be so, and keep them in the plan. This way you are building on the work the singer has already done without abandoning it entirely. Emphasize to the singer that the routine you develop together will be "tailor made" and will have a better fit than the prerecorded program.

Vocal Exercises: The Ingredients

Any vocal exercise can be broken down into several basic elements. These may include:

- Pitch and rhythmic pattern (e.g., the melody of the exercise)
- Linguistic (or sound) content (isolated phonemes, syllables, words, phrases, straw phonation, etc.)
- Dynamic range (variations in loudness)
- Degree of accent (e.g., legato to staccato)

As you design exercises, consider how each of these elements can be selected and combined to create an exercise that will help the singer acquire, develop, and perfect a coordination or conditioning target. The complexity of the task should be within the singer's current capability, and should increase as the singer's skill increases.

In most cases, the singing voice rehabilitation setting will not be the time to bring out your most complex and elaborate agility and coloratura drills. In all likelihood, most of the singers you work with will not be highly trained, advanced level classical singers. Some will have had no training at all (even though they may function at a very high level professionally); others will be at a beginning or intermediate level at best. Many may have had training that is not aligned with their chosen vocal style. They will need your help to effectively compensate for the functional impact of the voice problem, and this is usually best accomplished with more structured, simplified exercises. It's not that more complex and elaborate exercises never have a place in singing voice rehabilitation—they certainly do for the more advanced singers. Rather, I am advising caution in turning reflexively to exercises that may be familiar to you from your graduate studies in vocal performance or as a professional singer, or your experience teaching singers who do not have an injury.

Pitch and Rhythmic Patterns

Pitch/rhythmic patterns may be infinite in variety, but those most useful to you will likely include sustained single pitches, glides, scales, and arpeggios.

Sustained Pitches. Sustaining single pitches one at a time strengthens vocal fold adductors (thyroarytenoid, interarytenoids, lateral cricoarytenoid) (Stemple, 1984; Stemple, Lee, D'Amico, & Pickup, 1994) and also has the advantage of removing the complexity of pitch change from the vocal task (Figure 11–1). The singer is challenged to continuously coordinate lung pressure/airflow, vocal fold vibration, and vocal tract shape to maintain a steady and consistent sound. The pitch can be sustained without loudness or phoneme variation to isolate the ability to adapt breath support to changing lung volume (e.g., increase expiratory action as the lungs empty).

Pitch Glides/Sirens. Pitch glides allow the vocal folds to stretch and contract in a continuous fashion while coordinating breath support with the changing length and thickness of vocal folds, but without the degree of pitch precision that would be necessary in a scalar pattern. The focus is on continuous, gradual pitch change. This can be an excellent way to encourage adaptation of the breath support strategy under a condition of changing vocal fold length and thickness. The steady change in pitch (fundamental frequency, or F0) also results in gradual change in the interaction of F0 and harmonics with the formant frequencies of the vocal tract, so the singer starts to experience how adjustments of the throat and articulators enhance or undermine the sound. Figure 11–2 provides examples of pitch glides. Depending on the pitch interval of the glide, the pattern of intrinsic laryngeal muscle activation (relative engagement of TA/CT) may be fairly stable (as in a 1-3-1 glide) or may require gradual transition from TA to CT (or vice versa, depending

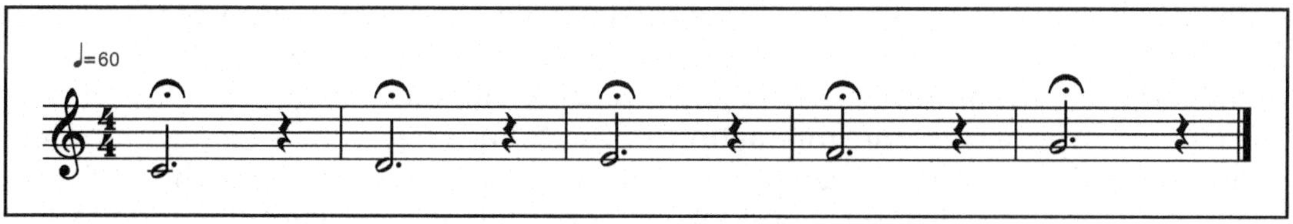

Figure 11–1. Example of sustained phonation on single notes.

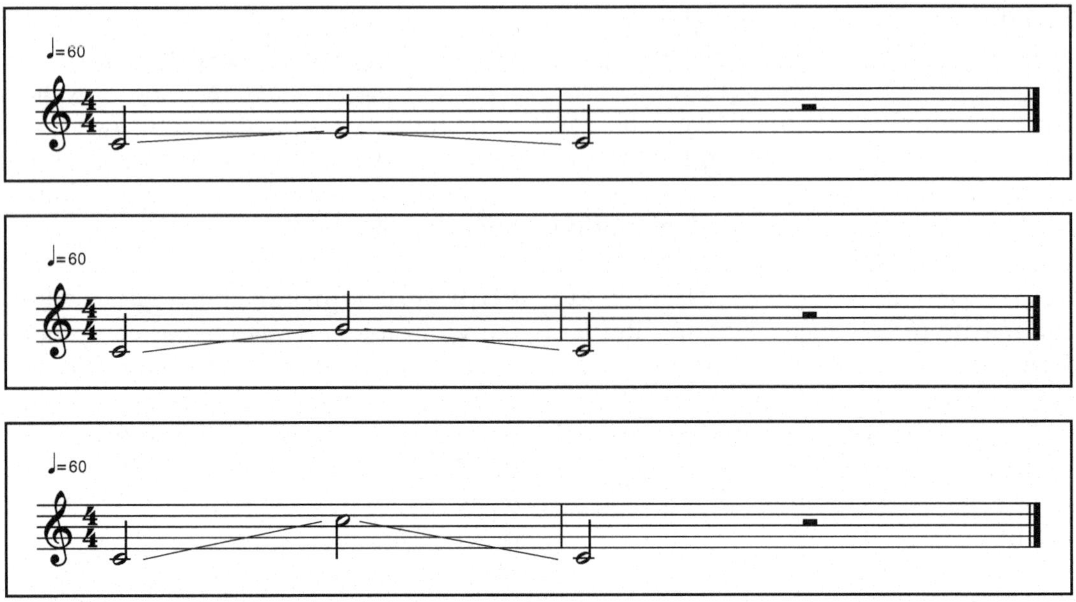

***Figure 11–2.** Examples of pitch glides of increasingly wide intervals.*

on the direction of the glide), as when spanning an octave or more. For singers who have little or suboptimal training, it is usually easier to accomplish this coordination on glides versus scalar patterns. Thus, the glide can provide a stair step on the way to scales or other more complex pitch patterns. The wider the glide's pitch interval, the more complex the task, so start at an interval you think the singer can achieve, and adjust to a narrower or wider interval as needed.

Scales. With scales (chromatic or diatonic), the singer must combine all the skills previously outlined for sustained pitches and glides, but with greater precision in adjustments of intrinsic laryngeal musculature (primarily the interaction of TA and CT) and resonance strategy. Figure 11–3 provides examples of scalar patterns).

A typical tendency is for the singer to (unconsciously) focus on the laryngeal coordination (e.g., changing pitch with laryngeal gestures alone) at the expense of coordination relative to breath support and resonance. In other words, the breath support or resonance technique established in a gliding pattern may go out the window once the scalar pattern is introduced. This can result in a tone that is inadequately supported and/or lacking optimal resonance. This phenomenon can be ameliorated by ensuring mastery of gliding patterns first, but an additional stair-step can be achieved by practicing the scales at a slow tempo, starting with shorter scale patterns (such as 12321), and/or cuing the singer to add a "microglide" between each step of the scale. Once this is executed smoothly, you can then gradually fade out the glide. Alternating glides and scales over the same

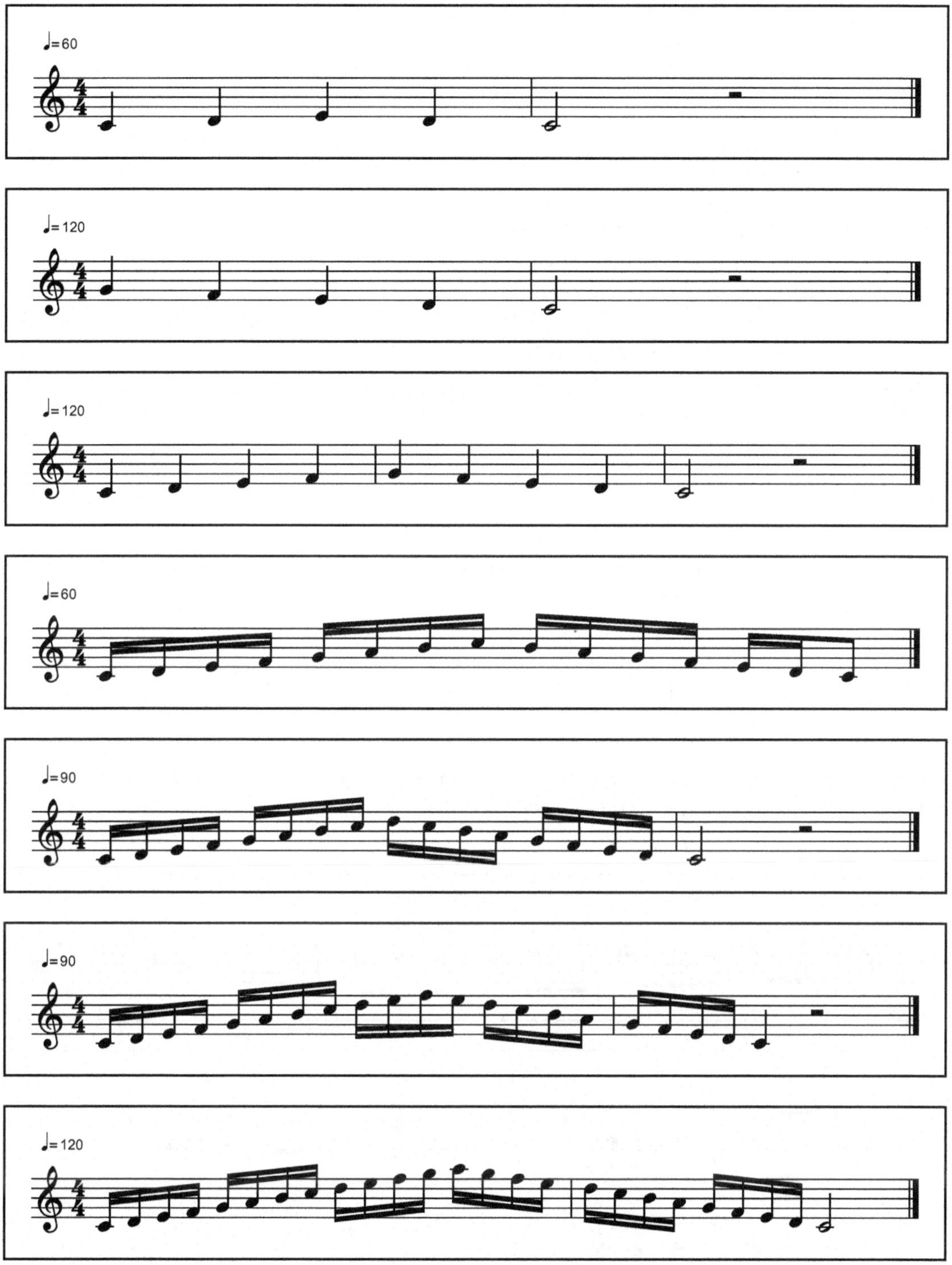

***Figure 11–3.** Examples of scale patterns of increasing pitch range and complexity.*

interval (e.g., 1-3-1 glide alternated with 12321 scale; Figure 11–4) is another way to promote carryover of coordination.

As the singer develops more precision, increase the tempo as well as the length and complexity of the scale. Figure 11–5 depicts examples of embellished scales. Depending on what kind of music the singer typically sings, consider expanding beyond the typical chromatic and major diatonic scales to include minor scales, pentatonic scales, blues scales, or scale patterns from various world music, such as ragas from Indian classical music.

Arpeggios. With arpeggios, the complexity of the vocal task increases even more due to the wider interval between notes. Also, the pitch range of arpeggios expands fairly quickly in the hierarchy. Figure 11–6 shows examples of arpeggios. As with scales, alternation of the arpeggio with a less complex task (such as a glide) will help to promote carryover.

Beyond the Basics. Pitch patterns aren't limited to sustained notes, glides, scales and arpeggios. The possibilities are limited only by your imagination. A great way to add complexity while simultaneously facilitating carryover into repertoire is to extract a fragment from a song and turn it into a vocalise. Figure 11–7 shows an example. This has the added advantage of

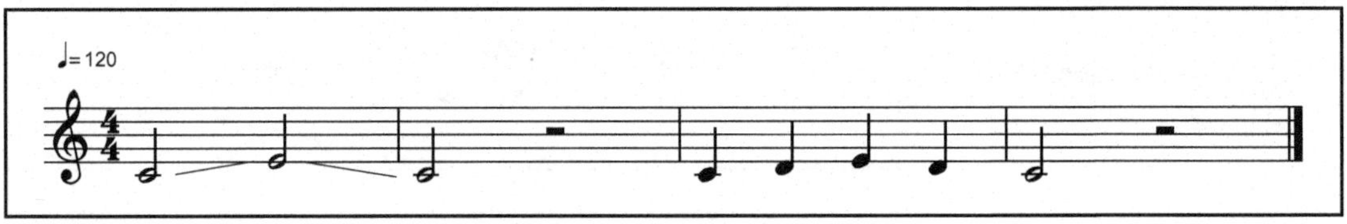

***Figure 11–4.** Example of alternating glide and scale over the same interval to promote carryover of coordination from a simple to a more complex task.*

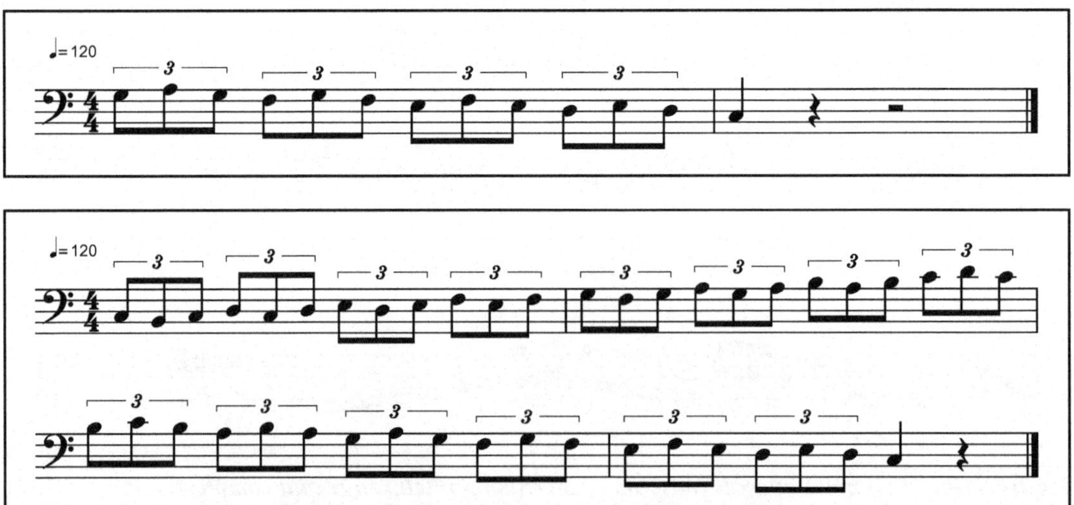

***Figures 11–5.** Examples of embellished scales.*

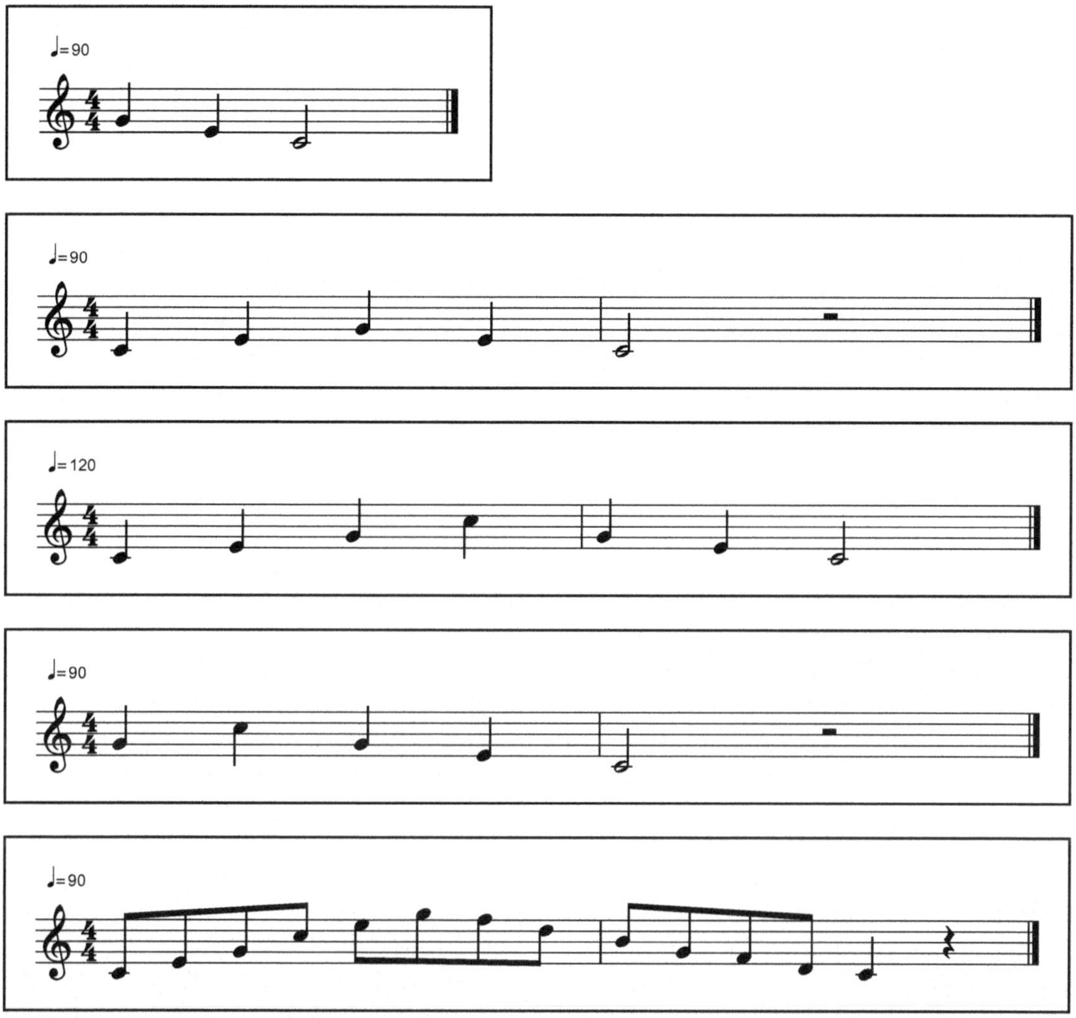

Figure 11–6. Examples of arpeggio patterns of increasing pitch range and complexity.

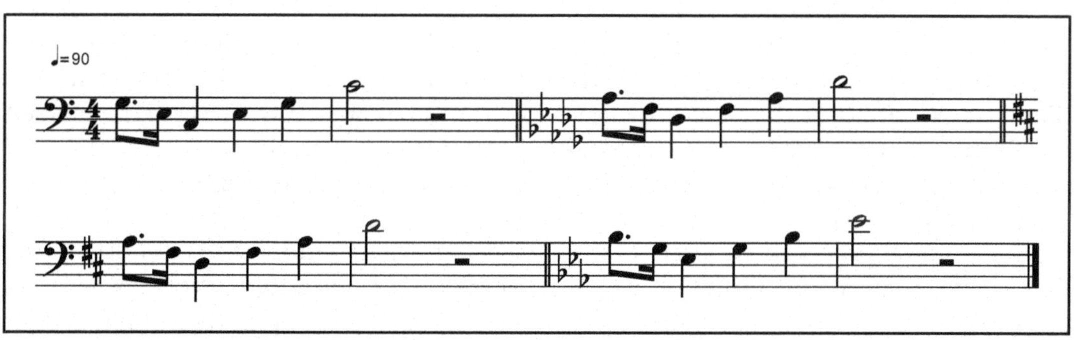

Figure 11–7. Extracting the first phrase of "The Star Spangled Banner" to create a vocalise.

incorporating repertoire work into rehabilitation fairly early in the process.

Linguistic (Sound) Content

Once you've decided on a pitch/rhythmic pattern, you will need to determine what linguistic material or sound the singer will sing. This might include:

- Straw phonation or trills
- Phonemes (vowels or consonants)
- Syllables
- Words
- Phrases

The words and phrases might be linguistically meaningful or nonsense. As with the selection of pitch pattern, your choice of linguistic content should be based on the specific coordination and conditioning objective.

Semi-Occluded Vocal Tract (SOVT) Sounds. Semi-occluded vocal tract (SOVT) sounds are an excellent choice for designing the sound component of a vocal exercise. This category of sounds includes lip and tongue trills, raspberries (labio-lingual trills), voiced fricatives (such as /β/, /z/, and /v/), nasal consonants (/m, n, ŋ/), "Y-buzz" (which is a sustained /j/ sound; Lessac, 1997), lip-rounded vowels (/o/ and /u/) (Stemple, 1984), and phonating through straws of varying length and diameter. What all of these sounds have in common is that they create a degree of resistance somewhere in the vocal tract and generate oral pressure that interacts with the lung pressure in such a way that optimal vocal fold vibration can be achieved.

This is particularly true for phonation through a small-diameter straw (e.g., coffee stir straw), which engages the respiratory muscles quickly and effectively, promoting optimal breath support. In addition, the positive oral pressure created by the straw decreases the forcefulness of vocal fold collision and "spreads" the vocal folds so that only the edges vibrate (Titze, 2001). In effect, the straw teaches the singer to adjust glottal resistance to match the impedance at the glottis with that of the straw and to lower the phonation threshold pressure (PTP). If the coordination is off, he or she will not be able to produce a sound. Lowering PTP is accomplished either by optimizing the balance of TA/CT (resulting in a more "squared up" vocal fold edge) or by narrowing the epilarynx tube to increase vocal tract inertance (Titze, 2010). The increased length of the vocal tract associated with phonating through the straw in and of itself increases vocal tract inertance (Titze & Laukkanen, 2007). As noted in Chapter 9, vocal tract inertance is a key component in achieving optimal voice production in which the vocal tract actually reinforces vocal fold vibration. By practicing with the straw, the vocal tract "learns" how to use the epilarynx tube to achieve the same coordination when the straw is removed (Titze, 2010).

Clearly, the benefits of SOVT as a component of vocal exercise are numerous, particularly in the arena of singing voice rehabilitation. The efficiency of vocal fold vibration achieved with SOVT, decreased forcefulness of vocal fold collision, and lowered phonation threshold pressure allow for vocal conditioning while minimizing exacerbation of vocal fold edema or traumatic vocal fold lesions. SOVTs are also beneficial in hypofunctional conditions such as vocal fold paresis or atrophy, as the entrainment of breath flow and vocal fold vibration promotes unloading of supraglottic hyperfunction, and an optimal TA/CT ratio assists in maximizing glottic closure without excess effort. For a review of research related to SOVT, see Kapsner-Smith, Hunter, Kirkham, Cox, and Titze (2015) and Titze and Verdolini Abbott (2012).

Vowels. Unless you come across a singer whose repertoire is entirely comprised of SOVT sounds, the ideal interaction of airflow, vocal fold vibration, and vocal tract that is facilitated by a semi-occluded vocal tract must ultimately be accomplished when singing words. Regardless of style, most of the sustained sound in singing occurs on vowels. Thus, working on optimizing vocal coordination by singing exercises on vowels is a central consideration in developing the vocal exercise regimen.

When choosing vowels, whether in isolation or as a part of syllables, words, or phrases, consider how resonant voice is accomplished (as described in Chapter 9). The goal is to achieve vocal production in which the vocal tract assists the vocal folds to produce acoustic energy. This is largely realized through the interaction of the source (fundamental frequency and harmonics generated by the vocal folds) with the resonant frequencies of the vocal tract (formant frequencies). See Chapter 9 for discussion of vocal tract formants and how they can be manipulated by the singer. First and second formant frequencies for different vowels are illustrated again in Figure 11–8.

Recall from Chapter 10 that different kinds of singing employ different resonance strategies and choose vowel content accordingly. For the inverted megaphone mouth shape of classical singing, lip rounding assists in boosting vocal tract inertance. This doesn't mean you should only choose vowels that are inherently rounded (/u, o, ɔ/, for example), but it does mean that vowels that naturally have lip retraction (/i/) may benefit from "cheating" toward a more rounded lip position. Combining lip rounding with narrowing of the epilarynx tube results in acoustic energy in the singers' formant cluster (2,500–3,500 Hz). According to Titze and Verdolini Abbott (2012), narrowing of the epilarynx tube is primarily accomplished indirectly through adjustments the singer makes to achieve a "ringing" quality in the voice. In the megaphone mouth shape of belting (regardless of the specific genre), the second harmonic is reinforced by the first formant, necessitating selection of vowels with relatively high first formant frequencies.

Understanding the acoustic underpinnings of vowel selection and formant tuning is a critical component in designing vocal exercises and customizing to the individual singer, but don't forget that your ear is possibly the most valuable tool in your arsenal for shaping voice. Each singer is different and you will likely need to experiment with different sounds to find the one that is most facilitating. Once this is achieved, use the facilitating vowel to shape those that are more challenging. For example, if the singer demonstrates better resonance on closed vowels, start with /i/ or /u/ and gradually move toward more open vowels, and vice versa.

Combining Sounds Into Syllables, Words, and Phrases. Sequencing sounds into syllables, words, and phrases brings the articulators into the vocal exercise regimen—a must for vocal performance, which almost always requires singing on words.

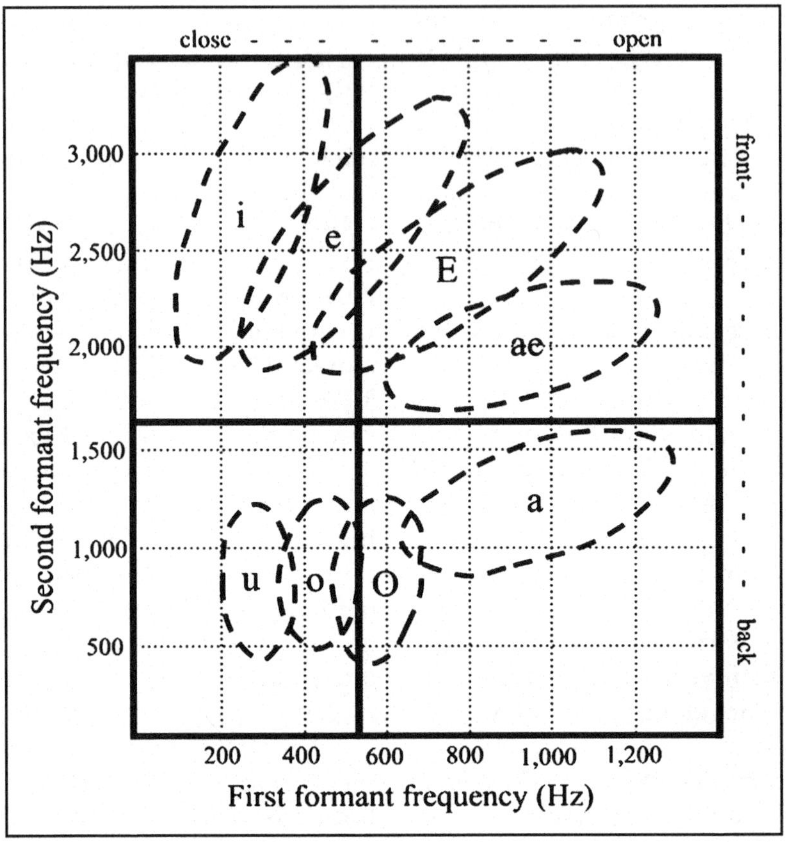

***Figure 11–8.** Vowel chart illustrating first and second formant ranges. Reproduced with permission from Inside View Press. Miller, D. (2008).* Resonance in singing. *Princeton, NJ: Inside View Press.*

Alternating or sequencing vowels is a good way to introduce the combination of articulation and phonation into vocal exercises. For example, producing the diphthong sequence /ɑiɑiɑi/ with the jaw stabilized allows the tongue to stretch while the sequence /uɑuɑuɑ/ promotes lip and jaw movement. Both encourage independence of articulation and phonation (i.e., phonation should not be impacted by the articulatory movement). This type of sequencing can also help in maintaining the vertical larynx position in the face of articulatory movement. In these tasks, the singer must adjust the resonance strategy to the changing vocal tract shape in such a way that the articulatory movement doesn't negatively impact the quality of the sound. However, since the singer doesn't have to contend with the interruption of airflow that occurs once consonants enter the picture, the task is simpler than CV syllables.

As with all steps of designing vocal exercises, the introduction of consonant and vowel combinations should be undertaken purposefully and with an understanding of the properties of the sounds and potential impact on phonation. Used strategically, consonants can prepare and entrain the system for optimum breath-phonation coordination and source-filter interaction.

We have already explored the benefits of semi-occluded vocal tract sounds in optimizing vocal production. These sounds can assist the singer in achieving the same coordination on vowels. For example, initiating a syllable with /z/, /v/, or a tongue trill positions the vocal tract favorably to assist vocal fold vibration and will virtually guarantee that the singer has engaged breath support, as these sounds cannot be produced without airflow. Incorporating /m/, /n/, or /ŋ/ into syllables provides a sensory and mechanical template for resonance that can launch the vowel. Using unvoiced consonants such as /k/ will challenge the singer to sustain coordinated phonation in the context of interrupted voicing. Other unvoiced consonants have characteristics that benefit coordination of breath and phonation, encouraging smooth onset or maintaining airflow when voicing ceases (as with /h/, /s/, /ʃ/, and /f/). For example, starting with /s/ and transitioning to /z/ helps ensure breath flow is engaged prior to onset of phonation. Voiced plosives (/b/, /g/, /d/) require a brief buildup of subglottic pressure that can increase TA engagement and improve glottic closure. Some consonants tend to raise the larynx (/g/), while others may encourage a lower larynx position (/b/).

Syllables can be sequenced in myriad ways. Repetition of the same syllable creates an articulatory oscillation (/lalalala/). Interrupting this oscillation with another sound (/lagalaga/) adds complexity, demanding a change in the motor program that moves the singer closer to the type of phonatory and articulatory acrobatics of performance. Sequencing place of articulation in this manner can also promote release of maladaptive muscle tension in articulators by requiring them to move flexibly instead of rigidly locking into place.

From here, it is just a hop, skip, and a jump to adding words and phrases to the exercise regimen. As always, selection should be made in accordance with the goal. This will be explored further in the next chapter.

Dynamic Range

Vocal exercises can be executed at varying levels of loudness. Changes in loudness represent changes in lung pressure, but changes are also going on in the larynx. These include variations in phase closure (open cycle becomes longer with low loudness and closed cycle becomes longer with increased loudness), amplitude of vibration (increases with loudness), and thickness of vocal fold vertical edge (thinner for soft phonation, thicker for loud phonation). Ideally, the singer should be able to control loudness with optimal adductory motor control. Titze and Verdolini Abbott (2012) describe how this occurs in the messa di voce gesture:

> If sound quality is to remain constant . . . there must be a gradual abductory gesture during the crescendo and a reversed adductory gesture during the decrescendo. This combination of increasing vibrational amplitude, together with fine-controlled valving to maintain a constant voice quality, is the ultimate test of laryngeal control. (p. 278)

Another way of targeting loudness control—thus increasing this finely-controlled valving to avoid the extremes of breathy or pressed vocal quality—is to use a shared numerical reference of 1 to 10, with 1 being the softest and 10 being the loudest (Edwards, 2014, attributed to Jeannette LoVetri). An exact measurement is not important, as long you and the singer are in agreement with the range. Have the singer experiment with varying levels of loudness to promote adductory control to gain a consistent sound quality across dynamic range and tasks.

Degree of Accent

Vocal exercises can be executed with varying degrees of separation between notes, ranging from the extremes of legato (smooth and connected with no separation between notes) to staccato (detached by rapid and repeated initiation and release on every note; Figure 11–9).

Legato singing requires the singer to maintain adducted vocal folds while making fine adjustments of TA/CT activation. The goal is to do this primarily by controlling lung pressure and airflow, avoiding compression in the larynx. Staccato singing "elicits clean and rapid voice onset, establishing a dominant mode of vibration" and "trains adductor/abductor muscles simultaneously with tensor muscles during pitch change" (Titze, 2001, p. 51).

The rate of vocal fold adduction/abduction in staccato singing is the same as the rate of the abdominal movement (Titze & Verdolini Abbott, 2012), and thus the singer must achieve very precise coordination between respiratory mechanics and laryngeal movement. In between these extremes of temporal separation lies marcato, in which phonation is continuous, but with a rhythmic pulsing (Figure 11–10).

In this mode of production, the pulsation is achieved by rhythmic movements

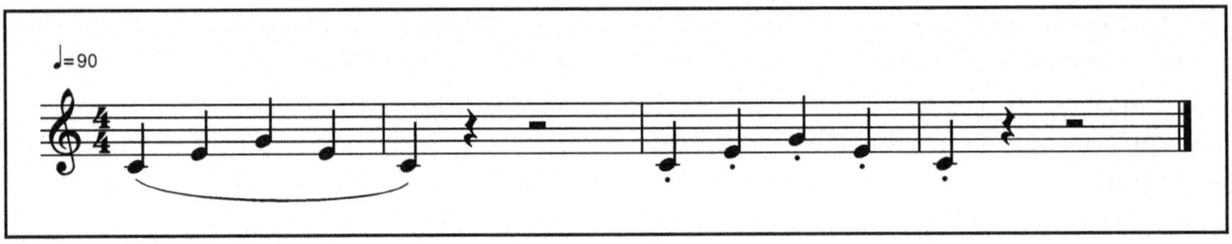

***Figure 11–9.** Example of legato versus staccato articulation.*

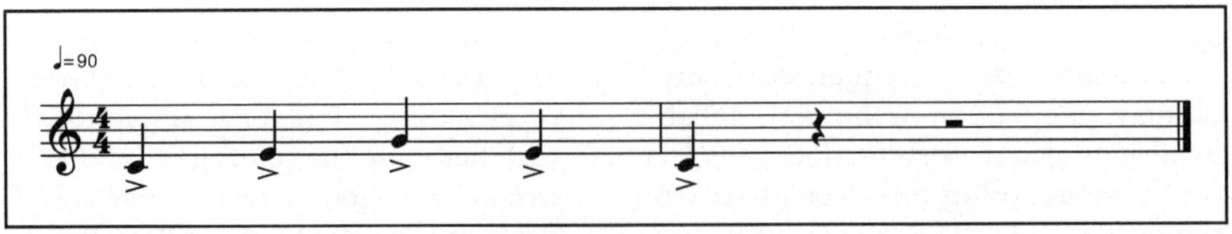

***Figure 11–10.** Example of marcato articulation.*

Swelling Test/Soft Phonation Exercises

Bastian, Keidar, and Verdolini-Marsten (1990) found that soft phonation staccato and legato exercises can be useful in detecting vocal fold swelling. In combination with soft (pianissimo) phonation, staccato exercises can provide a useful informal assessment of swelling in the context of singing voice rehabilitation, or as a regular vocal practice. Titze and Verdolini Abbott (2012, p. 281) suggest using such tasks quantifiably in an assessment measure they refer to as "inability to produce soft voice." They suggest having singers rate themselves on a 1 to 10 scale, 1 being the best. The rating is determined by counting the number of instabilities that occur in performing a soft phonation task, such as singing "Happy Birthday" as high and softly as possible (one of the tasks used by Bastian et al., 1990).

I typically use this strategy in the clinical context by having the singer execute a staccato 5-3-1 arpeggio on /hu/, /ho/, or /ha/ as softly as possible, starting at a comfortable pitch and gradually ascending chromatically until he or she either cannot phonate on the top note (phonation ceiling), or cannot ascend any higher (pitch ceiling). The aspiration (/h/) helps ensure that the onset is coordinated with the breath. It is often necessary to cue the singer to sing as softly as possible and avoid pushing or straining to ensure that an accurate ceiling is reached. It may take multiple attempts with your guidance for the singer to accurately execute the task—the urge to "muscle it" to achieve phonation can be strong.

Measuring the ceiling at the beginning of rehabilitation and at regular intervals throughout the process provides a useful, quantifiable measure of pitch range as a reflection of phonation threshold pressure. This is particularly helpful in cases of phonotrauma. If the underlying injury resolves, the ceiling on the test exercise should increase to what may be considered a baseline for the singer's healthy voice. If the singer experiences a sudden lowering of the ceiling on the test exercise, it may indicate an increase in inflammation, reinjury, or worsening injury. If the lowered ceiling persists, repeat stroboscopy will help ascertain whether an adjustment in intervention is needed.

of the abdomen. This can be highly effective in leading the singer to achieve prosodic stress or accented singing through breath control versus forceful adduction of vocal folds and supraglottic compression (Titze & Verdolini Abbott, 2012) and in fact forms the basis for the accent method of voice therapy (Kotby, 1995).

Putting It All Together

Now that you have all the ingredients, you can start putting them together into different recipes. As you do so, consider sequencing (starting gently and gradually building intensity and agility), the underlying injury, the singer's technical level and style, and the overall rehabilitation goals. The exercises should be designed to build vocal range, stamina, agility/ flexibility, and stability. Remember the underlying principles of each ingredient and how it will combine with others.

Here's an example: The benefits of sustaining single pitches have been described above. Once this skill is mastered, changing loudness level (crescendo/ decrescendo) increases the complexity of the task by requiring intrinsic laryngeal musculature (adductors and cricothyroid) to adjust degree of engagement in the face of changing lung pressure. By combining sustained phonation on single notes with SOVT sounds (particularly phonation through a small straw) and dynamic range (messa di voce), you quickly achieve optimal vocal fold vibration with fine control of intrinsic laryngeal musculature. The design of the exercise is illustrated in Table 11–1.

According to Titze (2001), this exercise ensures a gradual, medial to lateral vibration of the layers of the vocal fold, facilitates the singer's ability to match the tension in the thyroarytenoid muscle with that of the ligament, and trains the interaction of respiration and phonation by promoting coordination of intrinsic laryngeal musculature in the face of changing lung pressure. Progressing through the notes of a major scale one note at a time provides a variation on Stemple's adductory power exercise (described below). Phonating through the straw facilitates optimal vocal tract inertance. Once mastered, the singer can take the more advanced step of achieving this coordination while phonating on a vowel, choosing the vowel according to the resonance objective. This combination of benefits is a rationale for using this exercise with virtually any singer but is especially beneficial in promoting resolution of traumatic lesions (minimizing collisional adductive force during vibration) while ensuring necessary exercise. If the singer has significant vibration impairment, particularly if glottal closure is impaired, this exercise might prove too challenging. If so, adapt the ingredients. Instead of phonating through a stir straw, try phonation through a drinking straw. Too easy? Find a middle ground by having the singer partially occlude the drinking straw by squeezing it with thumb and forefinger, or by submerging the straw in a cup of water. See Table 11–2 for additional examples of assembling vocal exercises in a strategic manner.

Table 11–1. *Strategic Design of Vocal Exercise*

Pitch and Rhythmic Pattern	***Linguistic/Sound Content***	***Loudness Level***	***Degree of Accent***
Sustained single notes	Small straw phonation	Full dynamic range: messa di voce	Legato/ unaccented

Table 11–2. *Examples of Vocal Exercise Designs With Rationale*

<table>
<tr><th>Pitch and Rhythmic Pattern</th><th>Linguistic/Sound Content</th><th>Loudness Level</th><th>Degree of Accent</th></tr>
<tr><td>1-5-1 glide</td><td>Lip, tongue, or labio-lingual (raspberry) trill</td><td>Moderate</td><td>Legato/ unaccented</td></tr>
<tr><td colspan="4">Indication: Stretching vocal folds
Rationale: Assists singer in monitoring breath support (if breath flow stops, trill will stop); SOVT optimizes source-filter interaction (see chapter section on SOVT sounds)
Progression: Move to scalar pattern, glide over wider range, or continue 1-5-1 glide with vowels</td></tr>
</table>

<table>
<tr><th>Pitch and Rhythmic Pattern</th><th>Linguistic/Sound Content</th><th>Loudness Level</th><th>Degree of Accent</th></tr>
<tr><td>Two-octave pitch glide up and down</td><td>/i/ or /u/</td><td>Moderate</td><td>Legato/ unaccented</td></tr>
<tr><td colspan="4">Indication: Stretching vocal folds; more challenging than previous exercise
Rationale: Spans lowest to highest range, separates and unites registers to encourage mixing; stretches vocal folds starting with ligament and then muscle (Titze, 2001)
Progression: Move to scalar or arpeggiated pattern over same range</td></tr>
</table>

<table>
<tr><th>Pitch and Rhythmic Pattern</th><th>Linguistic/Sound Content</th><th>Loudness Level</th><th>Degree of Accent</th></tr>
<tr><td colspan="2">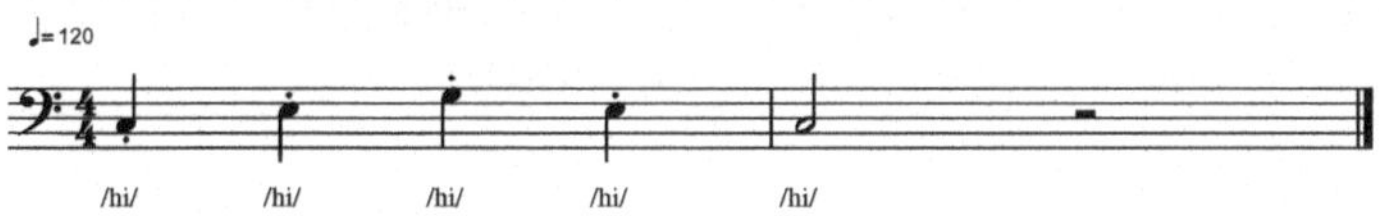</td><td>Moderate</td><td>Staccato</td></tr>
<tr><td colspan="4">Indication: Rapid coordination of respiration-phonation while avoiding mechanical stress to vocal folds
Rationale: Ascending and descending arpeggio spans moderate range so singer is not excessively taxed by extremes of TA/CT dominance; /h/ promotes clean onset coordinating breath-phonation; closed front vowel provides good options for formant tuning; staccato promotes precise coordination between respiratory mechanics and laryngeal movement for clean onset and pitch precision, training intrinsic laryngeal muscles holistically
Progression: Execute pattern twice, alternating staccato/legato to promote generalization of precision accomplished with staccato, or continue with staccato but over a wider interval (e.g., 1-3-5-8-5-3-1)</td></tr>
</table>

<table>
<tr><th>Pitch and Rhythmic Pattern</th><th>Linguistic/Sound Content</th><th>Loudness Level</th><th>Degree of Accent</th></tr>
<tr><td colspan="2">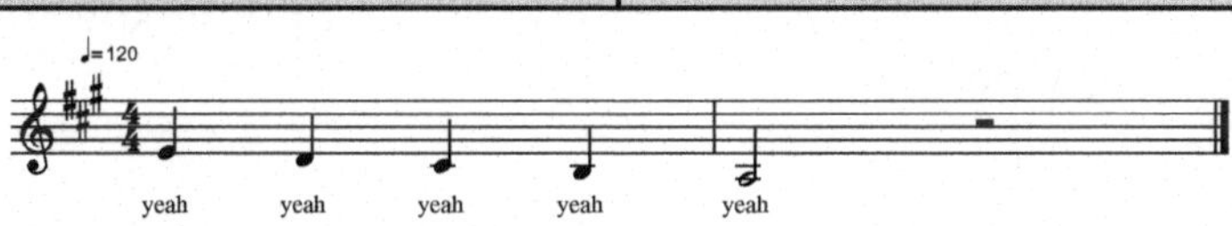</td><td>Moderate and constant with cues</td><td>Legato</td></tr>
<tr><td colspan="4">Indication: Belting
Rationale: Descending pitch pattern allows singer to start and stay in TA-dominant register to facilitate belting; repetition of /j/ initial in combination with /æ/ vowel promotes tongue and jaw</td></tr>
</table>

continues

Table 11–2. *continued*

mobility; /æ/ vowel has high first formant and promotes lip retraction, facilitating interaction of H2/F1 for belt; "yeah" is a frequently occurring word in CCM music; cuing singer to maintain loudness level of 5 to 6 on a 1 to 10 scale (10 being loudest) and to keep each note at the same loudness level facilitates optimal mix of TA/CT and avoids "pushing" as range gets higher

Progression: Move to more complex pitch pattern such as arpeggio (e.g., 1-3-5-3-1)

Pitch and Rhythmic Pattern	***Linguistic/Sound Content***	***Loudness Level***	***Degree of Accent***
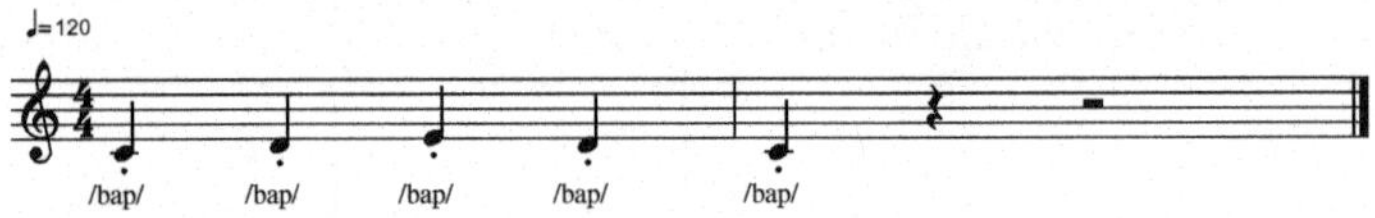		Moderate	Staccato

Indication: Improving glottic closure and/or achieving TA-dominant register

Rationale: Narrow range of pitch pattern minimizes need to negotiate register transition so that singer can focus on technical goal; initial voiced plosive positions vocal folds in adducted and "squared up" orientation to promote TA activation; unvoiced plosive at end accomplishes staccato by devoicing and articulation rather than abdominal movement, sets up complete glottic closure for next repetition of syllable; open back vowel keeps vocal tract in relatively neutral position; moderate loudness level encourages TA dominance; short duration of vowel (staccato) minimizes risk that singer will revert to incomplete closure or inadequate TA activation during sustained portion

Progression: Execute pattern twice, the second time sustaining /a/ for descending portion of exercise to see if singer can maintain TA activation and glottic closure on sustained vowel

STOCKING YOUR VOCAL EXERCISE PANTRY

As you've no doubt gathered by now, the possibilities for inventing vocal exercises are seemingly limitless, and a full exploration is clearly beyond the scope of this book. If you apply the principles herein and the examples from the next chapter, you will have a pretty good start, but the acquisition of new ingredients will be a lifelong endeavor for you. Pursue it actively! Table 11–3 lists some additional resources for finding specific exercises.

Vocal Function Exercises

Developed by Dr. Joseph Stemple, vocal function exercises (VFEs) are a series of systematic, isometric exercises that are designed to improve strength, endurance, and flexibility relative to respiration, phonation, and resonance (Stemple, Lee, D'Amico, & Pickup, 1994). Vocal function exercises have become a staple of voice therapy for both the speaking and singing voice since they were introduced by Dr. Stemple (Stemple, 1993), and the efficacy of these exercises both for speaking and singing voice has been demonstrated in numerous studies (Thomas & Stemple, 2007). Specific studies have demonstrated vocal improvement in aging patients (Gorman, Weinrich, Lee, & Stemple, 2008; Tay, Phyland, & Oates, 2011) and musical theater singers (Guzman, Angulo, Munoz, & Mayerhoff, 2013), but the exercises are widely considered to be beneficial in almost all populations, and they are regularly used by singing teachers and SLPs alike.

The exercise protocol consists of four exercises to be completed twice per day. The exercises are described as follows (Stemple et al., 1994):

1. Sustain /i/ as long as possible on a comfortable note
2. Glide from the lowest to the highest note in the frequency range using /o/
3. Glide from the highest to the lowest note in the frequency range using /o/
4. Sustain the musical notes C, D, E, F, and G above middle C for as long as possible using /o/. Repeat these notes two times.

The syllables "whoop" and "boom" are also recommended for Exercises 2 and 3, respectively (Stemple, 2006). The final exercise is often referred to as "adductory power" as it is considered to promote adductory strengthening (Lee & Stemple, 2007). A tutorial in vocal function exercises can be reviewed in DVD format (Stemple, 2006).

The exercises are often adapted and modified, particularly by singing teachers (LeBorgne & Rosenberg, 2014). I often use other SOVT sounds, such as straw phonation or trills instead of /o/ (by reason of the aforementioned benefits of such sounds), and I have the singer complete the adductory power exercise over each note of a one-octave diatonic major scale, with or without messa di voce. I also vary Stemple's Exercises 2 and 3 by having the singer complete the full-range glides ascending and descending in one gesture. I typically incorporate these variations on VFEs into the overall exercise regimen rather than having the singer complete them separately.

Table 11–3. Resources for Vocal Exercises

Speaking and singing exercises	Alison Behrman and John Haskell: *Exercises for Voice Therapy* (published by Plural Publishing); J. C. Stemple and E. R. Hapner, *Voice Therapy Clinical Case Studies*, 4th edition (published by Plural Publishing)
Classics of vocal pedagogy	Nicola Vaccai: *Practical Method of Italian Singing* (published by G. Schirmer, distributed by Hal Leonard) Mathilde Marchesi: *Marchesi Vocal Method* (published by G. Schirmir) Estelle Liebling: *Vocal Course* (published by Hal Leonard) Laure-Cinthie Damoreau: *Classic Bel Canto Technique* (published by Dover Publications)
Contemporary singing	Marci Rosenberg and Wendy D. Leborgne: *The Vocal Athlete: Application and Technique for the Hybrid Singer* (published by Plural Publishing) *So You Want to Sing: A Guide for Professionals* series from the National Association of Teachers of Singers (published by Rowman & Littlefield) • Karen Hall: *So You Want to Sing Music Theater* • Matthew Edwards: *So You Want to Sing Rock 'n' Roll* • Additional volumes pending http://www.nats.org/So_You_Want_To_Sing_Book_Series.html Jan Sullivan: *The Phenomena of the Belt/Pop Voice* (published by Logos Limited)
Vocal pedagogy programs	Jo Estill: Estill Voicetraining, https://www.estillvoice.com/ Jeannette LoVetri: Somatic Voicework: The LoVetri Method, http://www.thevoiceworkshop.com/somatic.html Mary Saunders-Barton: Bel Canto/Can Belto, http://belcantocanbelto.com/workshops Lisa Popeil: Voiceworks Method, http://www.popeil.com/

REFERENCES

Bastian, R. W., Keidar, A., & Verdolini-Marsten, K. (1990). Simple vocal tasks for detecting vocal fold swelling. *Journal of Voice, 4*, 172–183.

Edwards, M. (2014). *So you want to sing rock 'n' roll*. Lanham, MD: Rowman and Littlefield.

Gorman, S., Weinrich, B., Lee, L., & Stemple, J. (2008). Aerodynamic changes as a result of vocal function exercises in elderly men. *Laryngoscope, 118*(10), 1900–1903.

Guzman, M., Angulo, M., Munoz, D., & Mayerhoff, R. (2013). Effect on long-term average spectrum of pop singers' vocal warm-up with vocal function exercises. *International Journal of Speech Language Pathology, 15*(2), 127–135.

Kapsner-Smith, M. R., Hunter, E. J., Kirkham, K., Cox, K., & Titze, I. R. (2015). A randomized controlled trial of two semi-occluded vocal tract voice therapy protocols. *Journal of Speech, Language, and Hearing Research, 58*, 535–549.

Kotby, M. N. (1995). *The accent method of voice therapy*. San Diego, CA: Singular.

LeBorgne, W. D., & Rosenberg, M. (2014). *The vocal athlete*. San Diego, CA: Plural.

Lessac, A. (1997). *The use and training of the human voice: A bio-dynamic approach to vocal life*. Mountain View, CA: Mayfield.

Miller, D. (2008). *Resonance in singing*. Princeton, NJ: Inside View Press.

Saxon, K., & Schneider, C. (1995). *Vocal exercise physiology*. San Diego, CA: Singular.

Stemple, J. (1984). *Clinical voice pathology, theory and management*. Columbus, OH: Merrill.

Stemple, J. C. (1993). *Voice therapy: Clinical studies.* St. Louis, MO: Mosby Yearbook.

Stemple, L. (2006). *Vocal function exercises: DVD.* San Diego, CA: Plural.

Stemple, J., Lee, L., D'Amico, B., & Pickup, B. (1994). Efficacy of vocal function exercises as a method of improving voice production. *Journal of Voice, 8*, 271–278.

Tay, E., Phyland, D., & Oates, J. (2011). The effect of vocal function exercises on the voices of aging community choral singers. *Journal of Voice, 26*(5), 19–27.

Titze, I. R. (2001). The five best vocal warm-up exercises. *Journal of Singing, 57*(3), 51–52.

Titze, I. R. (2010, March 5). Posting on AHSA SIG3 listserve. sid3voice@list.healthcare.uiowa.edu

Titze, I. R., & Laukkanen, A. M. (2007). Can vocal economy in phonation be increased with an artificially lengthened vocal tract? A computer modeling study. *Logopedics Phoniatrics Vocology, 32*, 147–156.

Titze, I. R., & Verdolini Abbott, K. (2012). *Vocology: The science and practice of voice habilitation.* Salt Lake City, UT: National Center for Voice and Speech.

Thomas, L., & Stemple, J. C. (2007). Voice therapy: Does science support the art? *Communicative Disorders Review, 1*(1), 49–77.

CHAPTER 12

Customizing Vocal Exercises for Singing Voice Rehabilitation

We have now explored how motor learning and exercise physiology principles apply to vocal coordination and conditioning. We have reviewed the ways in which the voicing subsystems interact with each other and how we can optimize this interaction to produce desirable vocal sounds with minimal vocal expense. We have discussed the physiologic and acoustical differences between different styles of singing and the ramifications for voice habilitation and rehabilitation. We have stocked our vocal exercise pantry with the ingredients we need and developed rationales for combining them to create a variety of vocal exercises. Now it's time to integrate all this knowledge and information to customize vocal coordination and conditioning exercises on an individual basis.

In this section, we survey some of the most common functional and structural voice disorders and ideas on how to best achieve resolution or adaptive compensation through vocal exercise and technique. Voice disorders are too complex and their individual presentations too numerous for us to exhaustively encompass all scenarios and rehabilitation options within these pages. My intention is to provide you with a jumping-off point—a foundation on which to build your skills, insight, intuition, and proficiency. Each singer you work with will teach you something new to add to your store of resources.

MUSCLE TENSION DYSPHONIA

For many of the singers you work with, muscle tension will be a component of the voice problem, either as the primary diagnosis or as a secondary factor that arises from the body's attempts to compensate for an underlying structural or functional deficit. In all likelihood, you will need to address the muscle tension directly as part of the rehabilitation plan.

Anchoring the Larynx

In the grand scheme of body structures and systems (and compared with other musical instruments), the larynx is tiny, with a small, mostly cartilaginous skeleton that houses the vocal folds and diminutive muscles that animate and position them. The vocal folds in turn interact with the air from the lungs and with the vocal tract to produce pitch range and acoustic power that are quite astonishing considering their size. In singing, the structures of the larynx must rapidly and repeatedly adjust and reposition to accomplish the target sound, then with split-second timing reposition for the next target again and again. If these movements are not perfectly executed, the system may quickly become unstable, resulting in undesirable sounds, inefficient production, and maladaptive muscle tension.

The hand is another structure in the body that is relatively small and must execute exquisitely fine-tuned motor movements, such as writing. When we undertake such a task, the body's wisdom guides us to automatically provide a means of bracing the hand and fingers for the fine movement, placing our forearm or wrist on the writing surface. Phonosurgery is another such fine-motor manual endeavor. When executing micromanipulations of tiny instruments to operate on vocal fold lesions that may be the size of a grain of rice, the laryngologist sits in a special chair that supports the arms so that the hands and fingers can maneuver freely.

The larynx is constantly seeking this type of bracing to execute the athletic moves required for singing, often finding it in adjacent real estate such as the tongue and jaw. Although well equipped to provide the necessary bracing in terms of relative strength, these structures are poor candidates for the job as they are highly involved in shaping the resonator and positioning the larynx. Thus, bracing in these structures typically leads to maladaptive muscle tension that interferes with vocal quality and production. If one can achieve more appropriate bracing (or anchoring), the maladaptive articulatory tension will, in many cases, release. For this reason, it is important to consider a primary exploration of anchoring before directly addressing the maladaptive muscle tension, particularly in the tongue and jaw.

Fortunately, there are a number of locations in the body that can be recruited very effectively for providing laryngeal bracing or anchoring. Relatively small gestures in the head and neck and/or engagement of larger structures of the

Allocation of Effort

A key concept relative to anchoring for laryngeal stabilization (and when working with any maladaptive muscle tension) is allocation of effort. Maladaptive tension arises out of the effort the task demands. Singing is effortful. One can't simply say, "Relax that" without determining why the effort is called for and how it can be more effectively distributed. Thus, it will be most meaningful to direct the singer to take the effort currently being expended in a detrimental manner and consciously and constructively redirect it. The anchoring strategies presented here provide an avenue for accomplishing this reallocation. They will be especially helpful in singing situations that are more complex and demanding, such as singing at high pitch, for long duration of phonation, and when agility is required.

torso, pelvic floor, or even the lower body (hips and legs) are among the options for stabilizing the larynx. A number of strategies are described below. This sample menu is by no means exhaustive but provides a variety of ideas for you to incorporate into your "pantry" relative to releasing maladaptive muscle tension and stabilizing the larynx. These approaches may be used in isolation or in combinations. Have the singer execute exercises or repertoire while in various positions and assess the impact on muscle tension and sound quality. Once you find an effective position, the goal will be to gradually achieve the same alignment and engagement in a standing posture (or whatever performance posture is typical for the singer). Tips for accomplishing this are included below. When you understand the underlying principles of these alignment and stabilization strategies, you can use your imagination guided by your knowledge to adapt, modify, and invent for each individual singer.

Head and Neck Anchoring

Head and neck anchoring primarily involves engaging the powerful sternocleidomastoid (SCM) muscles to create a "scaffold" for the larynx anteriorly and posteriorly, with the engaged SCMs forming the anterior portion and the cervical spine forming the posterior portion. The optimal engagement of the SCMs assists a desirable orientation of the cervical spine with the occipital skull. "Imagine a string going from the crown of the head into the ceiling" is a common description of this alignment, and such a cue can sometimes be enough to achieve the necessary bracing of the larynx. This can be enhanced with gentle backward pressure on the forehead without allowing the head to move backwards. You can either apply this pressure yourself with the tips of your fingers, or cue the singer to do so. The goal is for the singer to feel the engagement of the SCMs and resulting alignment and gradually try to achieve the same engagement without the external pressure. This and other strategies for head and neck anchoring are described in the work of Jo Estill (Klimak, 2003). This strategy may be contraindicated in singers with excessive neck tension as it may exacerbate the problem. In such cases, it is often better to reallocate effort lower in the body, as described below.

Klimak (2003) lists several subtler gestures that also utilize the muscles of the soft palate and superior pharyngeal constrictor, such as flaring the nostrils, simulating sucking on a straw that is occluded, simulating a biting gesture, or simulating the onset of a sneeze.

Torso Anchoring

Bracing or anchoring the torso can provide laryngeal stability both by engaging the length of the spine to achieve an effect similar to that described above for the cervical spine and also by freeing the abdominal and respiratory muscles to make them more available for effective breath support. Torso anchoring utilizes the muscles of the upper and lower back, chest, abdomen, and pelvic floor to stabilize the larynx. These core strength muscles are important for general balance and stability of the body. Activating them for singing can help take the load off the larynx.

Using the Shoulder, Chest, and Upper Back Muscles for Anchoring. Engaging the muscles of the back (particularly latissimus dorsi) and the pectoralis muscles of the chest assists in anchoring the torso for laryngeal stability. This element of anchoring is also featured in Estill training (Klimak, 2003). To elicit the gesture, have the singer stand with arms at his or her side. Cue the singer to gently pull the shoulders down. "Move the shoulders away from the ears" can be a useful prompt. Alternatively, have the singer hold the arms at right angles, with elbows out to the side and fingers pointed upward. Push down on the singer's biceps while cuing the singer to resist your attempt to move the arms downward, or simply have the singer simulate this gesture by imagining the maneuver.

You can get the muscles of the arms and shoulders even more involved in torso anchoring by using a fitness ball. Have the singer hold his or her arms out in front with the fitness ball suspended between the hands and the wall. Make sure the singer is standing in such a way that the ears, shoulders, hips, and feet are in a straight line. Then have the singer push the ball into the wall with the arms without changing this alignment (Figure 12–1). This gesture engages the arms, shoulders, chest, and upper back. Make sure the singer is not using the whole body to push the ball by leaning into it—only the arms should move when alternating the relaxed versus engaged posture.

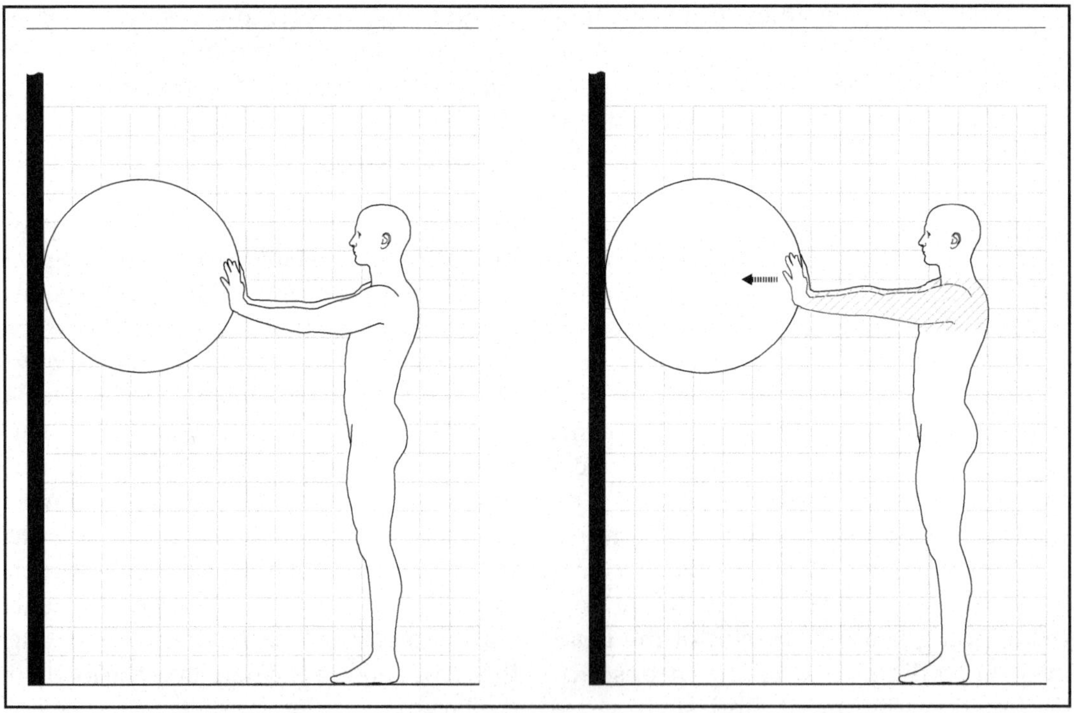

***Figure 12–1.** Using the shoulder, chest, and upper back muscles for anchoring with assistance of fitness ball. The "relaxed" posture is shown on the left and the "engaged" posture on the right. Shaded areas indicate location of engagement. Illustration by Bud Northern Design.*

Using the Lower Back, Lower Abdomen, Pelvic Floor, and Lower Limbs for Anchoring

There are a number of strategies for eliciting engagement of the lower back, lower abdomen, and pelvic floor to assist with torso and laryngeal stability. The large muscles of the lower limbs (gluteals, quadriceps, hamstrings) can assist with this anchoring as well. In all exercises, the goal is to engage core strength and maintain the position of the torso over the pelvic floor. For additional information and tips on mobilization of the pelvis and improving stability, see Gilman (2014).

Wall Squat. Have the singer stand with the back to the wall with the knees bent and the feet positioned 12 to 18 inches from the wall (Figure 12–2A). The back of the head, shoulder blades, and hips should be touching the wall. The curves of the neck and back will not touch the wall but should not be arched. The ear, shoulder, and hip should be in a straight line when viewed from the side. Depending on body morphology and head shape, the back of the head may need to be supported to achieve this alignment and avoid hyperextending the cervical spine backward. You can use a small towel or washcloth to create a "pillow" for the

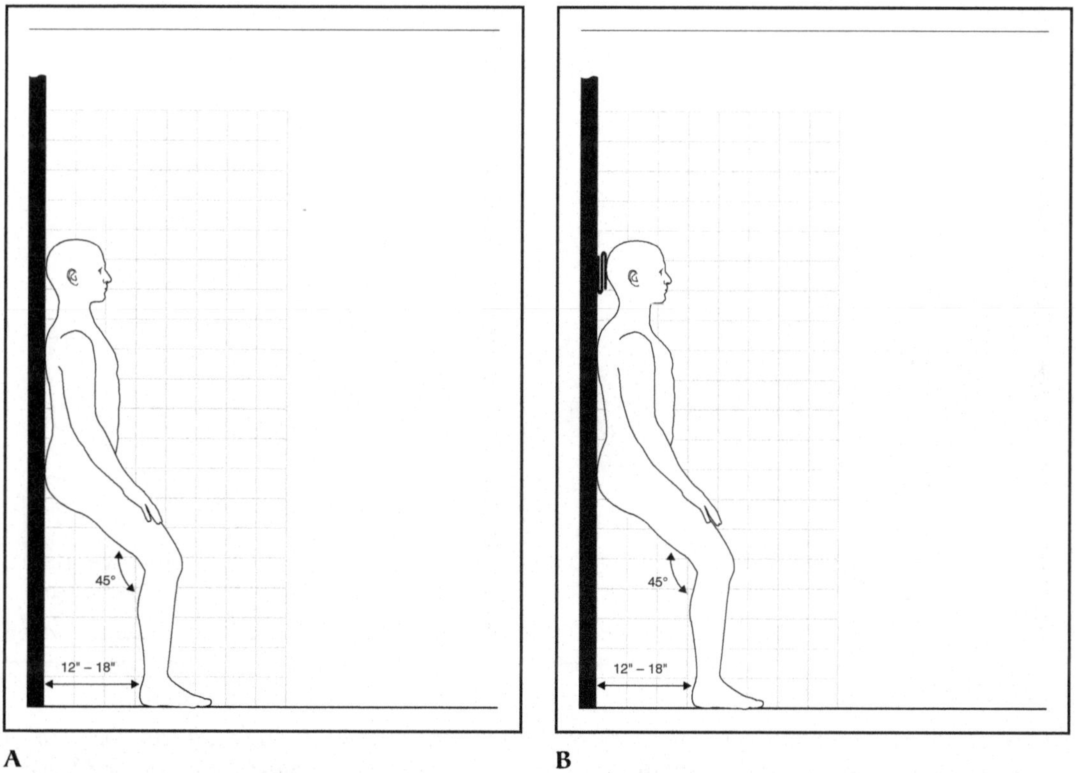

***Figure 12–2. A.** Torso anchoring using the wall to support squat position. **B.** Illustrates supporting the head to maintain optimal alignment. Illustrations by Bud Northern Design.*

back of the head, folding it to achieve the desired thickness (Figure 12–2B). Cue the singer to "let the wall hold you" or to imagine lying supine against the wall.

Seated "Pushback." Have the singer sit on the edge of the chair, with the torso and thighs forming a right angle and the thighs and calves forming a right angle (Figure 12–3A). It is helpful to position the chair against a wall. Depending on the chair height and length of the singer's legs, the angle of the torso and thighs might be slightly greater or less than 90 degrees. The ear, shoulder, and hip should be aligned when viewed from the side. Cue the singer to gently push back with the heels without changing the alignment of the head and torso (Figure 12–3B). The toes should remain on the floor (e.g., should not be lifted up). This gesture of pushing backward with the heels will engage the muscles of the lower abdomen, lower back, pelvic floor, and legs. It is important that the engagement remain moderate—pushing back too much can result in clenching the abdomen, and this tension may radiate upward in the body

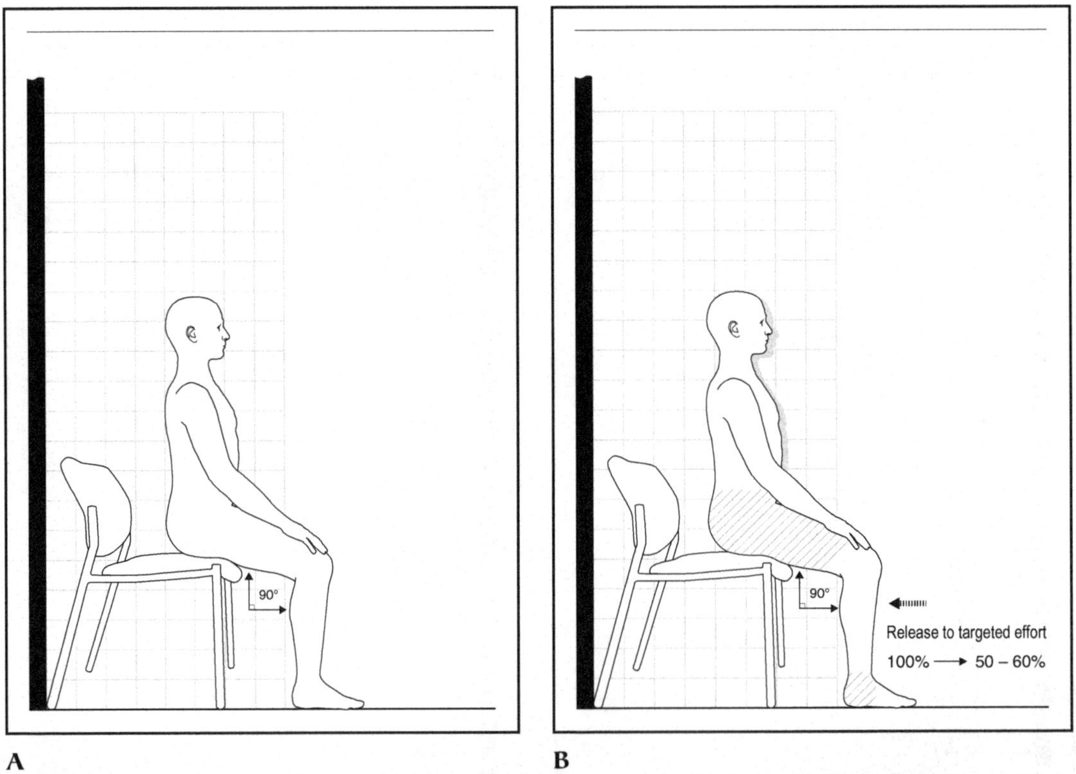

***Figure 12–3. A–B.** Torso anchoring with seated pushback. Shaded areas indicate location of engagement when pushing back with the heels to 50% to 60% effort. Illustrations by Bud Northern Design.*

to the abdomen, neck, or even the jaw. To avoid this, cue the singer to push back with 100% effort, then release to about 50% to 60% so that he or she can experience the range of engagement. Maintaining 50% to 60% of maximum effort should be effective, but adapt as needed based on results. Encourage the singer to explore and note the sensations associated with this gesture to aid in establishing a reference sensation for the engagement, and then have him or her try singing while this engagement is activated.

Sitting/Bouncing on the Fitness Ball. Have the singer sit on the fitness ball. The torso should be directly over the pelvic floor, which should be centered on the ball (Figure 12–4A). If the singer is in a lordotic posture, cue him or her to roll or tuck the hips forward until the back is straight, and the ear, shoulder, and hip are aligned when viewed from the side (Figures 12–4B and C).

To enhance the target engagement, have the singer gently bounce on the ball while singing (Figure 12–4D).

To further enhance the engagement, after a few bounces, cue the singer to "hold the top of the bounce" (Figure 12–4E). This requires even more activation of the muscles of the lower abdomen and back and can really help to cement the reference sensation. Depending on the singer's degree of core strength, this gesture may or may not be achievable, and even with good core strength, he or she may only be able to hold it for a few seconds before releasing. It is important to avoid leaning forward as in Figure 12–4F, which results in reliance on leg muscles versus core strength, and may confuse the target sensation. Holding the "top of the bounce" position is a more challenging movement, so if the singer cannot achieve the maneuver, simply abandon it in favor of one of the previous steps.

Ball-Assisted Squat. Have the singer stand with the fitness ball between the back and the wall with the legs extended at about a 45-degree angle (Figure 12–5A). The ball should fit into the curve of the back. The ear, shoulder, and hip should be in a line when viewed from the side. Have the singer slowly roll down into a squat, maintaining this alignment, feeling the engagement of the lower abdomen, lower back, pelvic floor, and leg muscles (Figure 12–5B). The singer should try singing in the squat position, and then experiment with going back and forth between the standing and squatting positions to establish a reference sensation for the engagement.

To enhance, cue the singer to gently push back with the heels while in the squat position, as in the seated pushback above (Figure 12–5C).

Getting Upright. Ultimately, the goal is to find an anchoring strategy that is effective, and then to achieve the same engagement in a performance posture. Once the singer can consistently execute the gesture successfully, have him or her transition to a squat position without the assistance of the chair or ball and gradually stand out of the squat, maintaining the anchoring engagement (Figure 12–6).

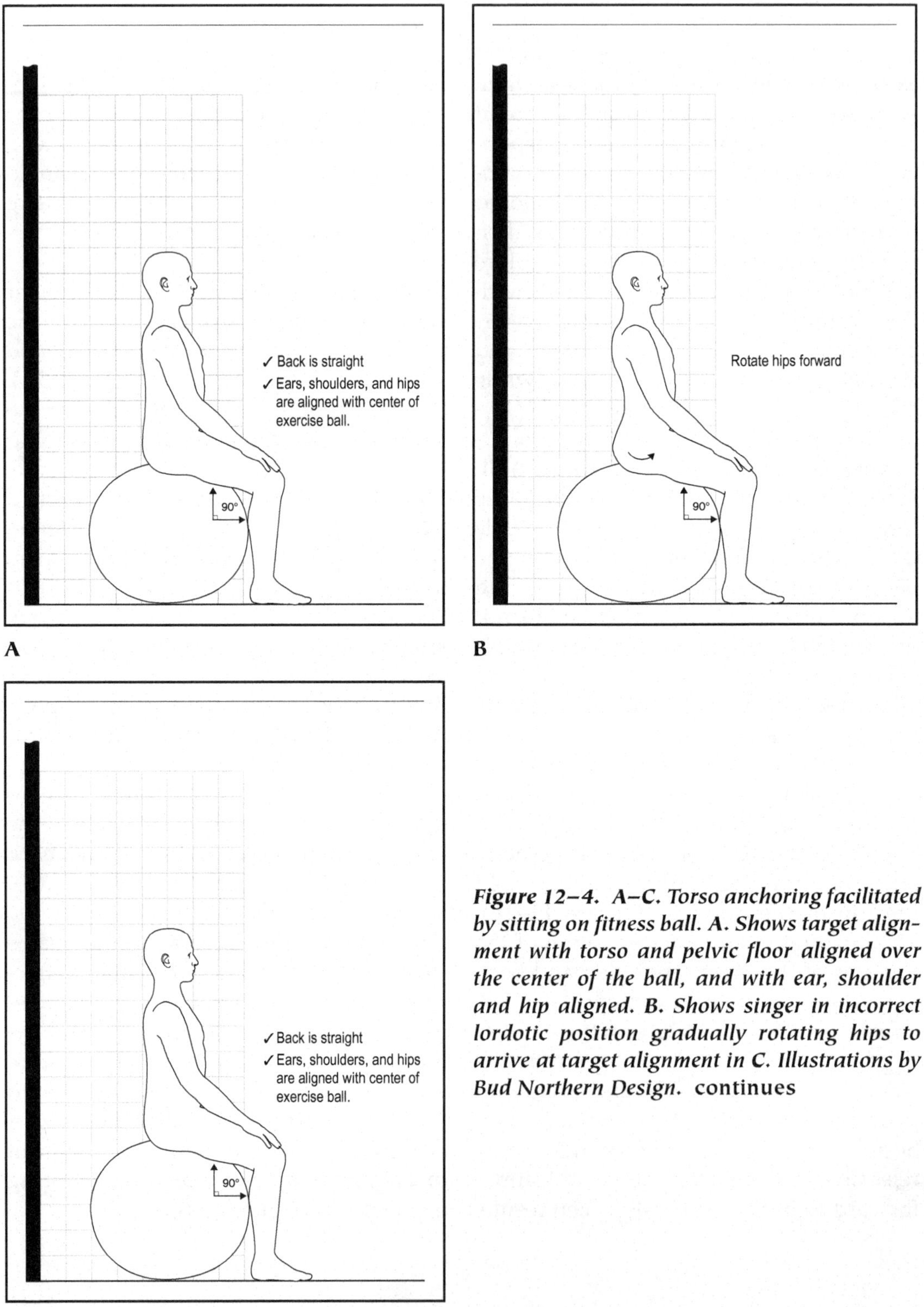

A

B

C

Figure 12–4. A–C. *Torso anchoring facilitated by sitting on fitness ball.* ***A.*** *Shows target alignment with torso and pelvic floor aligned over the center of the ball, and with ear, shoulder and hip aligned.* ***B.*** *Shows singer in incorrect lordotic position gradually rotating hips to arrive at target alignment in* ***C.*** *Illustrations by Bud Northern Design.* continues

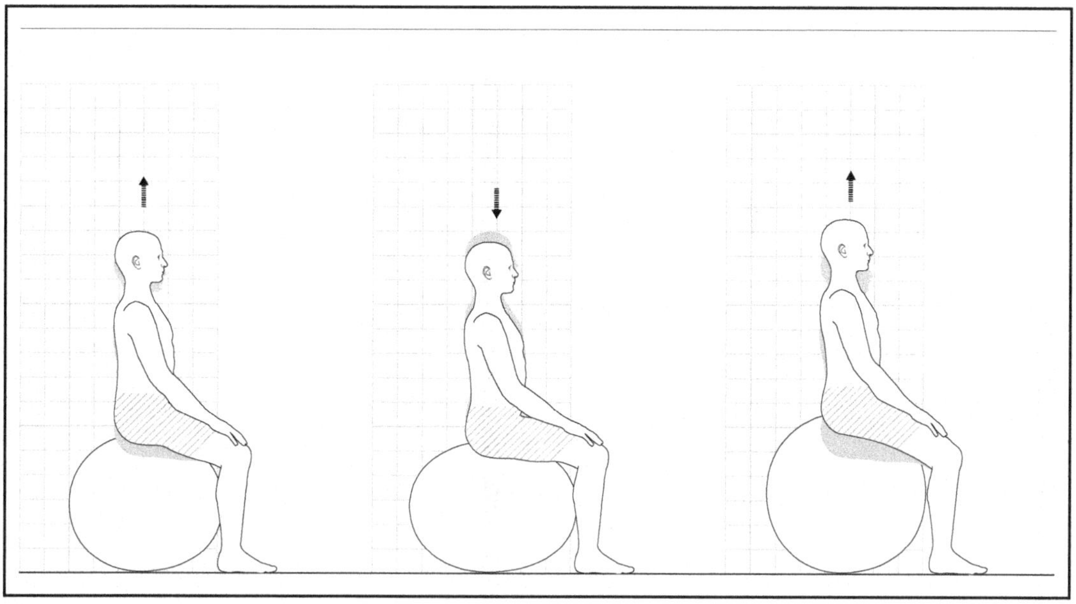

D

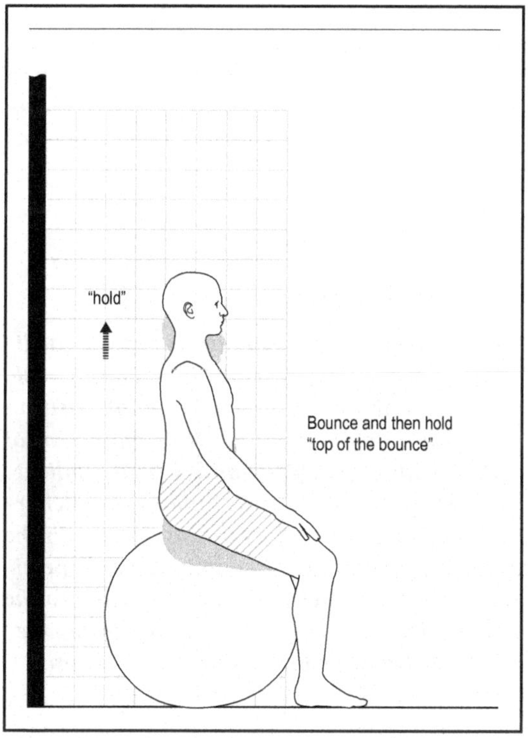

E

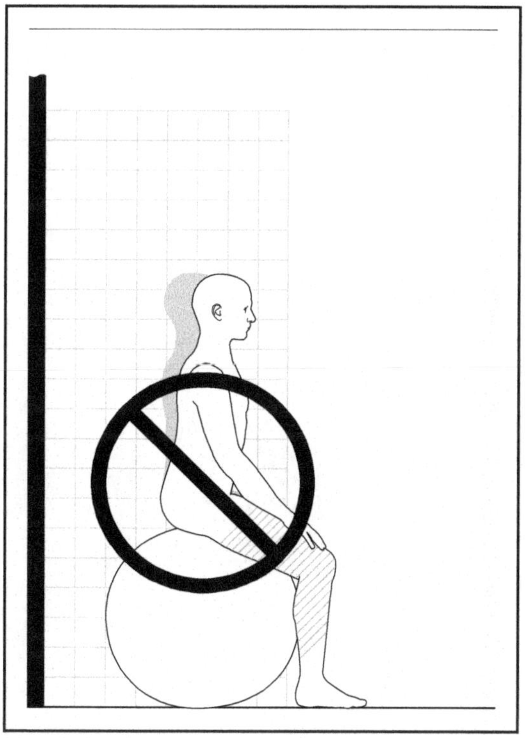

F

Figure 12–4. continued *D. Bouncing on fitness ball to enhance torso anchoring. E. Enhancing torso anchoring by holding "top of the bounce" position. Shaded areas indicate location of engagement. F. Avoid leaning forward when attempting to hold "top of the bounce" position. Illustrations by Bud Northern Design.*

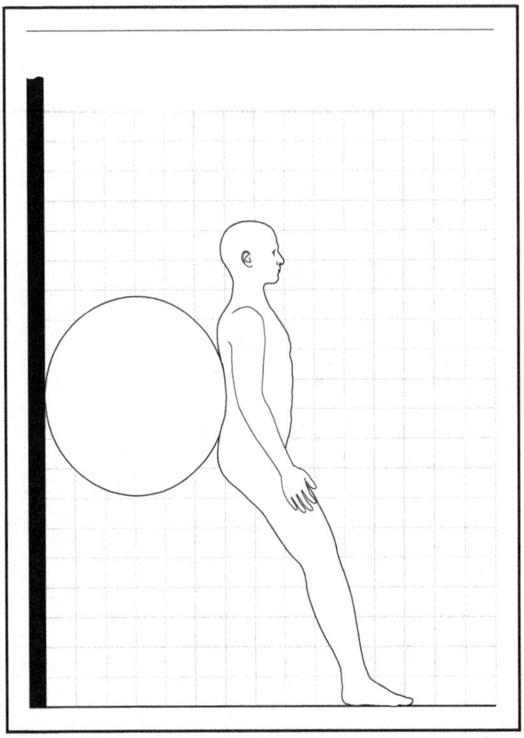

A

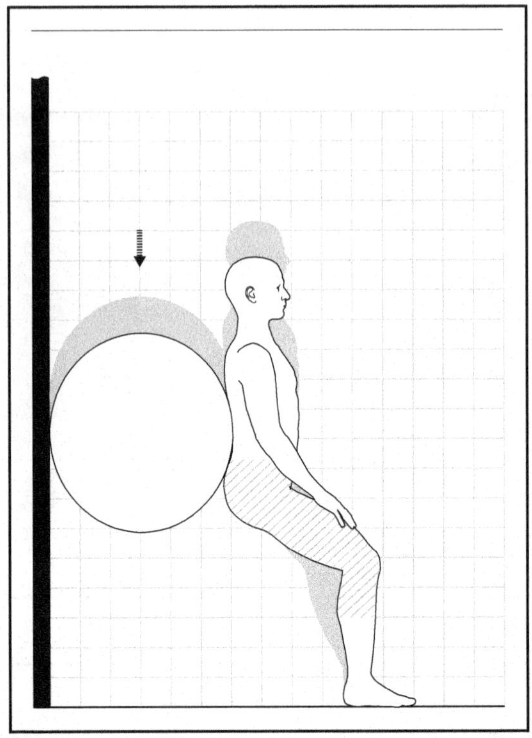

B

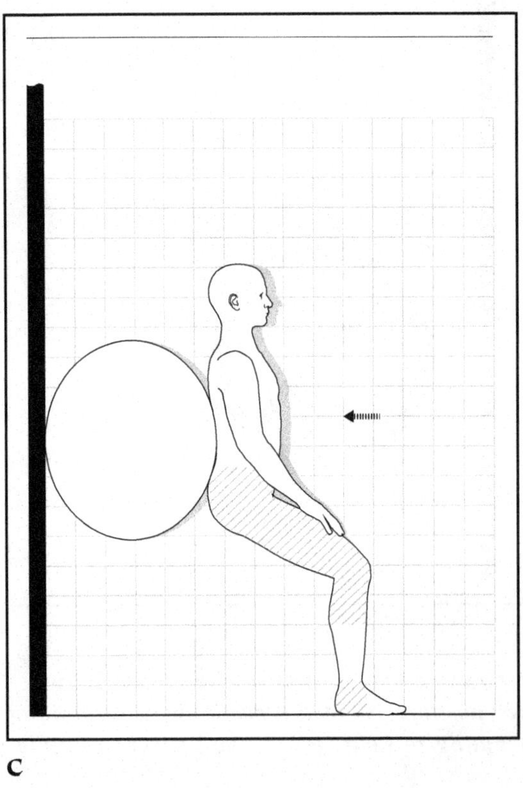

C

Figure 12–5. ***A–B.*** *Using fitness ball to facilitate squat position, starting in standing position (A) and rolling down to squat position maintaining alignment (B). Note alignment of ear, shoulder, and hip. Shaded areas indicate location of engagement.* ***C.*** *Enhancing anchoring in squat position by pushing back with the heels, engaging lower abdominal, back, pelvic floor, and leg muscles to push the ball into the wall. Shaded areas indicate location of engagement. Illustrations by Bud Northern Design.*

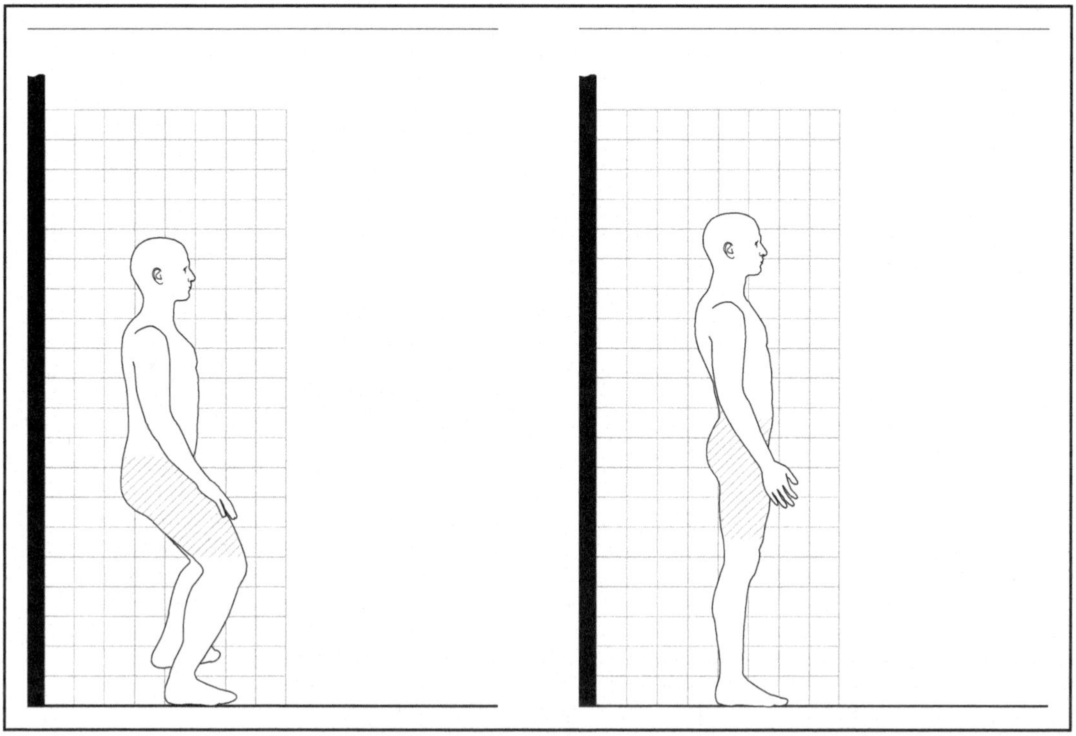

***Figure 12–6.** Transitioning from squat to standing position while maintaining anchoring in the lower body. Shaded areas indicate location of engagement. Illustrations by Bud Northern Design.*

Tongue Tension

The tongue is a powerful, intricately muscled structure and is often a first resort as a locus of effort in singing. Unfortunately, its direct attachment to the larynx makes it a poor choice for effective anchoring, as tension in the tongue will inevitably result in increasing laryngeal effort. Tongue tension often invites the jaw to get in on the endeavor, too. Sometimes what appears to be jaw tension is primarily a reflection of tongue tension.

See Table 12–1 for strategies to reduce maladaptive tongue tension. Strategies are presented in order of degree of external assistance, from greatest to least. Those that provide the greatest external assistance will provide the most structure and are appropriate for severe tongue tension. Note that vowels will naturally be distorted by protruded tongue positions. If the singer can easily execute the exercises that are less structured, proceed directly to those exercises. Work in a pitch range that is amenable to the positioning. You may have to alternate strategies depending on pitch range. For example, the singer may easily accomplish /jaɪ/ syllables without holding the tongue in low or middle range, but may need to hold the tongue to get it to release in the high range. Once the singer is proficient at a given level, move on to a less structured task, then ultimately fade the strategy altogether.

All of the exercises in Table 12–1 require the tongue to release its "locked"

Table 12–1. Strategies for Reducing Maladaptive Tongue Tension

Strategy	Tips and Cueing
Use a piece of gauze or paper towel (never tissue) to gently hold the tip of the tongue (moistening the gauze or towel can make this exercise more tolerable for those who have a sensitive gag reflex). The tongue should be protruded well over the lower lip, but without pulling on it. Sing on /ɑ/ or /æ/. As the tongue becomes less resistant to the protruded position, have the singer try singing on /jaɪ/, exaggerating the excursion of the base of the tongue in articulating the diphthong.	The tongue should be in a relatively flat and relaxed position, with the tip pointing down toward the chin, not lifted. Monitor for retraction or lifting of the tongue, which will tell you that the tongue is resisting the position. Cue the singer to both watch for retraction in the mirror and feel for it in the hand that is holding the tongue. When the singer can easily sing on /ɑ/ or /æ/ while holding the tongue, transition to repetitions of /jaɪ/. All the articulation should be accomplished by the movement of the back of the tongue *without* assistance from the jaw. Gradually release the tongue to rest in the mouth to sing on sustained vowels or continue on to /jaɪ/ without holding the tongue, as described below.
Position the tip of the tongue behind the bottom front teeth and protrude the tongue dorsum out and over the bottom front teeth. Sing on /ɑ/ or /æ/.	If the tongue attempts to retract, cue the singer to gently push the tongue forward, maintaining contact between the tongue tip and bottom front teeth. Gradually release the tongue to rest in the mouth.
Hold a drinking straw horizontally under the tongue. The straw should rest on the bottom teeth with the tongue gently laying over it and protruding out of the mouth. Sing on /ɑ/ or /æ/.	This position will likely be challenging at first. Having the singer hold the end of the straw will prevent it from dropping. The tongue should remain in a wide, flat position, not curled. If the straw bends under the tongue, the singer is using too much downward pressure. Once the singer can consistently sing with the straw under the tongue, have him or her gradually remove the straw and attempt to continue singing on vowels with the same degree of release.
Sing pitch patterns (such as 1-2-3-2-1) on the syllable /jaI/, repeating the syllable on each note, exaggerating excursion of the base of the tongue in articulating the diphthong. The tip of the tongue should rest against the bottom front teeth.	As above, the articulation should be accomplished only by moving the base of the tongue, without assistance from the jaw. Gradually transition from the diphthong to sustained vowels, starting with /ɑ/.
Alternate /ŋ/ with /ɑ/ with jaw stabilized.	Articulation should be accomplished with tongue movement only.
"Raspberry" (labio-lingual trill) or tongue trill.	The tongue is forced to release in order to vibrate to produce the trill. If the singer is unable to produce the trill, probe to see if he or she is successful with an unvoiced trill. If so, this tells you that the tongue tension is tied to phonation. Have the singer start the trill unvoiced and gradually add voicing. If tension is severe, you may need to start by prolonging the unvoiced trill and attempting phonation very briefly. Gradually increase the duration of the voiced trill as proficiency increases.

Table 12–1. *continued*

Strategy	*Tips and Cueing*
Hum with the tongue protruded	The tongue should be protruded over the lower lip and the lips should be closed around it. Have the singer experiment with how far the tongue is protruded to see what effect differing positions have on the sound quality and degree of release. The tongue should remain relatively flat, without elevating the tip or curling the sides. When the singer can execute the task reliably, move on to alternating /m/ and /a/ with the tongue still protruded. Gradually allow the tongue to relax back into the mouth, maintaining the release that was accomplished with the protrusion.

Note. *Visual feedback from a mirror will be helpful in all strategies, enabling the singer to monitor the position of the tongue and identify when the tongue attempts to retract. Strategies are presented in order of degree of external assistance from more to less.*

position and move freely. The singer may notice a sensation of fatigue in the base of the tongue after completing exercises. This is normal and should resolve over time. If the singer is experiencing pain, the strategy is not working. Regroup and continue to explore strategies for tongue and other possible loci of tension until you find one that works.

Edwards (2014) recommends use of nonsense words like "glockida" and "diddle daddle deedle daddle do" to promote tongue movement. Executing these sequences with the jaw stabilized isolates tongue movement from the jaw.

For further discussion and additional tips relative to reducing tongue tension and optimizing tongue mobility, see Rosenberg and LeBorgne (2014), Gilman (2014), and LeFevre (2011).

Jaw Tension

The jaw is another powerful articulator that can be a component of maladaptive muscle tension. See Table 12–2 for strategies to reduce jaw tension. Remember that tongue tension can masquerade as jaw tension, so if the jaw strategies do not result in a decrease in laryngeal effort and improved vocal quality, consider going back to the tongue tension reduction strategies. As noted above, you may need to adjust the strategies depending on pitch range. For additional strategies for releasing jaw tension, see Gilman (2014).

> Temporomandibular joint dysfunction (TMJ or TMD) is a common disorder with a prevalence of 5% to 12% (National Institute of Dental and Craniofacial Research, 2014). If you work with a singer who reports chronic jaw pain, consider referral to a physical therapist (PT) with expertise in head and neck disorders. The PT may in turn refer to a dentist or oral surgeon.

Laryngeal Tension

Laryngeal tension may result from inadequate coordination of phonation subsystems. If this is the case, the tension should

Table 12–2. *Strategies for Reducing Maladaptive Jaw Tension*

Strategy	***Tips and Cueing***
Hold the mandible with the hand. The thumb and index finger should be positioned to create a "c" shape spanning the mandible, with the thumb and index finger spanning the lower jaw and the chin nested between them. Drop the jaw and gently allow the weight of the hand to hold the jaw in an open position. Sing on sustained vowels.	You can either have the singer hold his or her own jaw, or use your hand to demonstrate and assist. The jaw should not be forcefully opened, nor should it open to the fullest possible extent (which could exacerbate tension). Be careful to ensure that having the hand on the jaw does not result in tucking the chin or tilting the head downward.
Hold the tip of the tongue against the roof of the mouth. Gently move the jaw up and down in isolation and while singing on /n/ or /l/.	The excursion of the jaw does not need to extend to the full range of motion. The goal is for the singer to experience a sensation of soft and mobile jaw vs. stiff or tight jaw. If you notice a lot of deviation in the tracking of the jaw during this exercise, the singer may have TMD. Consider referral to PT as noted in this chapter.
Engage a gentle "chewing" motion in isolation and during phonation using nasal consonants.	Again, the range of motion should be moderate, targeting gentle mobilization.
Waggle the jaw from side to side or up and down while singing sustained vowels.	Watch for stiff movement from one fixed position to the next. The movement of the jaw should be continuous, smooth, and loose. The waggling may be assisted manually.
Sing pitch pattern (such as 1-2-3-2-1 or 5-4-3-2-1) on "blah," repeating the syllable on each note.	Cue the singer to use a lot of jaw and tongue movement, even allowing the cheeks to puff out when producing the syllable.
Sing on /wau/ or /jal/, emphasizing excursion of jaw.	In contrast to the tongue exercises earlier, the goal here is to encourage excursion in the jaw.

Note. *Visual feedback from a mirror will be helpful in all strategies, enabling the singer to monitor the position and movement of the jaw. Strategies are presented in order of degree of external assistance from more to less.*

resolve with improved breath support and optimizing source-filter interaction. SOVT sounds are particularly beneficial for reducing laryngeal tension and effort.

Laryngeal tension is often a reflection of maladaptive muscle tension in another location. Consider the role that tongue or jaw tension may be playing and be sure to address those areas appropriately. The anchoring strategies enumerated above are also facilitating for reducing laryngeal tension.

Although laryngeal tension is often secondary, there may be times when you find it beneficial to address the larynx directly. Sometimes the problem results from inappropriate laryngeal height. Remember from Chapter 10 that a low larynx is needed to achieve the long resonator of classical singing and a high larynx for the shorter resonator of belting. If the singer is a belter but has been taught to lower the larynx, a somatic argument may ensue, resulting in laryngeal tension. Conversely, if a singer in classical style has not learned to adequately lower the larynx and is attempting to sing with the larynx in the more neutral speech posture, laryngeal tension could be the outcome.

Have the singer monitor laryngeal position by placing the thumb and index finger in the thyrohyoid space. High larynx position can be elicited by elevating the chin or even tilting the head backward in isolation and while phonating. A spoken "yeah?" with upward inflection can also elicit higher larynx position, as can articulating /gi/. For low larynx, have the singer inhale with a yawning gesture, feeling the larynx drop with the yawn, and then attempt to maintain this lower posture during phonation. Another way to lower the larynx is to explore the movement of the larynx when articulating /b/. The larynx drops as we start this phoneme. Once the singer feels the movement, have him or her try to hold the onset of /b/. When the position is established, the singer should try to maintain the lower larynx position during phonation. For further information on facilitating low larynx for classical singing, see LeFevre (2015). For additional ideas on unloading laryngeal constriction, see Edwards (2014).

Upper Body Tension

Maladaptive muscle tension can manifest itself in the neck, shoulders, arms, and even the upper torso. Often the tension takes the form of a holding or clenching gesture. If the tension results from poor alignment or inadequate stabilization of the head, neck, or torso, application of the strategies enumerated earlier in this chapter may effectively release the upper body tension. If the tension is more isolated, mobilizing the area in question serves to bring the singer's awareness to the location of the tension and will often help to release it. Some strategies for mobilizing the upper body to reduce tension are listed below. For additional ideas and techniques for addressing upper body tension, see Gilman (2014).

Reducing Upper Body Tension

Have the singer practice the technique first in isolation. Try incorporating breathing awareness into the movements (e.g., "Inhale as you raise the shoulders, exhale as you release them down"). Gradually transition to phonation while still executing the movement, progressively increasing the complexity of the task.

Instruct the singer to:

- Tilt the head forward and backward and/or from side to side
- Rotate the head from side to side, looking first over one shoulder, then the other
- Raise and lower (shrug) the shoulders, either together or one at a time
- Swing the arms like a pendulum in parallel or reciprocally, "swim" the arms backward or forward, raise and lower the arms like a jumping jack, or hold the arms overhead
- Twist side to side from the waist, letting the arms swing with the side-to-side motion

Throwing objects or simulating a throwing gesture can also be beneficial (and engages core strength for stability). You can use a small foam ball or beach ball. Be sure to arrange the space to reduce risk of breaking objects.

- Have the singer throw the ball across the room, first with one arm, then the other, or with both arms.
- Have the singer throw the ball into the air and then catch it as it comes down.
- Play catch with the singer, throwing the ball back and forth between you.

Abdominal Tension

Abdominal clenching is very common for a variety of reasons. People often try to hold the abdomen in to make it look flatter and avoid "letting it all hang out." The abdomen is an area of the body where we naturally hold tension when concentrating or when feeling tense or stressed. In my experience, abdominal clenching frequently arises from misunderstandings about the mechanics of breath support or from overemphasis on breath support in the training process.

Suggestions for releasing abdominal tension are provided below. For additional ideas and techniques, see Gilman (2014). For tutorials on teaching the mechanics of breath support, see Gilman (2014) and Edwards (2014).

> Breath support gets blamed for a world of sins in singing. Of course optimizing breath support is essential for successful singing, but if the problem lies elsewhere and the singer is instructed to "support more," excessive abdominal tension may result. For example, the problem may be inappropriate laryngeal height, inadequate resonance, or unfavorable interaction of source-filter. Any one of these may contribute to an undesirable sound, and none will be corrected by trying to "support more."

Releasing Abdominal Clenching

Most of these techniques use gravity or passive motion to facilitate release of the abdomen. Have the singer practice the technique first in isolation while exploring the sensations associated with releasing the abdomen, creating a sensory reference. Gradually start to incorporate phonation, maintaining the abdominal release, and progressively increase complexity.

Instruct the singer to feel how gravity assists inhalation or exhalation in the following positions:

- Bend over from the waist, letting the arms fall toward the floor.
- Bend from the waist over a chair, holding the arms or seat of the chair for support.
- Bend from the waist over a fitness ball, placing the hands on top of the ball for support.
- Lie supine on the floor.

Instruct the singer to feel how resistance and recoil assist inhalation or exhalation in the following tasks:

- Hold a beach ball or fitness ball against the abdomen and feel how the abdomen pushes the ball away on inhalation and how the recoil of the ball pushes the abdomen in on exhalation.
- Stand with the fitness ball suspended between the abdomen and the wall, exploring the same sensations.
- Pulse /s/, /f/, /θ/, or /ʃ/ rhythmically without clenching, feeling the alternation of engagement and release of the abdomen.

Relaxation and Stretching Exercises

Relaxation and stretching exercises serve multiple purposes. I include them in this section as they can be useful for targeting maladaptive muscle tension during nonphonation tasks. In addition, bringing attention to various parts of the body that are involved in phonation serves to increase the singer's general somatic awareness. Finally, when included in the regular vocal exercise regimen, relaxation and stretching exercises function as a brief period of transition between whatever activity the singer has been engaged in and working on vocal exercises, which can help the singer to be more focused while practicing.

There are numerous resources for relaxation and stretching exercises. See Rosenberg and LeBorgne (2014, Chap. 2) for additional ideas. I have listed below the series that I typically have singers execute as part of their practice regimen. For all exercises, cue the singer to let the arms and hands do the reaching (keeping head and neck upright). Monitor for breath holding and remind the singer to breathe through the movements. Encourage slow, relaxed movements versus rushing through the exercises. It is important to ascertain whether the singer has any neck or disc injuries prior to engaging in numbers 9 and 10. If the singer has such a history, these exercises may be contraindicated and it will be advisable to consult an appropriate physician or physical therapist before assigning them.

Relaxation and Stretching Exercises

For all exercises, cue the singer to let the hands and arms do the reaching, keeping the head and neck upright; to breathe through the movement and avoid holding the breath; and to execute the exercises slowly rather than rushing through them.

1. Massage the face (forehead, temples, cheekbones, jaw, chin, etc.) with the fingertips.
2. Massage the back of the neck by letting the fingers run from the top of the neck to the bottom.
3. Reach the hand across to the opposite shoulder (e.g., massage the right shoulder with the left hand) and massage the shoulder blade, top of the shoulder, and side of the neck. It may help to support the elbow with the other hand. Repeat on the other side.
4. Massage the base of the tongue/floor of the mouth by "walking" the thumbs around the soft area right behind the chin.
5. Massage the larynx directly. Put the thumb on one side of the larynx and the fingers on the opposite side. Gently pull the thumb and fingers slowly down the larynx from the hyoid bone to the cricoid cartilage over a count of 5 seconds 5 to 10 times. [Note: demonstrate the appropriate degree of pressure for the singer. He or she should feel pressure, but it shouldn't feel like choking or gagging.]
6. Stretch the face. Scrunch the face with eyes closed, lips pursed and forehead furrowed, then open the eyes widely, raise the eyebrows, and smile a big smile.
7. Gently soften the jaw open while inhaling and soften the jaw closed on the exhale.
8. Stick the tongue all the way out with the tip pointed at the chin, then slowly let it relax back into the mouth.

9. Turn the head all the way to the right looking over the right shoulder. Roll the head down and to the left (as if drawing a half-circle across the chest with the chin) until looking over the left shoulder. Follow the same path to return to the right. Be sure not to let the head fall backward while looking over the shoulder.
10. Let the right ear drop down toward the right shoulder and hold the stretch for a few seconds. Return to the center, then let the left ear drop down toward the left shoulder. Return to the center. Keep the head facing forward without turning toward the shoulder and avoid pushing the head down.
11. Roll the shoulders back five times, then forward five times.

Calling in Reinforcements

For some singers, the underlying basis for the maladaptive muscle tension may exceed what can be resolved with voice rehabilitation alone. In such cases, referral to a physical therapist who is knowledgeable and experienced in addressing such problems can be extremely efficacious. You may find it helpful to research the practices in your area to learn of their specialties and experience so that you can identify appropriate clinicians. If the singer continues to struggle with unloading muscle tension despite your best efforts (especially if they are experiencing pain), consider referring to PT. I have done so many times and have seen excellent results. In some cases, I have continued voice therapy concurrently with PT and in other cases have suspended voice therapy for a period to allow the PT to advance recovery, resuming voice therapy afterward. For information on physical therapy in the United States, visit the American Physical Therapy Association at http://www.apta.org/

STRUCTURAL PATHOLOGIES

See Chapter 3 for a review of the wide range of diagnoses that fall into this category. The shared result of structural pathologies that involve the membranous vocal folds is impairment of vocal fold vibration, changes in vocal fold mass, and (in most cases) impaired glottal closure, all of which can contribute to maladaptive muscle tension as the body attempts to compensate. These factors have important implications from the perspective of singing voice rehabilitation.

Many of the singers that you work with (possibly even the majority) will have a diagnosis of phonotraumatic injury, ranging from mild edema to severe vocal fold scarring and everything in between. Depending on the severity, this type of injury is often quite responsive to behavioral voice rehabilitation. Since these injuries result from phonotrauma, they tend not to enlarge or become more severe if the contributing factors are adequately addressed (and may in fact shrink or completely resolve). For vocal fold hemorrhage, voice rest is the first course of treatment, often followed by voice rehabilitation.

Malignant lesions, leukoplakia, and recurrent respiratory papillomatosis typically do not vary in size and severity with voice use—they "grow" on their own. In the case of polypoid corditis, enlargement is often a function of continued smoking. Surgery is usually the first course of treatment in such cases. The surgical interventions with which such lesions are treated can result in vocal fold scarring. Behavioral voice therapy following surgery may help optimize healing and effective compensation.

Granulomas usually involve the cartilaginous portion of the vocal fold, but if large enough, can affect posterior glottic closure and can cause painful phonation, which can lead to maladaptive muscle tension.

Impact of Impaired Vocal Fold Vibration

Impaired vocal fold vibration impacts vocal quality, particularly if the source signal becomes less periodic because of the interference of the lesion. The voice may be rough, hoarse, or diplophonic. The vocal fold stiffness caused by structural pathologies diminishes the amplitude and extent of mucosal wave, decreasing the harmonic energy the vocal folds can generate and necessitating greater lung pressure to initiate and sustain vocal fold oscillation. Structural pathologies often result in patterns of vibration that may be inconsistent, resulting in unstable and unreliable voice (pitch and phonation breaks), and may affect how well and how consistently glottal configuration can be controlled, which will make achieving optimal register and transitioning between registers more difficult.

Impact of Changes in Vocal Fold Mass

Structural pathologies result in increased vocal fold mass, which can lead to lower fundamental frequency and loss of high range. Such pathologies are often not symmetrical, and the resulting asymmetry in vocal fold mass can cause aperiodic and inconsistent vibration, diplophonia, and unstable and unreliable voice in general.

Impact of Impaired Glottal Closure

Impaired glottal closure results in changes in vocal quality (breathiness, hoarseness, and/or roughness are typical). In addition, when vocal folds cannot completely adduct, the interaction of source-filter may be compromised as the vocal folds will not valve airflow in a normal way (e.g., the valve will be "leaky"). This leaky valve will also have an impact on breath support. The singer will typically report problems coordinating breath support, or a decreased ability to sustain phonation. Register negotiation may also be impaired if the ability to reliably control subglottic pressure is diminished. Depending on the size and location of the lesion(s), impaired closure may only be evident in specific pitch ranges. If lesions are on the vibrating edge, they become more prominent as the vocal folds thin and stiffen with an increase in pitch. The singer may note difficulty phonating in high range, delayed onset of phonation, or quality changes in high range.

Rehabilitation Targets and Approaches

Obviously, the goal in rehabilitation for phonotrauma is to optimize vocal fold vibration, improve glottic closure, and reduce maladaptive muscle tension. Fortunately, we have an excellent resource to accomplish this: resonant voice. Recall from previous chapters that the vocal tract has the capacity to help the vocal folds vibrate better. Therefore, use of SOVT exercises will be essential in rehabilitation of structural pathologies. The objective will be to gradually entrain the vocal tract to achieve the inertive benefits of SOVT after the occlusion has been removed. These exercises not only optimize compensation for the underlying injury but may help to resolve the inflammatory component (Verdolini Abbott et al., 2012).

The severity of vibration impairment may dictate which SOVT sounds the singer can produce. Phonation through a stir straw may be too challenging in cases of severe vibration or closure impairment, at least initially. Experiment with different sounds to find one that the singer can easily achieve. As the injury resolves, the singer may be able to "graduate" to small-straw phonation to more fully capitalize on vocal tract inertance.

The complexity of the exercise should be based on the singer's current function (e.g., start with patterns that the singer is able to accomplish successfully and gradually increase complexity, as illustrated in the previous chapter and the case studies in this chapter). Pitch patterns such as glides and narrow scales can be a good place to start, promoting gentle stretching of the vocal folds. When the singer can accomplish the task on SOVT sounds, gradually transition to vowels and syllables based on the principles we explored in the last chapter.

Optimizing respiratory coordination is also important, especially if the singer does not have a firm foundation in breath support technique. However, *over*emphasis on breath support without effectively recruiting the vocal tract can exacerbate traumatic injuries by creating excessive subglottic pressure and increasing mechanical stress on the vocal folds. Thus, strategies aimed primarily at adduction and high subglottic pressure (such as Valsalva maneuver) are contraindicated. Phonotrauma often benefits from a "top-down" approach: optimizing the configuration of the vocal tract improves vocal fold vibration, which in turn improves the ability of the vocal folds to interact with airflow in an optimal way.

Voice Therapy After Phonosurgery

A period of complete or modified voice rest is typically recommended after phonosurgery, although the range of duration is quite broad. A survey of otolaryngologists by Behrman and Sulica (2003) found that 0 to 14 days was the range for recommendation of complete voice rest and 0 to 24 days for modified voice rest, with an average of 1 week. Complete voice rest typically encompasses all behaviors that result in vocal fold adduction, including speaking and singing, but also throat clearing, coughing, crying, laughing, and heavy lifting.

The benefits of active recovery and tissue mobility following surgery are well supported by research in the realm of orthopedics, and the principles underlying such recommendations may apply to wound healing for voice. Current research is limited as to determining whether this is in fact the case, but a recent study purports that the right kind of vocal fold mobilization may be beneficial in resolving edema (Verdolini Abbott et al., 2012)—with emphasis on *the right kind of exercise*. In this study, the effective exercises were drawn from resonant voice practices, as previously noted. For this reason, it is my opinion that singing exercises should be introduced into the rehabilitation regimen as soon as possible, ideally in the first or second session, 2 to 3 weeks following surgery. These exercises should initially be very gentle and low impact using SOVT sounds spanning a conservative pitch and loudness range, gradually expanding and increasing duration, pitch range, and intensity as tolerated over the ensuing weeks.

NEUROLOGIC ETIOLOGIES

Vocal Fold Paralysis and Paresis

As noted in Chapters 3 and 4, vocal fold paralysis (complete vocal fold immobility) or paresis (weakness) may be transitory or permanent. Behavioral voice rehabilitation is typically not the first course of treatment for paralysis. Surgical intervention usually involves vocal fold augmentation in the short term and medialization thyroplasty or reinnervation in cases of complete denervation of the recurrent laryngeal nerve (RLN). Following surgery, singing voice rehabilitation can often yield improvements in vocal function, quality, and stamina. In cases of paresis in which the ability to adduct the vocal folds is intact, voice therapy may be a first course of treatment.

Impact of Vocal Fold Paralysis or Paresis

Loss of vocal fold innervation via the RLN not only results in loss of mobility but also leads to loss of muscle tone. This means that even when the position of the vocal fold and glottic closure are surgically improved, the paralyzed vocal fold will not function normally. The inability to engage the thyroarytenoid muscle affects the vertical dimension of glottic closure, making it difficult to achieve a "squared up" edge. This has obvious implications for register control but also for overall vocal stability. The paralyzed vocal fold will not be as effective at building up subglottic pressure, which causes an asymmetry in glottal resistance that may lead to diplophonia, pitch and phonation breaks, and decreased duration of phonation. If the superior laryngeal nerve (SLN) is intact, pitch range may be functional but likely not normal. The lowest end of the range may be lost due to inability to contract TA to shorten the vocal fold, and high range may be decreased due to inability of the posterior cricoarytenoid muscle to assist CT in stretching the vocal fold by stabilizing the arytenoid cartilage on top of the cricoid cartilage (Titze & Verdolini Abbott, 2012). If transient RLN paralysis is suspected, voice rehabilitation may be effective during the recovery to minimize maladaptive compensation.

In cases of complete, permanent denervation of the SLN, vocal fold mobility may be intact, but the cricothyroid muscle will be impaired, resulting in severe pitch range limitations. Since stretching and stiffening the vocal folds is also a function of CT, SLN paralysis can also have subtle effects on adduction, particularly relative to symmetry. This is an unambiguously devastating diagnosis for a singer, with poor prognosis for continuing singing.

Vocal fold paresis for either the RLN or SLN results in symptoms that are similar to those associated with paralysis but are usually much more subtle. Often the singer can learn to compensate adequately to continue singing.

Rehabilitation Targets and Approaches

The goal of rehabilitation in cases of vocal fold paralysis or paresis is to recruit respiration and vocal tract configuration to maximize vocal fold function (the locus of the impairment) while minimizing compensatory muscle tension. Targets will include ensuring adequate breath support without overwhelming the ability of the vocal folds to resist airflow, using resonant voice techniques to assist vocal fold vibration, and muscle tension reduction strategies as needed.

Since innervation of the vocal folds is compromised, decreased vocal stamina is likely, and the singer will often report vocal fatigue. Overload may help to increase strength and stamina and achieve effective compensation but must be implemented carefully to avoid exacerbating muscle tension or creating phonotrauma. Exercises should be constructed to incrementally increase range and duration of phonation, and recovery time should be carefully monitored. Capitalizing on vocal tract inertance with SOVT exercises can help to boost stamina by taking some of the load off at the laryngeal level.

Exercises should target the specific malfunction. For example, if glottic closure is impaired, include elements that will promote the interaction of TA and lung pressure to optimize vocal fold adduction. Using CVC syllables that begin with /b/ and end with /p/ can be advantageous (such as /bip/, /bup/, bæp/). If TA is compromised, there will likely be a "sweet spot" in the pitch range at which vocal fold tension will optimally assist in glottic closure. Use this pitch zone as your starting point, pivoting up and down from this point as illustrated in Case Study 2 to entrain adaptive coordination through an ever widening range. If the singer demonstrates excessive supraglottic compression, SOVT exercises can also be helpful in unloading the hyperfunction while optimizing vocal tract assistance to the glottis. As always, the complexity of the task should start with what the singer can successfully achieve and gradually increase.

Spasmodic Dysphonia and Tremor

Spasmodic dysphonia (SD) and tremor present particular obstacles in terms of singing. Both have an effect on speaking and singing, which may have paradoxical presentation and treatment.

In spasmodic dysphonia, the spasms may be task specific (see Chapters 3–4 for further information). Singing is often more intact than speaking, and in fact, this indicator is part of the differential diagnosis for SD. The problem for the singer lies in the treatment of the disorder: injection of botulinum toxin into the affected muscle(s). The temporary paralysis of intrinsic laryngeal muscles with botulinum toxin can severely impair singing but may be necessary to achieve functional communication in moderate to severe cases. Collaboration between the singer, laryngologist, clinical singing voice rehabilitation specialist, and voice teacher is essential for determining the relative importance of speaking and singing activities and achieving the optimal balance of function for each. Optimizing interaction of phonation subsystems and minimizing maladaptive muscle tension through rehabilitation can help maximize the outcome.

Tremor can be challenging to treat relative to singing (see Chapters 3 and 17 for information on the etiology and medical treatment of vocal tremor). When treating tremor in the speaking voice, the goal is to shorten the duration of phonation during speech to mask the tremor (Barkmeier-Kraemer, 2013). Singing is all about sustaining phonation, rendering the tremor even more noticeable. This is further complicated in classical singing by the expectation for consistent vibrato. The tremor effectively results in a vibrato rate that is too slow and that sometimes encompasses a pitch deviation that is too wide, making the vibrato sound "wobbly." Usually, the tremor is less noticeable when singing staccato, but obviously the singer must be capable of legato singing to function. If the tremor is not too severe, sometimes the singer can learn to optimize coordination of phonation subsystems and employ stabilization elsewhere in the body in a manner that helps decrease the impact of the tremor. See the case study below for "Kathy" for strategies relative to vocal tremor.

VOCAL FOLD ATROPHY

Vocal fold atrophy is typically associated with birthdays—the more of them we have, the greater the risk. The general effects of aging on the voice and of vocal fold atrophy in particular are numerous and notable enough that the entirety of Chapter 17 is devoted to the subject. For information on the impact of vocal fold atrophy on singing as well as recommended targets and approaches for rehabilitation, see Chapter 17.

THERAPEUTIC USE OF REPERTOIRE

For singers who are currently working with a voice teacher and/or are already competent at applying technique to repertoire, it is feasible that you may discharge them from rehabilitation with minimal work on performance material. However, if these skills and resources are not present, it is appropriate—indeed, incumbent—to incorporate repertoire into the rehabilitation process.

I once heard someone explain the difference between voice lessons and voice rehabilitation in this way: "In voice rehabilitation, you only work on exercises, and in voice lessons, you work on exercises *and* repertoire." In my opinion, this could not be further from the truth (see Chapter 6 for a differing perspective on how voice habilitation and rehabilitation converge and diverge). Singing repertoire is the equivalent of "conversational level" in speaking voice therapy, which any clinician knows is the end goal regardless of disorder. Structured tasks from sounds to sentences are only the stair steps leading to real-life functionality. For singers, whatever kind of music they typically sing *is* their functional level.

This doesn't mean that repertoire is addressed in the same way in rehabilitation as it is in voice lessons, wherein the preparation (both technical and artistic) of all aspects of entire performances is addressed in depth and over time. If you have done your job as a singing voice rehabilitation specialist well, the exercises you have designed should have a positive impact on maximizing vocal function and improving vocal health (although it is important to realize that, depending on the nature of the injury, exercises do not always resolve the problem to a point of adequate function). Before discharging, you must ensure that the singer is capable of translating any improvements in vocal coordination and conditioning that have been acquired through rehabilitation exercises in such a way that these skills can be applied to repertoire.

Achieving this can take many forms and will vary from one singer to the next. As in all aspects of rehabilitation, the approach should be adapted to meet the needs of each individual singer. Establishing a translational sequence of steps to bridge vocalise and song can be very helpful. Extract a phrase from a song and have the singer first execute it using SOVT sounds, then using a facilitating vowel or syllable(s), then perhaps a vowel sequence that corresponds to the text, and finally proceed to the text itself. The sequence may be more or less structured depending on the singer's needs. Illustrate to the singer how this process can then be repeated on the next phrase, and the next, and so on until coordination is optimized for the entire song. Working from the other direction, you can extract a phrase or fragment from a song and turn it into a vocalise that becomes part of the regular exercise regimen, as described in Chapter 11. There are several examples of this in the following case studies. It is not necessary to work on every song in the singer's repertoire—only to ensure that the singer understands the principle and is capable of application.

MONITORING PITCH AND LOUDNESS RANGE AND VOCAL STAMINA

As indicated above, many vocal pathologies result in compromised pitch range. In developing the vocal exercise regimen, a component objective may be to increase pitch range to preinjury status, or at least to maximize the range. However, this goal must be addressed carefully to avoid exacerbating the injury or promoting maladaptive muscle effort. When it appears that a pitch ceiling has been reached—as evidenced by inability to phonate, delayed onset of phonation, or excessive strain—take the exercise down a step or two to a more comfortable level. Have the singer try approaching the higher pitch again with a technical adjustment (for which you have provided appropriate cueing or strategies). If the singer achieves the note successfully with the technical adjustment, continue upward, repeating the pattern until a true ceiling is reached that does not resolve with technical adjustment. Once the true ceiling has been identified, bring the singer back down to a comfortable pitch level again so that the exercise concludes with a successful attempt, thus reinforcing the motor learning you are trying to entrain. The same approach should be utilized for working on the low end of the range. Pitch range may vary considerably from one session to the next—the range should increase as the injury resolves and coordination and conditioning improve. Sometimes pitch range may decrease from one session to the next, which is an indication for adapting the exercise regimen. If the loss of range persists, consider repeat stroboscopy to determine whether the injury has worsened.

Dynamic range may also be compromised by vocal injury and may be a component of the rehabilitation goals as well. It can be beneficial to explore dynamic range in terms of effort rather than loudness, since soft phonation may be executed with a great amount of effort, and loud singing may be accomplished with minimal effort, depending on skill and coordination. Establishing a shared numerical reference for degree of effort (1–10, 10 being greatest) can be a useful construct for monitoring based on the singer's report and will also promote the singer's internal monitoring ability (LeBorgne & Rosenberg, 2014). Explore the span of dynamic range the singer can achieve and the associated effort in each session as described above for pitch range.

Finally, monitor the singer's vocal stamina across sessions. As noted in Chapter 11, overload can be a beneficial principle in optimizing vocal conditioning but must be used prudently in the face of vocal injury. Mild fatigue after a vocal workout is not unusual, especially if the singer is out of condition. However, the fatigue should resolve relatively quickly, at most within a day. If it takes longer for the singer to recover, it is time to consider adjusting the exercise regimen. Conversely, if the singer is tolerating the recommended duration of exercise, gradually increase to ascertain the true stamina "ceiling."

CASE STUDIES

The following case studies illustrate a variety of rehabilitation exercises. The exercises for each singer differ based on diagnosis, type of singing, vocal demands, and amount of vocal training. You will note that while certain exercises appear across multiple cases, the routine for each singer is tailored to his or her individual needs. As you review the cases, see if you can identify the basis for the selection of exercises in terms of what you know about the impact of injury on vocal function, coordination of the subsystems of phonation, shaping voice, and vocal exercise design.

Case Study 1: Professional Bluegrass Singer

"Randall" was a 51-year-old award-winning professional bluegrass singer with a vocally demanding performance and recording career. He was diagnosed with tonsil cancer 4 months prior to his evaluation at our clinic and had undergone chemotherapy and radiation treatment to the left tonsil and left neck nodes. As is typical, he experienced weight loss and general deconditioning associated with chemotherapy. He resumed performing once treatment was complete but noted significant voice changes, including loss of falsetto range, difficulty projecting in his low range, effortful phonation, vocal fatigue, xerostomia, and rough, strained vocal quality. "I can only sing about a fifth comfortably" (meaning over the range of a perfect fifth).

Stroboscopy revealed mild vocal fold atrophy (likely related in part to weight loss and deconditioning), as well as bilateral vocal fold sulci, moderate vibration impairment consistent with radiation changes, and compensatory supraglottic hyperfunction. The laryngologist also diagnosed allergic rhinitis and prescribed fluticasone. Hydration was adequate but frequent throat clearing was noted.

Although he had minimal vocal training, Randall was a very accomplished singer. However, during singing assessment, he demonstrated inadequate breath support, abdominal clenching, and significant vocal strain in the range from A3–A4. Above A4, he sang in falsetto, also with significant laryngeal strain and base of tongue tension. This muscle tension pattern was noted at the low end of his range as well, from about D3–A2.

Voice therapy was recommended with goals targeting vocal hygiene, vocal pacing, and improving vocal coordination and conditioning. He had nine voice therapy sessions over a period of 14 weeks. The design and evolution of Randall's vocal exercise regimen for speaking and singing are outlined in Table 12–3.

Table 12–3. *Case Study "Randall": Vocal exercise regimen for 51-year-old professional bluegrass singer with minimal vocal training. Diagnosis: Radiation changes to the vocal folds (associated with radiation for tonsil cancer, as described in the chapter text); bilateral vocal fold sulci; mild vocal fold atrophy.*

Session Number	*Exercises*
1	1. Reviewed treatment plan and goals 2. Listened to recordings that predated onset of dysphonia for baseline 3. Instruction on mechanics of low abdominal breathing (LAB)/breath support for singing. Practiced LAB in isolation; then exhaling on /s/ 4. Transitioned from /s/ to /z/ to promote sustained breath release with voicing 5. Adductory power phonating through drinking straw C3–G3 6. Speaking voice: Introduced resonant voice and breath support for speaking; /m/ was a facilitating launching sound. Worked on /m/ in isolation and /m/ initial syllables
2	1. Relaxation and stretching exercises 2. Adductory power phonating through drinking straw C3–C4 diatonically 3. Unstructured pitch glides through full-range phonating through drinking straw 4. 12321 on /m/ to establish reference sensation for resonant voice C3–E4 5. Pitch glides 5–1 on /hæ/ C3–A4. Strategies: Holding drinking straw horizontally under tongue to reduce tongue tension and facilitate lip retraction, and tilting head back 30 to 45 degrees to facilitate gentle laryngeal elevation. Abrupt transition from TA dominant to CT dominant at F4 6. 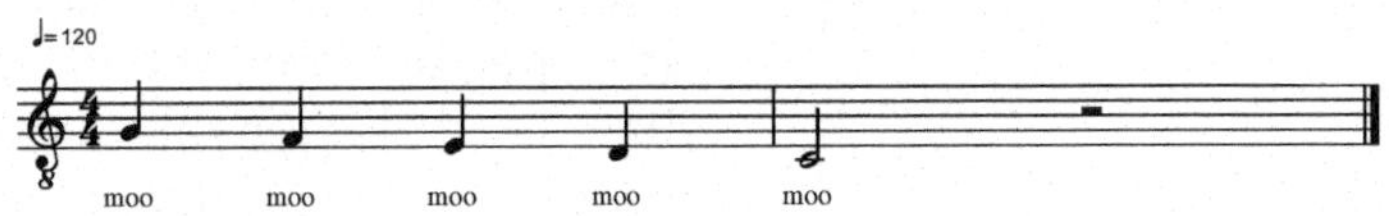 to explore low larynx position A3–A2; cue: "sing it like Elvis" 7. Speaking voice: Worked through hierarchy from syllable to words using /m/ launching sound
3	1. Relaxation and stretching exercises 2. Adductory power phonating through drinking straw submerged in water to increase resistance C3–C4 3. Paradoxical breathing pattern noted (contracting abdomen on inhale, expanding abdomen on exhale). Reviewed mechanics of abdominal breathing in isolation and exhaling on /s/ to "reset" coordination 4. Pitch glides through full-range phonating through drinking straw submerged in water 5. 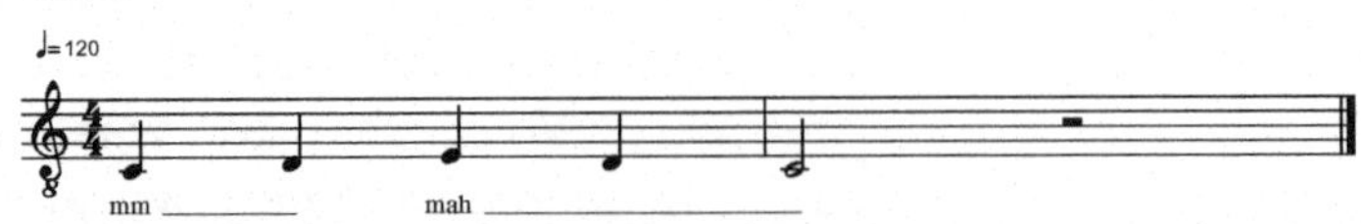 transferring resonance from /m/ to /a/ C3–E4 6. Pitch glides 5–1 on /hæ/ holding drinking straw under to reduce tongue tension and facilitate lip retraction, C3–F4 in TA-dominant register. Started with head back for laryngeal elevation, gradually moving head to upright position

Table 12–3. *continued*

Session Number	Exercises
3 *continued*	7. 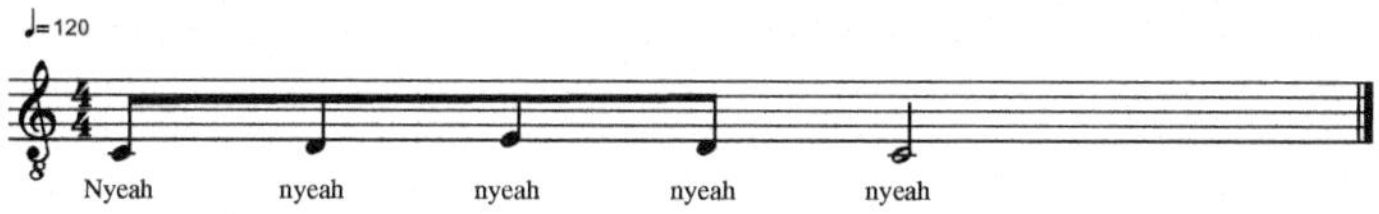 for "twang" resonance 8. 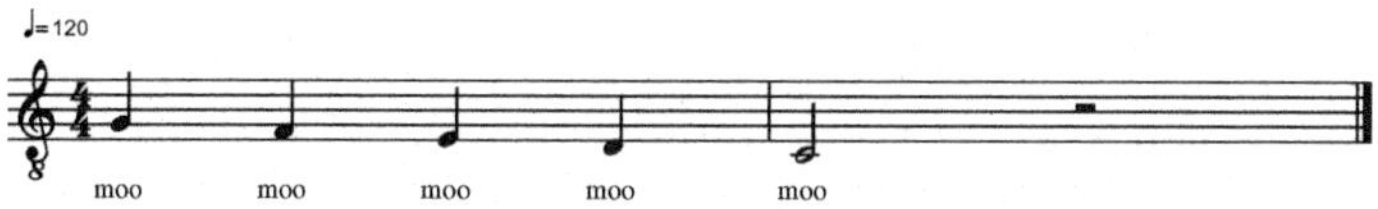 for low larynx position A3–A2; cue: "sing it like Elvis" 9. Speaking voice: Worked through hierarchy from syllable to phrases using /m/ launching sound
4	1. Relaxation and stretching exercises 2. At this point he was able to achieve adductory power phonating through small-diameter (stir) straw C3–C4 3. Pitch glides through full range on lip trill. Abdominal clenching noted during phonation. Released clenching when standing bent over from the waist. Practiced phonating glides in this position to establish sensory reference for abdominal release 4. Continued transferring resonance from /m/ to /a/, decreasing dependence on /m/ to launch resonance, B flat 2–E4 (alternating pattern as illustrated below): 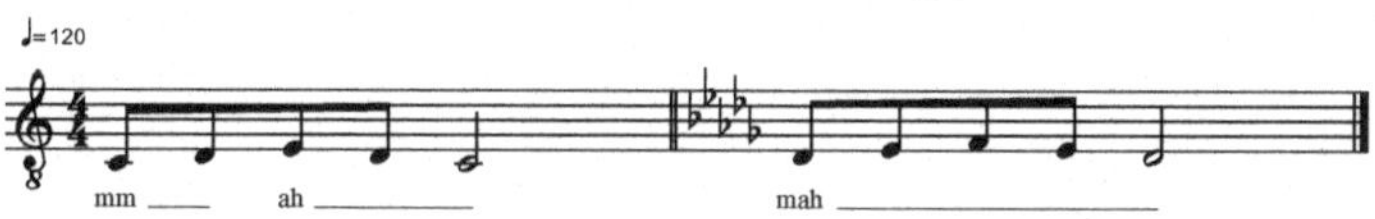 5. Pitch glides 5–1 on /hæ/ holding drinking straw under tongue as in previous sessions, C3–F4 in TA-dominant register. Occasionally tilted head back to facilitate laryngeal elevation. Abrupt transition from TA dominant to CT dominant at F#4. He was able to maintain TA-dominant mix to G4 by "stepping up" from F4 as illustrated: 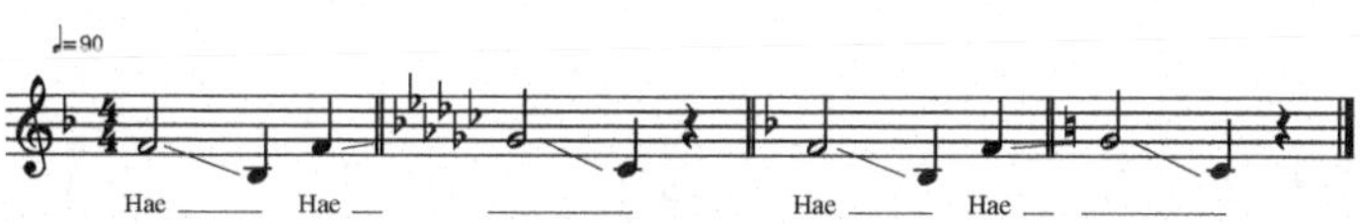 6. 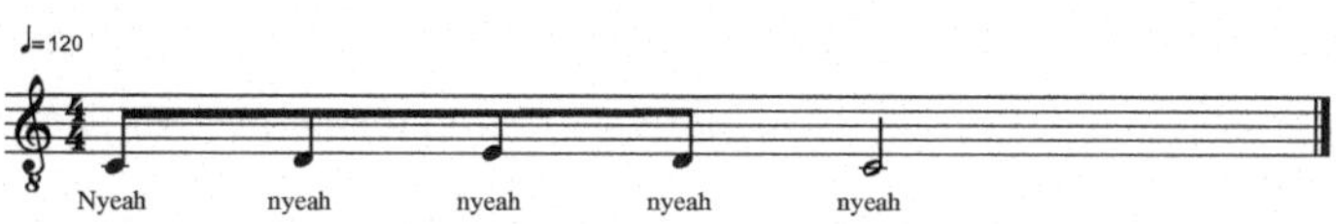 for "twang" resonance D3–E4 7. 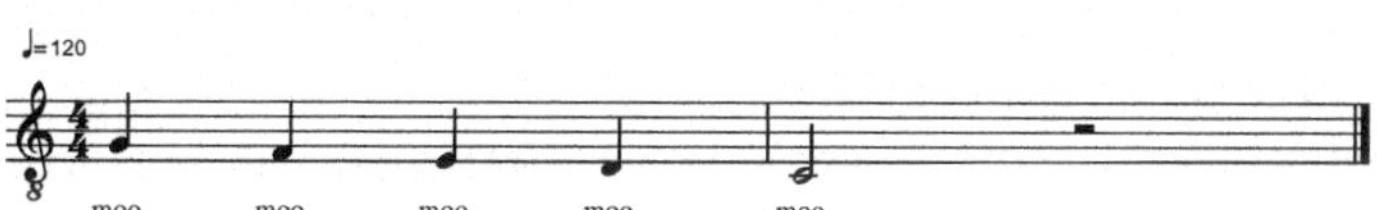 for low larynx position A3–A2 8. Speaking voice: Worked through hierarchy from syllable to sentences using /m/ launching sound

continues

Table 12–3. *continued*

Session Number	Exercises
5	Session was primarily devoted to vocal pacing strategies to prepare for pending increase in performance frequency and duration, minimal time on exercises 1. Adductory power phonating through small-diameter (stir) straw C3–C4 2. Pitch glides through full range on lip trill 3. Speaking voice: Worked through hierarchy from syllable to sentences using /m/ launching sound as in last session. Proceeded to structured conversation (responding to clinician questions)
6	1. Relaxation and stretching exercises 2. Adductory power phonating through small-diameter (stir) straw C3–C4 3. Pitch glides through full range on lip trill 4. 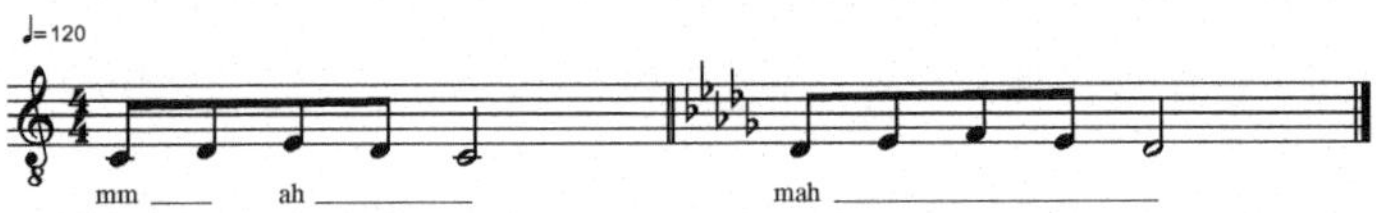 as in previous session 5. Pitch glides 5–1 on /hæ/. Achieved adequate lip retraction without needing to use drinking straw under tongue. Used "stepping up" from F4 as in previous session. Able to maintain TA-dominant mix to A4 6. 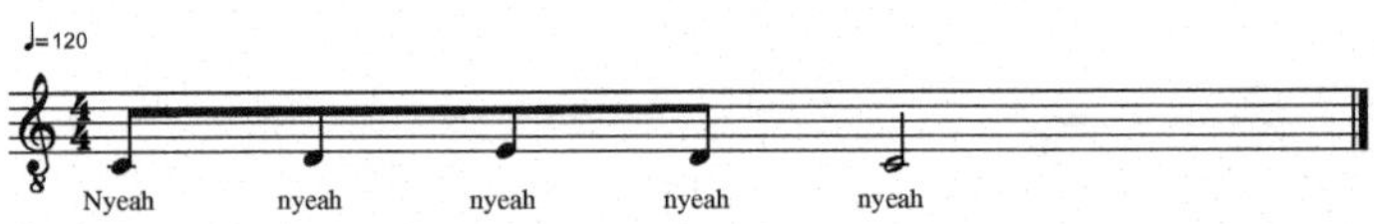 as in previous session. Worked from exaggerated to moderate degree of twang 7. New exercise for falsetto derived from fragment of song phrase, C4–D5: 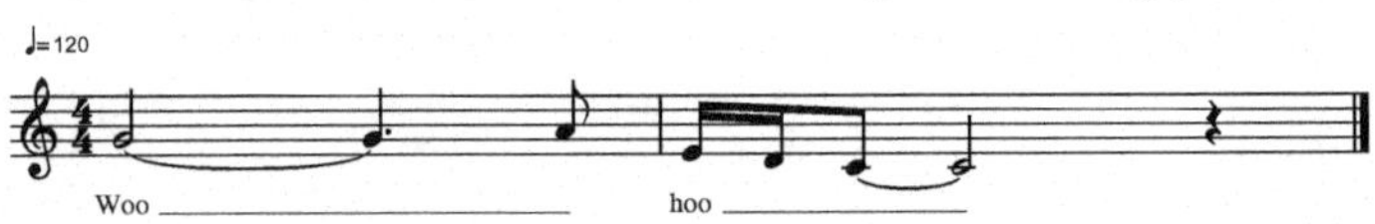 8. 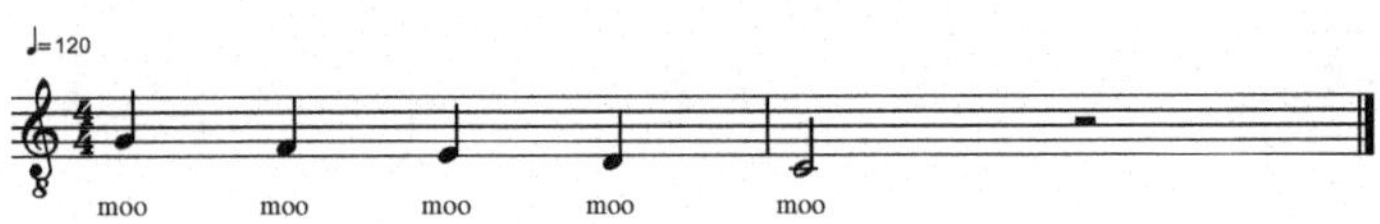 A3–A2 for low larynx position 9. Speaking voice: Paragraph reading recalibrating resonance with small straw as needed
7	Very fatigued after vocally demanding week performing and speaking at international bluegrass festival 1. Reviewed vocal pacing strategies 2. Worked on gentle SOVT exercises to optimize source-filter interaction and ameliorate inflammation 3. Relaxation and stretching exercises 4. Speaking voice: Worked through hierarchy from syllable to sentences using /m/ launching sound. Reviewed performance video. Pressed voice and inadequate breath support observed in stage banter during performance

Table 12–3. *continued*

<table>
<tr><th>Session Number</th><th>Exercises</th></tr>
<tr><td>8</td><td>
1. Relaxation and stretching exercises
2. Adductory power phonating through small-diameter (stir) straw C3–C4
3. Pitch glides through full range on lip trill
4. New exercise: B flat 2–F4
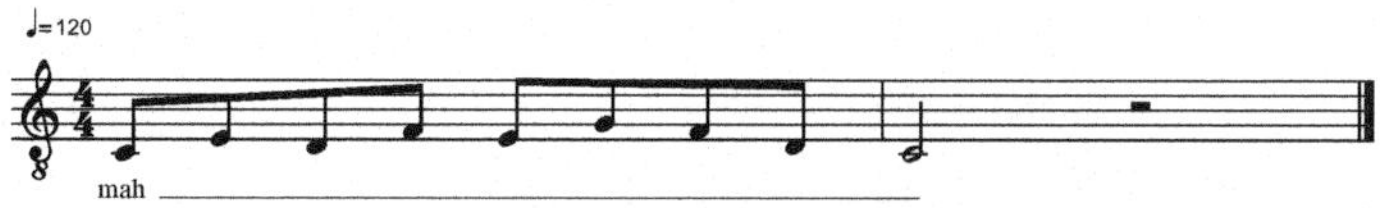

5. Pitch glides 5–1 on /hæ/ alternating with 5-4-3-2-1. Able to maintain TA-dominant mix to A4
6.
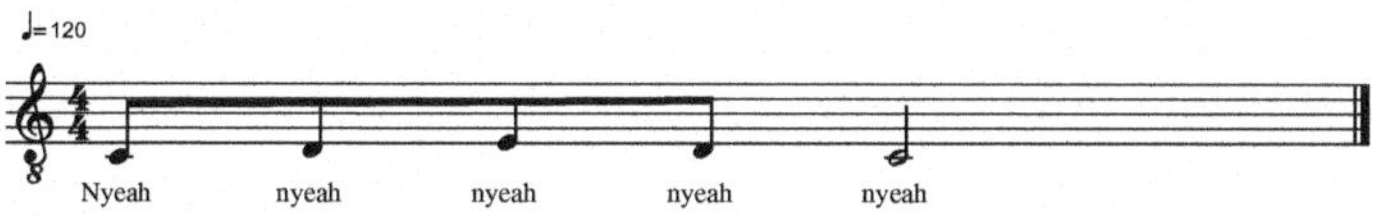

as in previous session
7.
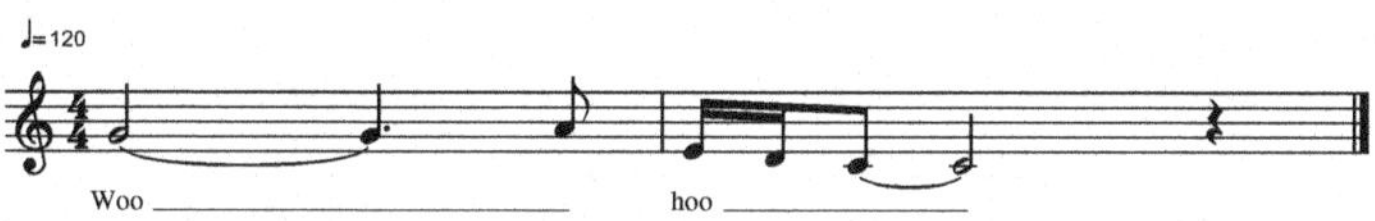

C4–D5 as in previous session
8.
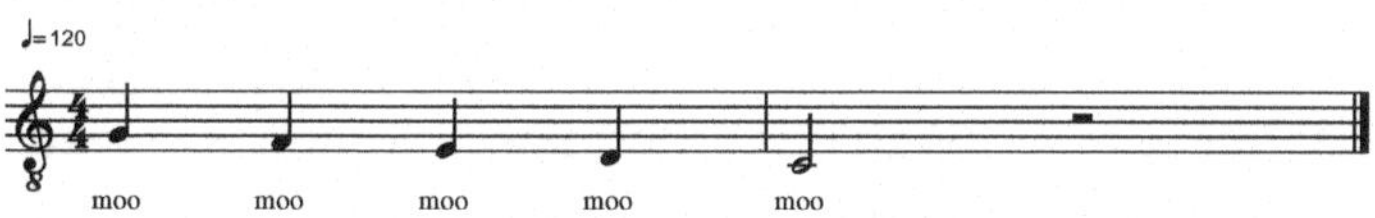

A3–A2
9. Added cool down: (a) laryngeal massage × 10; (b) descending pitch glides on lip trill, starting high and gradually working down to speaking range; (c) structured speaking exercises from syllable to sentence with /m/ initial
10. Speaking voice: Practiced "stage banter" typically used in concerts recalibrating resonance with small straw and attention to breath support as needed
</td></tr>
<tr><td>9</td><td>Relatively independent with vocal exercise regimen from last session. Improved speaking technique observed at conversational level. Worked on passages from songs to transfer skills by singing passages on lip trill or with small straw, then on vowels, using /æ/ and twang resonance where TA-dominant mix was required and /wu/ for falsetto passages. Discharged from therapy. Reevaluation with stroboscopy revealed sulci were still present but he was effectively compensating for underlying structural abnormality with improved glottic closure and vibration and decreased hyperfunction.</td></tr>
</table>

Note. *Vocal hygiene, medical management of seasonal allergies, and vocal pacing were addressed throughout the therapy process but are minimally included in this chart, which focuses on the evolution of the exercise regimen.*

Initially, he was not able to achieve stable phonation through a stir straw, likely the result of impaired vibration from radiation changes, vocal fold atrophy, excessive subglottic pressure, and pressed voice. For this reason, SOVT exercises using sounds with less resistance were used initially, gradually increasing resistance as source-filter interaction and breath support improved. Exercises were designed to address range and register concerns, improve vocal quality, and improve vocal stamina and ease of phonation. Note that both low and high larynx positions were targeted: low larynx to decrease pressing and improve extent of low range, high larynx to extend belt range with minimal strain. Additional exercises targeted falsetto in isolation since this was a component of his performance voice.

Randall was able to continue performing through his rehabilitation, although this was sometimes challenging. By the time he was discharged, he felt he was at 80% of his precancer vocal function and felt able to adequately meet performance demands with vocal pacing adjustments and regularly completing warm-up exercises.

Case Study 2: Amateur Choral Singer With Vocal Tremor

"Kathy" was a 65-year-old choral singer. She was diagnosed with essential tremor several years prior to being seen in our clinic. At first, the tremor was limited to head and hand movements but had recently started to affect her voice as well. Kathy had taken voice lessons on and off over the years and had sung as a classical soprano in community and church choirs for most of her adult life. She was very passionate about singing. At the time of her evaluation, she had been singing in a prestigious symphony choir for over 10 years. The choir had just finished the season and was getting ready for summer hiatus. At the last rehearsal, the director took her aside and expressed concern about her voice, saying that he wanted her to reaudition at the beginning of the next season. She was devastated by the possibility that she might have to leave the choir and was committed to doing everything she could for a successful reaudition.

Perceptually, her speaking voice was characterized by moderate tremor and mildly breathy and hoarse quality, with intermittent pitch and phonation breaks. When singing, the tremor became more pronounced with consistent tremulous pulsations at about 4 Hz. Considerable base of tongue, jaw, neck, and shoulder tension were noted, as well as mildly rough quality, inadequate oral resonance, and moderate laryngeal strain. CT-dominant registration was well developed, but her voice was often weak in her low range due to inadequate engagement of TA.

On stroboscopy, her vocal folds were smooth with mild bowing. She achieved complete glottic closure, although closure was sometimes light or incomplete associated with intermittent inadequate breath support. Anterior to posterior supraglottic compression with involvement of the base of the tongue was noted. Rhythmic trembling of the larynx and base of tongue was observed in all sustained phonation tasks.

Our laryngologist prescribed propranolol to help with the tremor. He also prescribed a nasal antihistamine for allergic rhinitis. Voice therapy was recommended. Since we only had about 8 weeks before her reaudition, I enlisted one of my colleagues to provide concurrent speaking voice therapy so that we could focus exclusively and intensively on singing in her sessions with me.

The course and evolution of Kathy's vocal coordination and conditioning through exercise are detailed in Table 12–4. The focus was on optimizing laryngeal stabilization using a variety of techniques outlined earlier in this chapter, combined with gradual transition from staccato to legato singing tasks. You will note the absence of adductory power exercises in her routine. Sustaining single pitches was contraindicated in her case as this type of exercise would make the tremor more evident. We also explored a variety of SOVT sounds to arrive at those that provided just the right amount of resistance to optimize source-filter interaction without exacerbating the tremor.

Kathy's tremor did improve with propranolol, but the side effects of gastrointestinal irritation and general fatigue made it impractical for her to take the full dose. Working with the laryngologist, she arrived at a tolerable dose that gave her the most benefit.

Kathy was one of the most dedicated and diligent singers I have ever worked with. Over the course of the summer, she regularly attended therapy sessions twice a week—once with me for singing and once with my colleague for speaking voice. She bought a fitness ball so that she could practice the stabilization strategies we worked on, and she religiously practiced exercises and her audition repertoire multiple times each day. As her audition approached, I encouraged her to schedule practice time in the church where the audition would take place so that she could get used to the environment and also to schedule "mock" auditions with friends and family in attendance. Although the tremor was still noticeable in her voice, she achieved a degree of vocal control that resulted in a successful reaudition, and she was able to continue the singing activities that brought her so much joy.

Table 12–4. ***Case Study "Kathy": Vocal exercise regimen for 65-year-old choral singer. Diagnosis: Mild vocal fold atrophy and essential tremor.***

Session Number	Exercises
1	1. Reviewed treatment plan and goals 2. Listened to recordings that predated onset of dysphonia for baseline 3. Explored a variety of head, neck, and torso anchoring strategies as outlined in this chapter. The most successful for her were bouncing on the fitness ball during phonation (see "Ball Bounce" and Figure 12–4D), and pushing the fitness ball against the wall (see "Shoulder Pull-Down" and Figure 12–1). We utilized these postures and others during most singing tasks throughout the course of her treatment. 4. Reviewed respiratory mechanics for singing, which she was already familiar with. Practiced low abdominal breathing pattern without phonation while executing the posture/anchoring strategies above 5. Attempted phonation with small-diameter straw. This tended to increase tremor. Phonation through drinking straw was better. Explored a variety of vowels. /a/ was most stable and facilitating for her 6. 5–1 glide phonating through drinking straw, C4–F5. Cues: Execute glide quickly, avoid sustaining top and bottom notes and focus on the siren quality
2	Posture/stabilization strategies from last session were utilized in all tasks 1. Added relaxation and stretching exercises 2. Fast 5–1 glide phonating through drinking straw, then on /wa/ C4–C6 3. 54321, 13531, and 1358531 patterns on /ha/ staccato C4–G5 4. 54321 on /ha/ staccato, gradually transitioning to legato F4–E5. At first, legato was implemented only on 2-1, then 3-2-1, etc. (as illustrated) until she could execute the entire 54321 phrase legato with minimal evident tremor: 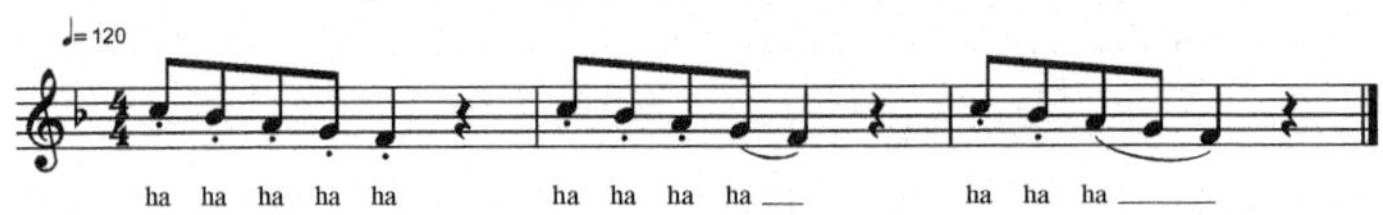 5. Worked on short phrases from her audition repertoire singing staccato on /ha/
3	Posture/stabilization strategies from previous sessions were utilized in all tasks. Added rolling hips back and forth while seated on fitness ball to explore reference sensation for engagement of lower abdomen, pelvic floor and lower back (see Figure 12–4B, C). 1. Relaxation and stretching exercises 2. 5–1 glide on /wa/. Some voice breaks noted on bottom note. Changed to /wu/, rearticulating the /wu/ on the bottom note (as illustrated), ultimately to C6 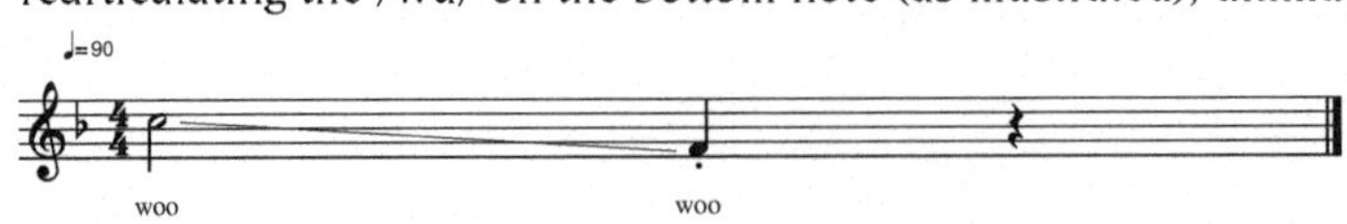 Vowel change and lip rounding resulted in improved oral resonance. Cues: Exaggerate lip-rounding, use phonation through a drinking straw as a reference 3. 54321 on /ha/ staccato, gradually transitioning to legato as in last session E4–E5, this time starting legato on 5-4, then 5-4-3, etc. until she could execute the entire 54321 phrase legato with minimal evident tremor. Repeated the exercise seated on fitness ball, gradually standing while maintaining engagement of lower abdomen, pelvic floor, and lower back. Vocal quality was somewhat weak below E4 due to inadequate engagement of TA.

Table 12–4. *continued*

Session Number	***Exercises***
3 *continued*	4. 13531 F4–F5 staccato on various vowels launching with /h/ (/ha/, /ho/, /hu/, /hɛ/, /hi/) sequencing to legato articulation as in previous sessions 5. 1358531 on /ha/ starting staccato and transitioning to legato F4–A5 6. Worked on passages from audition repertoire on /ha/ staccato, then legato. Cue to "think crescendo" helped maintain breath support and resulted in less evident tremor.
4	1. Introduced epigastric movement elicited with /k/ and /ʃ/ for additional stability (see Chapter 9) 2. 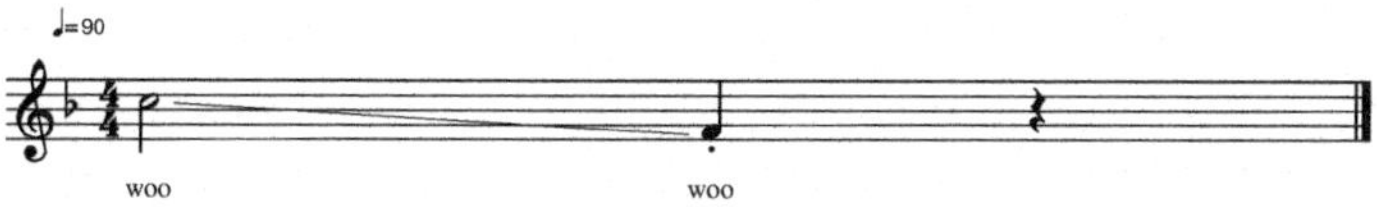 to C6 3. 54321 on /ha/ staccato to legato as in previous sessions D4–A5. Added new posture/stabilization strategy standing with fitness ball suspended between her back and the wall (see "Ball Assisted Squat" and Figures 12–5A–C) 4. Repeated staccato/legato sequences from last session using gentle engagement of epigastric area in pitch range D4–A5. Inadequate TA activation in low range as previously noted, resulting in decreased projection 5. Applied strategies to audition repertoire
5	1. Reviewed exercises and strategies from last two sessions 2. Worked on strengthening lower passaggio. Started by identifying pitch that elicited good amount of TA activation (B3). Proceeded to chromatic exercises, pivoting up and down, maintaining engagement of TA on ascending portion: 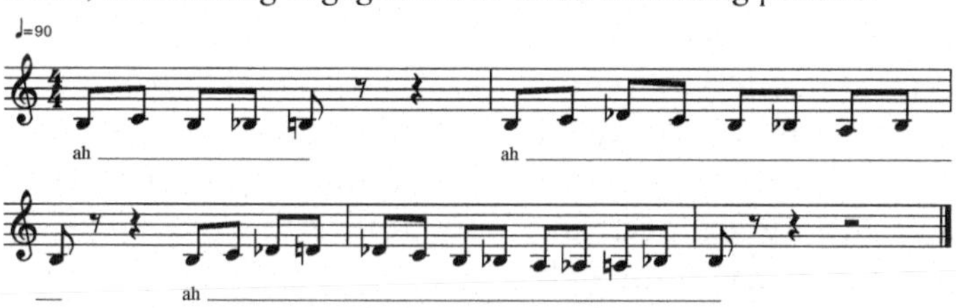 Cues to modify vowels facilitating (toward more closed vowel ascending and more open vowel descending) aided in stabilizing register 3. Worked on audition repertoire staccato-legato on /ha/, then on vowels corresponding to text, then on text. On sustained notes, practiced pulsing eighth notes with epigastric movement, then gradually faded pulsation while maintaining active engagement of the abdomen. Cue: "Think crescendo"
6	1. Reviewed exercises from previous sessions with decreased dependence on stabilization props. She was able to achieve engagement of torso for stability in standing position most of the time. 2. Continued to work on audition repertoire. In more complex passages, sang on /ka/ first to engage epigastric movement, then on words. Cues: "Think crescendo" and "think loud"
7	Reviewed exercises and strategies from previous sessions. Reviewed audition material. She was mostly independent in achieving legato singing with effective compensation for tremor. Discharged from therapy following successful audition.

Note. *Speaking voice was addressed concurrently with singing voice therapy with a different clinician as discussed in text.*

Case Study 3: Professional Classical Soprano Following Microflap Excision of Vocal Fold Cyst

At the time she was evaluated at our clinic, "Laurina" was a 38-year-old operatic soprano with a successful international career performing leading roles with major opera companies and symphony orchestras across the United States, Europe, and Asia. She had experienced an upper respiratory tract infection during an opera engagement 8 months earlier. She was seen by an otolaryngologist local to the performance who examined her with laryngoscopy and prescribed oral steroids. She was able to get through the performance but noted that her voice had been "up and down" since then. She saw another laryngologist during a subsequent performance and was diagnosed with a vocal fold polyp. Voice rest was recommended. She cancelled a recital engagement and her voice improved but was still not back to normal.

Laurina was a highly trained and skilled singer. Her vocal hygiene habits were excellent and she was generally mindful about vocal pacing, although she admitted sometimes feeling fatigued after prolonged periods of practice when preparing new repertoire.

Stroboscopy revealed a right vocal fold cyst near the vibrating edge resulting in hourglass closure with moderate to severe impairment of vocal fold vibration on the affected side. There was a small amount of contralateral edema. Surgical excision of the cyst was recommended, to be followed by voice therapy. The laryngologist informed her of the risk of the cyst rupturing with continued voice use, which could result in a more severe injury. She had a pending concert performance in 3 weeks that she didn't feel she could cancel. The repertoire was not particularly challenging and her role in the performance was relatively short. After that, she had a recital that she felt she could reschedule to a later date, and she would not have another opera engagement for 4 months. She decided to go ahead with the imminent concert and undergo surgery shortly afterward.

We started her postoperative course of voice therapy 2 weeks after the surgery. The course of Laurina's postoperative rehabilitation is detailed in Table 12–5. We began with low-intensity tasks, focusing on SOVT to facilitate healing. Over the course of her recovery, we gradually increased the duration of singing and complexity of the exercises. We reviewed the video from the concert she sang prior to her surgery, and some base of tongue and laryngeal tension were noted. She felt this had occurred gradually following her initial injury. Based on this finding, rehabilitation exercises included strategies for tension reduction. As an accomplished singer, Laurina was already in the habit of executing technically intricate exercises. However, after her surgery, she noted decreased agility. This was not a surprising development considering her injury and surgery. Exercises were developed to address this functional component, many of which were drawn from her regular vocal exercise regimen. Halfway through her therapy, she resumed voice lessons with her teacher, continuing lessons concurrently with voice therapy for the remainder of her treatment.

Table 12–5. Case Study "Laurina": Vocal exercise regimen for 38-year-old professional operatic soprano. Diagnosis: Status-post micro-flap excision of right vocal fold cyst.

Session Number	***Exercises***
1	Two weeks postsurgery 1. Relaxation and stretching exercises introduced 2. Adductory power on lip trill/raspberry A4–A3 diatonically 3. 1-3-1 glide on lip trill to C5. Strain noted at C5. Also trialed 1-5-1 glide, but she reported decreased ease of phonation with the wider interval, so it was discontinued. 4. "Swelling Test" (see Chapter 11 for details on soft phonation swelling test): 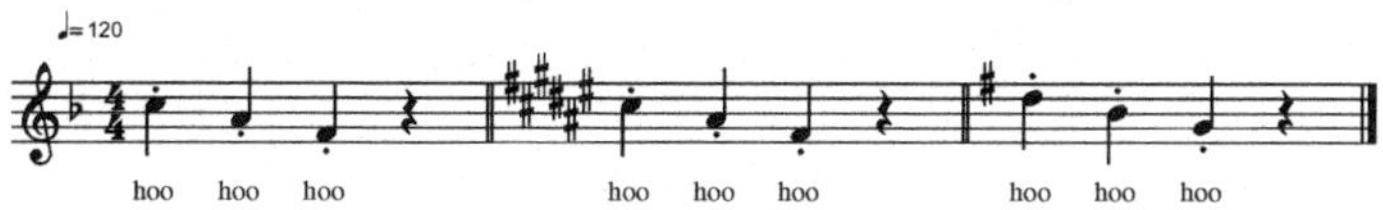 Ceiling was at A5 (e.g., no sound would come out at that pitch when attempted at minimal loudness). Breathy or delayed onset noted between beginning at F#4 5. 5-4-3-2-1 on lip trill to C5 (reported strain at this pitch) A total of about 10 minutes of the session was spent on vocal exercises. She reported that she didn't feel fatigued at the end, but that her voice felt "effortful and weak." Instructions for home practice: 5 to 10 minutes per day of gentle exercises
2	1. Relaxation and stretching exercises 2. Adductory power on lip trill A4–A3 diatonically, successfully repeated later in session on small-diameter straw 3. Unstructured ascending and descending glides on small straw in comfortable range 4. 1-3-1 glide on lip trill to F5. Strain noted at F5. Also attempted 1-5-1 glide again in same range without strain this time 5. Swelling test with ceiling at C6, some breathy onset noted between F#5 and C6 6. 5-4-3-2-1 and 1-3-5-3-1 on lip trill to A5 (reported strain at top pitch) 7. Speaking voice: Worked on "recalibrating" pitch and resonance with straw phonation at A3, followed by structured tasks with /z/ initial through sentence level Instructions for home practice: Practice 10 to 20 minutes per day as tolerated, divided into multiple sessions
3	1. Relaxation and stretching exercises 2. Adductory power on small straw from A4–A3, added crescendo 3. 1-5-1 glide on lip trill to C6 4. 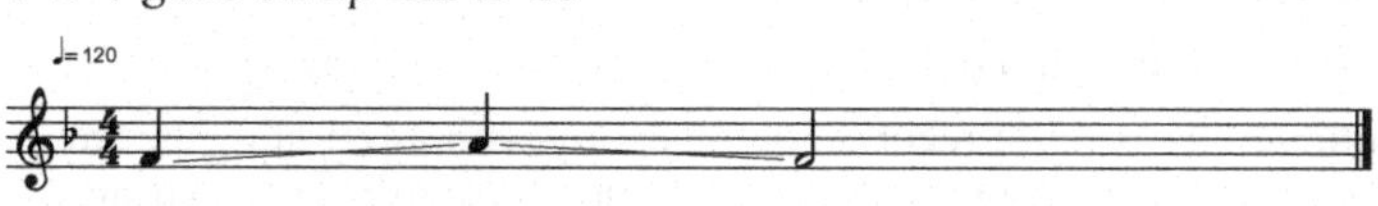 to A5 to initiate phonation on vowels 5. Swelling test with ceiling at D6, clean onset to B5 6. Speaking voice: Paragraph reading, mostly independent with "recalibrating" Instructions for home practice: Practice for 20 to 30 minutes per day as tolerated

continues

Table 12–5. *continued*

Session Number	***Exercises***
4	Worked on improving laryngeal stabilization strategy with "Ball Bounce" during exercises today (see Figure 12–4D) 1. Relaxation and stretching exercises 2. Adductory power on small straw from A4–A3 with messa di voce, repeated on /i/ from B flat 4 to B flat 3 3. 1-8-1 glide on lip trill to D#6 4. Swelling test ceiling at D#6 5. Five-note scale: 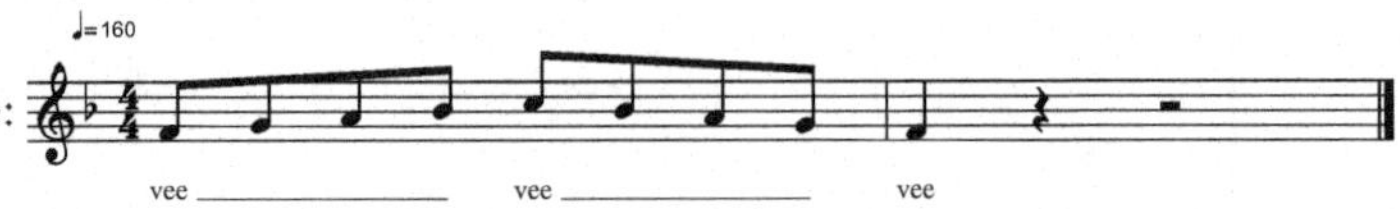 to B flat 5. Somewhat unsteady. Worked on transitioning from staccato to slow legato and then fast legato to promote reconditioning of agility: 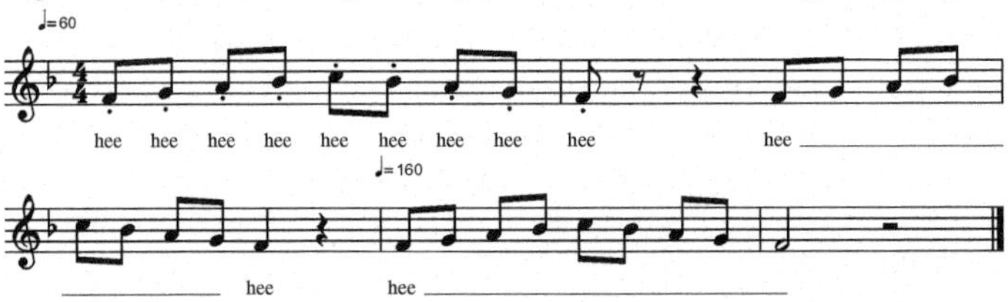 6. 1-3-5-3-1 on /jaɪ/ (as described in Table 12–1) for release of base of tongue tension, D4–A5 7. Added cool-down: Laryngeal massage; descending glides on lip trill to speaking pitch; structured speaking exercises with /z/ initial 8. Speaking voice: Independent in structured conversation Instructions for home practice: Increase practice to 30 to 40 minutes per day as tolerated, breaking practice time into multiple short sessions
5	1. Reviewed exercises from previous session 2. Added nine-note scale C4–D6 on various vowels utilizing the same sequence of staccato to legato that was employed in the five-note scale in the previous session Continued work on posture/stabilization strategies as in previous sessions helped decrease laryngeal tension and facilitated vocal agility. Instructions for home practice: Increase practice to 40 to 50 minutes per day as tolerated
6	1. Reviewed exercises from previous session 2. Swelling test ceiling F6 3. Continued to work on reconditioning agility with alternating staccato and legato as in previous sessions, and also alternating dotted rhythms with straight rhythms using a variety of vowels. Examples of dotted rhythms employed: 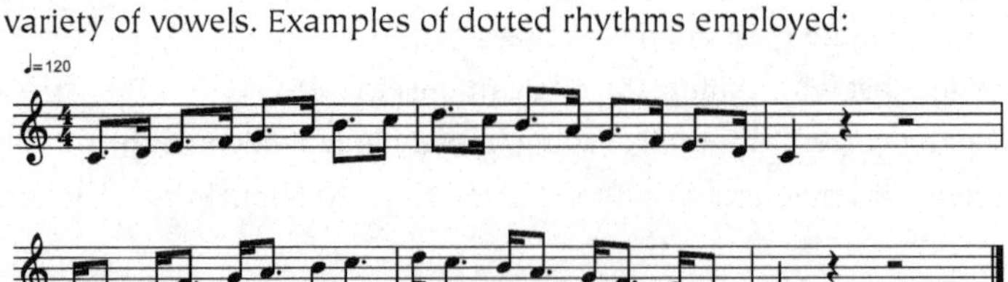 Also used this strategy in coloratura passages from repertoire

Table 12–5. *continued*

Session Number	*Exercises*
6 *continued*	4. Added 1-3-5-8-5-3-1 on /a/ to C6 Continued to work on posture/stabilization strategies as in previous session Instructions for home practice: Increase practice time to 50 to 60 minutes as tolerated, breaking into short sessions as needed; resume voice lessons with regular teacher for 30-minute lesson
7	Reviewed exercises from previous session 1. Swelling test ceiling F6 2. Continued alternating dotted rhythms with straight rhythms using a variety of vowels: 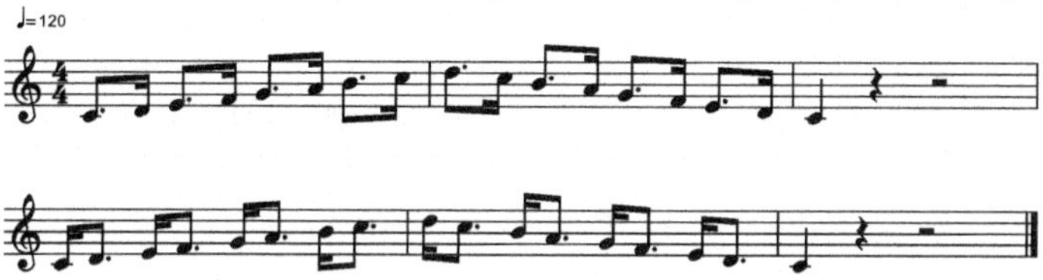 Also used this strategy in coloratura passages from repertoire 3. Added agility exercise from her typical vocal exercise regimen on a variety of vowels, A3–C6: 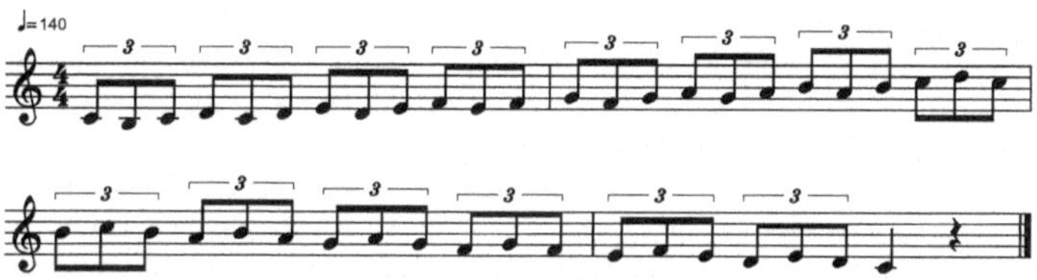 Instructions for home practice: Continue to practice for to 40 to 60 minutes as tolerated
8	Much of the session was devoted to discussion of vocal pacing strategies in preparation for resuming performing, including planning practice time. Reviewed some of the exercises from previous sessions. At this point, she was tolerating 45 to 60 minutes of vocal exercise daily and had resumed 60-minute voice lesson weekly. Speaking voice: Independent at conversational level
9	Reviewed current practice routine: 1. Relaxation and stretching exercises 2. Adductory power on small straw from A4–A3 with messa di voce, repeated on /i/ from B flat 4 to B flat 3 and then B flat 4–C6 3. 1-8-1 glide on lip trill to E6 4. Swelling test ceiling at F#6 5. Five-note scale × 3 on various vowels; smooth and agile to D6 6. 1-3-5-8-5-3-1 on /jaɪ/ (as described in Table 12–1) for release of base of tongue tension, B flat 3–F6 7. Nine-note scale alternating staccato/legato and dotted/straight as in previous sessions on vowels, A3–F6

continues

Table 12–5. *continued*

Session Number	*Exercises*
9 *continued*	8. 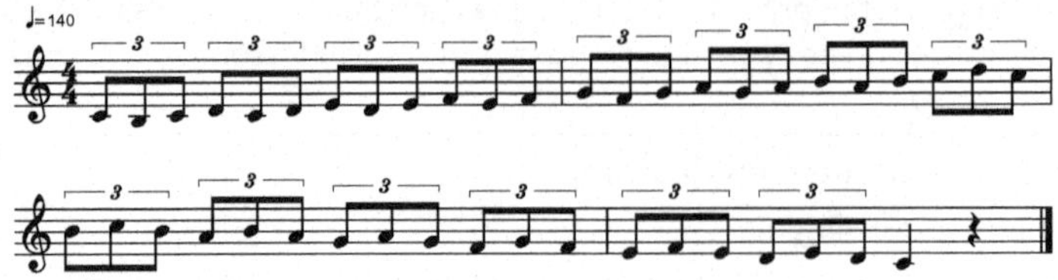 on vowels A3–F6 Then: 9. Added: 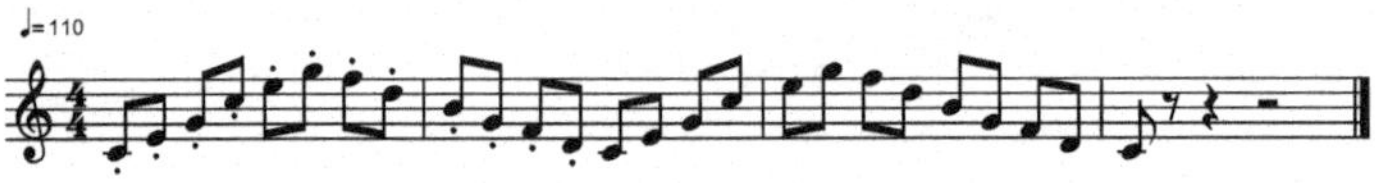 on vowels A3–F6 for agility, precision, range expansion 10. Worked through several passages from repertoire using posture/stabilization strategies and BOT tension reduction as in exercises 11. Cool-down
10	Continued to work on vocal pacing strategies and application of rehabilitation exercises to repertoire. Reevaluation with stroboscopy revealed straight and smooth left vocal fold edge, some residual irregularity on right edge, normal closure and vibration. She felt voice was 85% based on stamina. Discharged from therapy.

Note. *At the time she started her postoperative therapy, vocal hygiene and vocal pacing habits were already excellent, although we worked on planning practice time. Preoperative speaking voice was generally adequate and she required little in the way of speaking voice training during the rehabilitation process.*

At her 3-month postoperative evaluation, only a slight area of irregularity was noted at the location where the cyst had previously been, and the contralateral swelling had completely resolved. Closure and vibration were excellent. Fortunately, her first operatic performance 4 months after surgery was a role that she had performed many times and she felt she was adequately recovered and prepared in time for the performance.

Laurina had a relatively swift recovery. She continued her performing career successfully and, to my knowledge, without further incident. The speed at which she improved had a lot to do with the fact that she is a highly trained, gifted singer with excellent vocal technique. It is important to note that in cases of more severe injury with less technically advanced singers, or when there has been little preoperative groundwork, the postoperative therapy process is typically much more gradual, may span a longer period of time, and may take more sessions.

Case Study 4: Professional Rock Singer Following Vocal Fold Hemorrhage and Bilateral Vocal Fold Fibrotic Lesions

"James" was a 45-year-old rock singer. He was diagnosed with an acute right vocal fold hemorrhage following sudden voice loss after a particularly intense concert at an outdoor venue. He also had bilateral fibrotic vocal fold lesions. At the initial stroboscopy evaluation at our clinic, vibration was severely decreased on the right side and moderately decreased on the left and closure was incomplete. Complete vocal rest was recommended for 1 week following the hemorrhage. The laryngologist also prescribed a course of oral steroids to aid in determining his baseline swelling and to more clearly assess the underlying lesions. Stroboscopy was repeated 7 days later, at which time the hemorrhage had resolved by about 50%. The lesions appeared somewhat smaller following the steroid treatment but still spanned the middle third of the vocal folds. Modified voice rest with no singing was recommended. At the end of the third week, the hemorrhage had almost entirely resolved and voice therapy was initiated. Vibration impairment had improved to moderately decreased on the right and mildly to moderately decreased on the left, and closure had improved, although he still demonstrated considerable hyperfunction.

James was the headliner of his own band, which almost exclusively performed his original songs. The band rehearsed for 3 hours once per week and performed two to three times per month. Engagements were typically 2 to 3 hours long, often followed by interactions with the audience while working at a merchandise table. Optimizing vocal pacing was a major component of James's rehabilitation plan, with strategies as described in Chapters 14 and 16.

James had taken one semester of voice lessons in college and at one point used a vocal exercise CD geared toward rock singing, but he couldn't remember what the exercises were. He had not engaged in a regular vocal warm-up routine for several years.

Vocal hygiene goals included increasing hydration to 64 ounces per day and decreasing caffeine consumption to 16 ounces per day of coffee, as well as eliminating alcohol when performing. Contributing medical factors included GERD and allergic rhinitis, which were treated by the laryngologist.

The content and evolution of James's vocal exercise regimen are outlined in Table 12–6. Treatment spanned a period of 12 weeks. His songs frequently required rapid transition between TA-dominant register and falsetto, and exercises were included to entrain this skill. These exercises were designed by extracting song fragments, often replacing text with facilitating vowels or syllables, as described in Table 12–6.

Given his recent vocal fold hemorrhage, we recommended that he take a break from rehearsing and performing to minimize risk of further injury or recurrence of hemorrhage. By the end of his course of therapy, he had resumed performing activities, although with improved vocal pacing and regular practice of his new vocal exercise regimen.

Repeat stroboscopy revealed lesions that were smaller and somewhat softer, although he still had vibration impairment. The potential for further improvement with surgery was discussed, but he felt his voice was adequate to meet his needs and didn't want to take more time off from performing.

Table 12–6. ***Case Study "James": Vocal exercise regimen for 45-year-old professional rock singer/songwriter with minimal vocal training. Diagnosis: Status-post vocal fold hemorrhage; bilateral fibrotic vocal fold lesions. He was on complete vocal rest for 1 week following hemorrhage. Stroboscopy was repeated for each of the following 2 weeks to assess resolution of hemorrhage, during which he was on modified voice rest with no singing. Therapy started during the third week, at which point the hemorrhage was almost fully resolved.***

Session Number	***Exercises***
1	1. Reviewed treatment plan and goals 2. Listened to recordings that predated onset of dysphonia for baseline and reviewed typical rehearsal and performance schedule 3. Worked on establishing low abdominal breathing pattern. He was familiar with the technique but tended to use excessive abdominal clenching on exhalation. Eliminated clenching by practicing breathing pattern while bent over from the waist and lying supine on the floor. Practiced exhaling on /s/ and /ʃ/, gradually transitioning to voiced cognates
2	1. Reviewed breathing exercises 2. Adductory power on tongue trill C3–G3 diatonically 3. Full-range unstructured glide on tongue trill 4. 5–1 glide on tongue trill B flat 2–F4 5. Speaking voice: /z/ initial syllables and words
3	1. Adductory power on small-straw phonation C3–C4 diatonically 2. Full-range unstructured glide on tongue trill 3. 5–1 glide on tongue trill B flat 2–G4 4. 5–1 glide on /wu/ for falsetto F4–G5 5. Speaking voice: /z/ initial syllables through phrases Instructions for home practice: 10 to 15 minutes per day of exercises and 10 to 15 minutes of songs, as tolerated
4	1. Adductory power on small-straw phonation C3–C4 diatonically with crescendo 2. Full-range unstructured glide on tongue trill 3. 5–1 glide on tongue trill B flat 2–G4 4. 5–1 glide for falsetto alternating with 54321 as illustrated F4–G5: 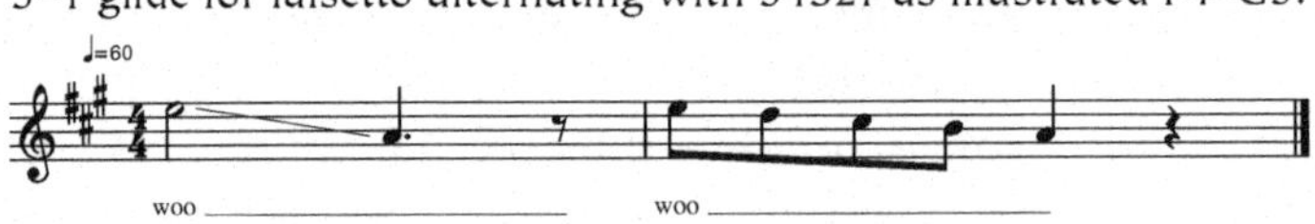 5. 8–1 glide on tongue trill to transition to low range C5–A2 6. Introduced "twang" resonance C3–G4 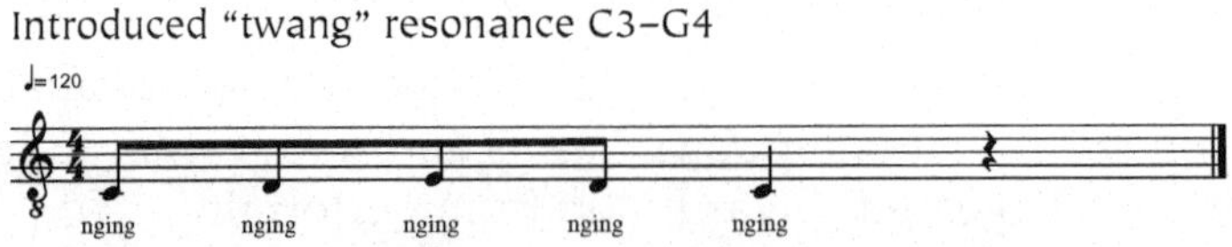 7. 5–1 on /jæ/ for belt C3–G4. Cues: Exaggerate lip retraction and slightly raise chin; increase vertical mouth opening as pitch increases while still maintaining retracted lip position; "think twang"

Table 12–6. *continued*

Session Number	Exercises
4 *continued*	8. Speaking voice: /z/ initial sentences; typical short phrases from daily communications ("that's right"; "let's go"; "how you doin'?"; etc.) Instructions for home practice: 10 to 15 minutes per day of exercises and 10 to 20 minutes of songs, as tolerated
5	1. Adductory power on small-straw phonation C3–C4 diatonically with messa di voce 2. Full-range unstructured glide on tongue trill 3. 5–1 glide alternating with 5-4-3-2-1 on tongue trill B flat 2–G4 4. 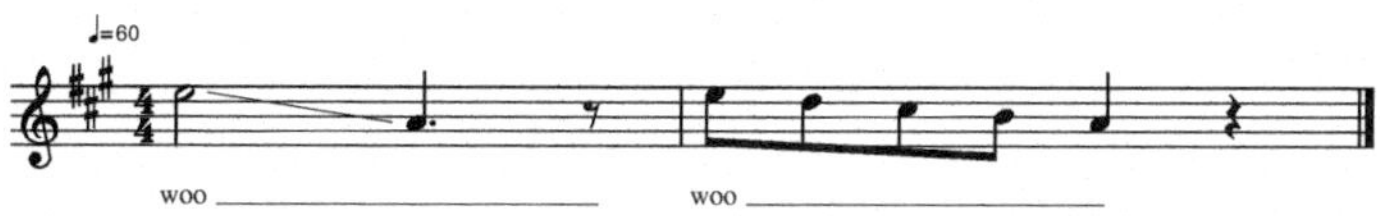 for falsetto F4–G5 5. 8–1 glide on tongue trill to transition to low range C5–A2 6. 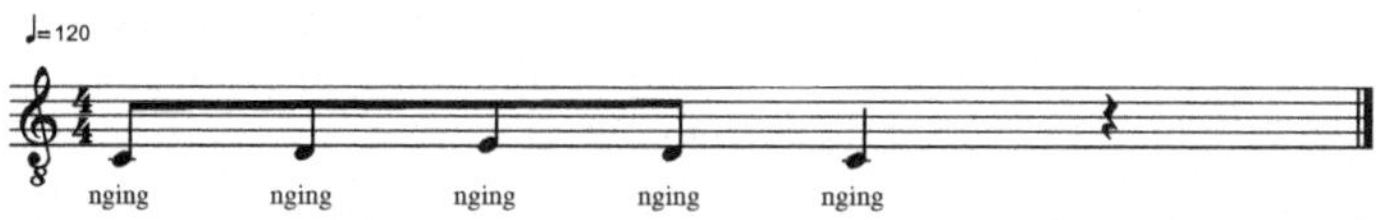 for "twang" resonance C3–A4 7. 5–1 on /jæ/ for belt C3–A4 with cues as in previous session 8. Speaking voice: Paragraph reading using lyrics from his songs Recommendation: Resume rehearsing with the band for no more than 45 minutes total singing Instructions for home practice: 30 to 40 minutes per day of exercises and songs
6	At this session, he presented with increased hoarseness associated with frequent sneezing and nasal congestion. He also admitted "overdoing it" a little when he resumed rehearsing with the band, singing for about 75 minutes. High range was constrained in pitch glides as compared with the previous session. Stroboscopy was performed during the session to determine whether he had recurrence of hemorrhage. No hemorrhage was evident, but he had viscous mucus in the nose and posterior pharynx and slightly increased vocal fold edema. The laryngologist was consulted. He prescribed nasal antihistamine for seasonal allergies. James was instructed to modify vocal exercise regimen until symptoms resolved.
7	1. Adductory power on small-straw phonation C3–C4 diatonically with messa di voce 2. Full-range unstructured glide on lip trill instead of tongue trill (he had previously not been able to coordinate lip trill) 3. 5–1 glide alternating with 5-4-3-2-1 on lip trill B flat 2–G4 4. 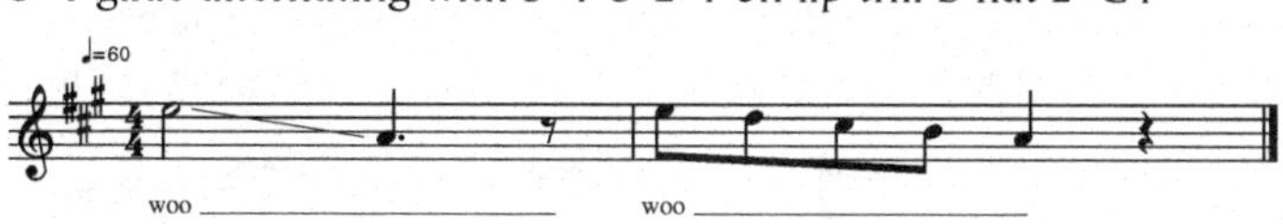 for falsetto F4–G5 5. 8–1 glide on lip trill to transition to low range C5–A2 6. 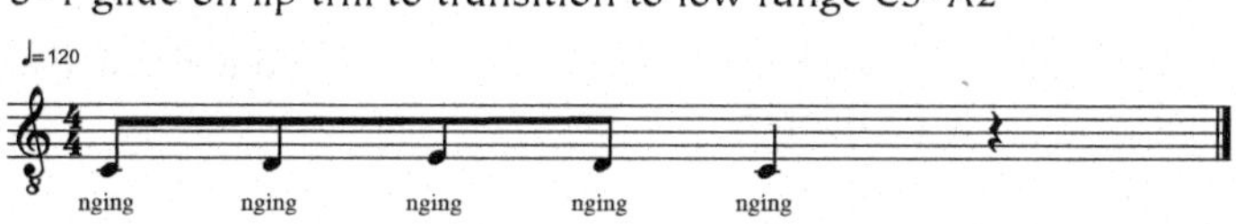 for "twang" resonance C3–G4

continues

Table 12–6. *continued*

Session Number	Exercises
7 *continued*	7. 5–1 on /jæ/ for belt C3–G4 8. Added: 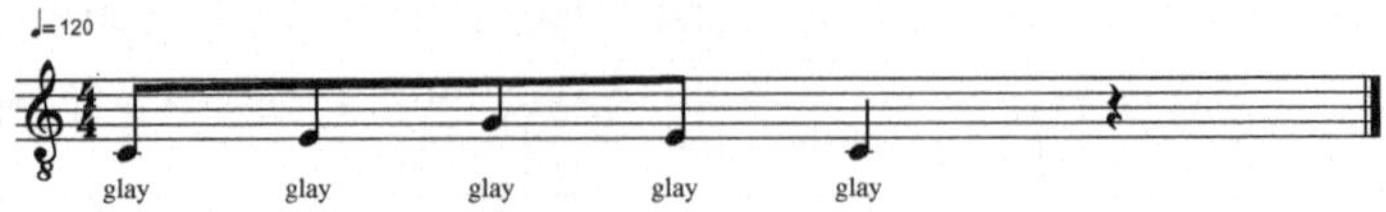 for belt and tongue mobility C3–G4 9. Introduced cool-down: Laryngeal massage; descending glides on tongue trill to speaking range; structured speaking tasks with /z/ initial, syllables through phrases 10. Speaking voice: Structured conversation/responding to clinician questions Recommendation: Resume rehearsing with the band for no more than 45 minutes total singing once per week Instructions for home practice: 30 to 60 minutes of exercises/songs as tolerated
8	He reported diligent adherence to recommended duration of rehearsal and was able to get through 45 minutes of singing with minimal fatigue. 1. Adductory power on small-straw phonation C3–C4 diatonically with messa di voce 2. Full-range unstructured glide on lip trill 3. 5–1 glide alternating with 5-4-3-2-1 on lip trill B flat 2–G4 4. 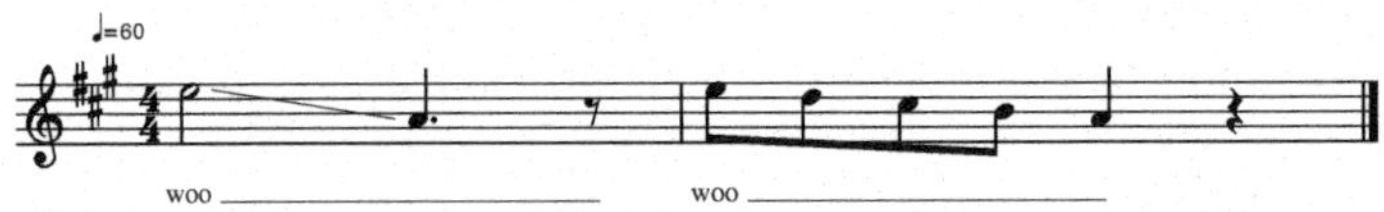 for falsetto F4–A5 5. 8–1 glide on tongue trill to transition to low range C5–A2 6. 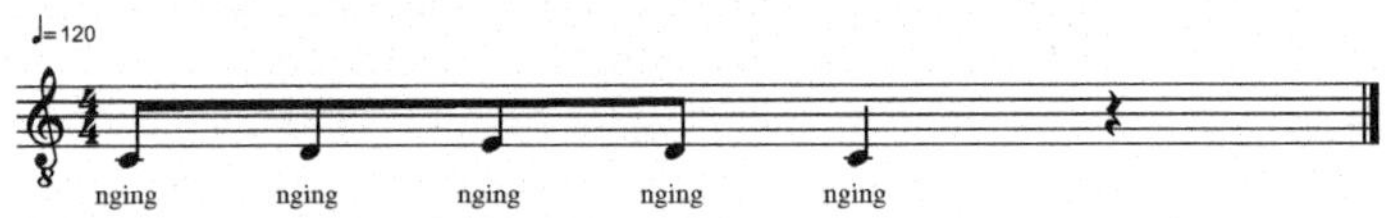 for "twang" resonance C3–A4 7. 5–1 on /jæ/ for belt C3–A4. Established shared reference for effort level of 1 to 10, 10 being the highest effort. Worked on varying effort randomly from 1 to 10 for dynamic control and to promote TA/CT balance for high belt 8. 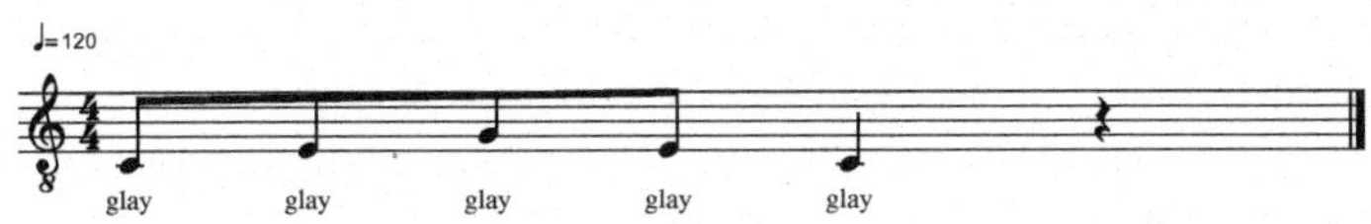 for belt and tongue mobility C3–A4 9. His songs frequently required rapid transition between TA-dominant register and falsetto. Introduced new exercise to entrain this skill, extracting fragment from one of his songs: 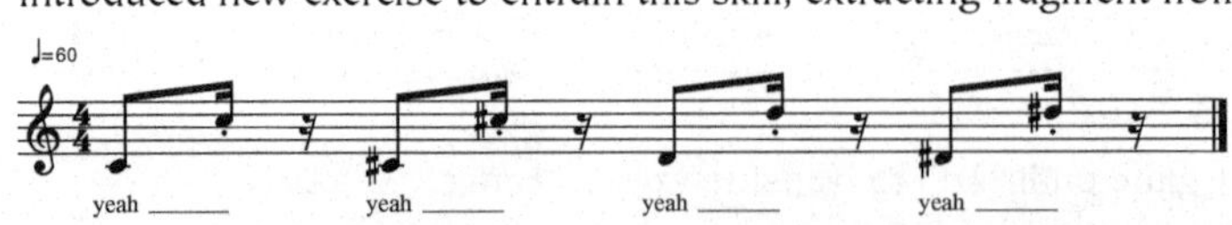 with TA dominant on the bottom note, staccato falsetto with "squeak" or "whimper" quality on the top note, F3–F5 10. Cool-down

Table 12–6. *continued*

Session Number	*Exercises*
8 *continued*	11. Speaking voice: Simulated radio interview Recommendation: Plan on resuming performance in 2 to 3 weeks. Continue home practice as previously noted.
9	1. Adductory power on small-straw phonation C3–C4 diatonically with messa di voce 2. Full-range unstructured glide on lip trill 3. 5–1 glide alternating with 5-4-3-2-1 on lip trill B flat 2–G4 4. 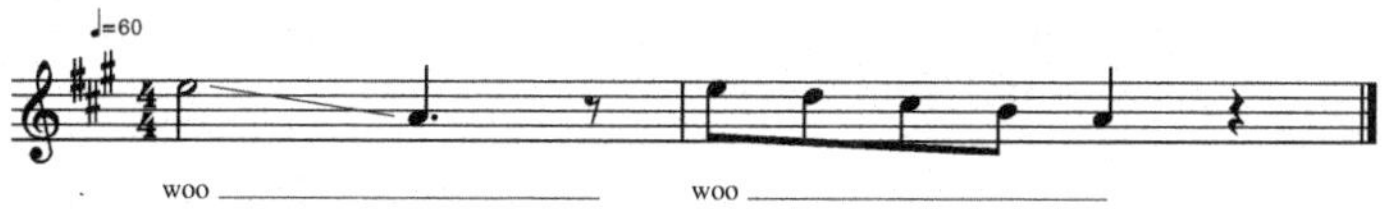 for falsetto F4–A5 5. 8–1 glide on tongue trill to transition to low range C5–A2 6. 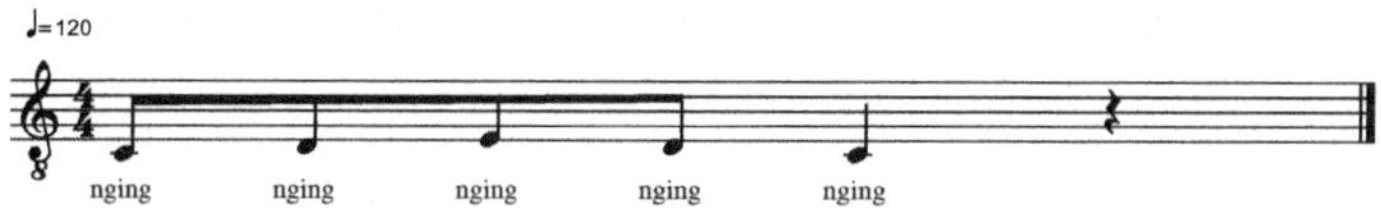 for "twang" resonance C3–A4 7. 5–1 on /jæ/ for belt, C3–A4 varying effort randomly from 1 to 10 from C3–F4; then keeping effort at 7 to 8 from F4–A4; good projection, no excessive strain 8. 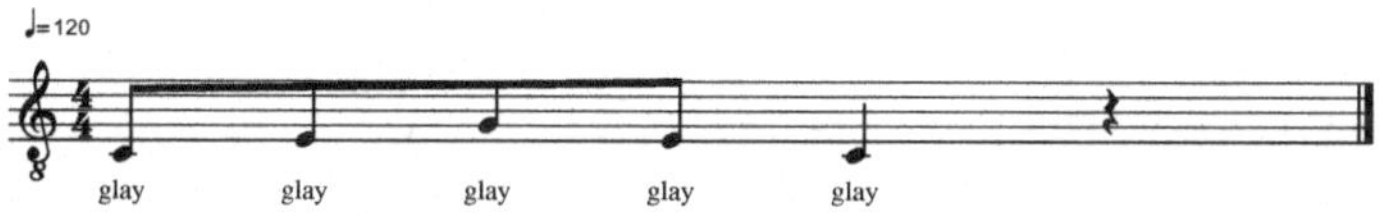 for belt and tongue mobility C3–A4 9. 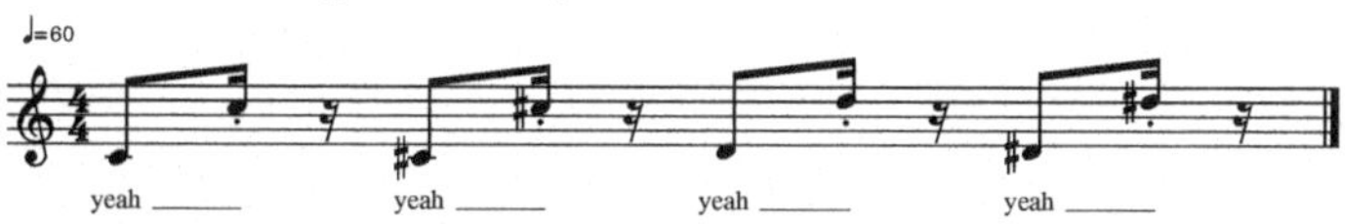 as in previous session, F3–A5 Continued to work on alternating TA-dominant register with falsetto: 10. Extracted song fragment alternating falsetto on first part of the exercise ("hoo") with TA dominant on second part ("ah"), B3–D5: 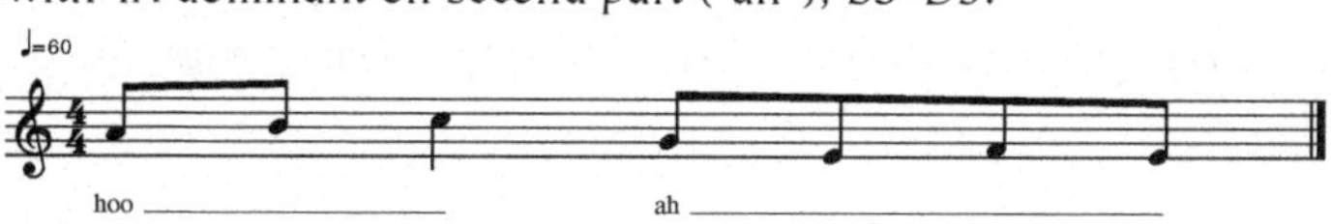 11. Worked on applying techniques to songs from set lists 12. Cool-down 13. Speaking voice: Simulated after-show "meet and greet" with audience/fans
10	He reported that he tolerated a 2-hour performance well. 1. Adductory power on small-straw phonation C3–C4 diatonically with messa di voce 2. Full-range unstructured glide on lip trill 3. 5–1 glide on lip trill B flat 2–G4 4. 5-4-3-2-1 on /wu/ for falsetto F4–A5 5. 8–1 glide on tongue trill to transition to low range C5–A2

continues

Table 12–6. *continued*

<table>
<tr><th>Session Number</th><th>Exercises</th></tr>
<tr><td>10
continued</td><td>
6. 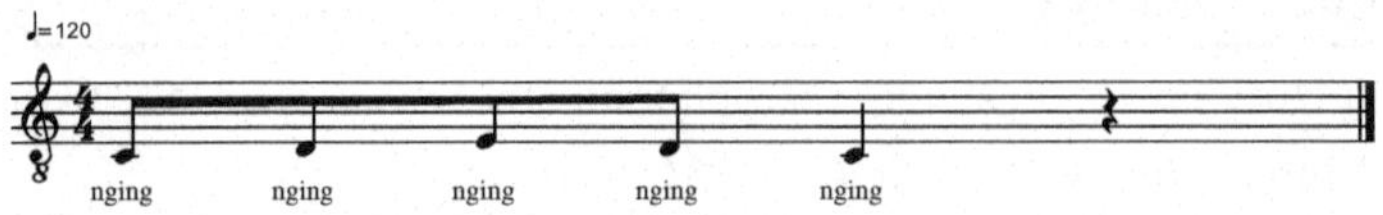

for "twang" resonance C3–B flat 4
7. 5–1 on /jæ/ for belt C3–A4 varying effort randomly from 1 to 10 from C3–F4; then keeping effort at 7 to 8 from F4–A4
8. 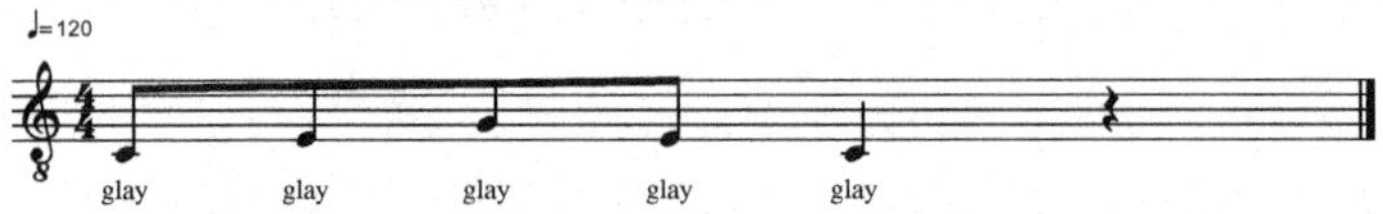

C3–A4 for belt and tongue mobility
9. 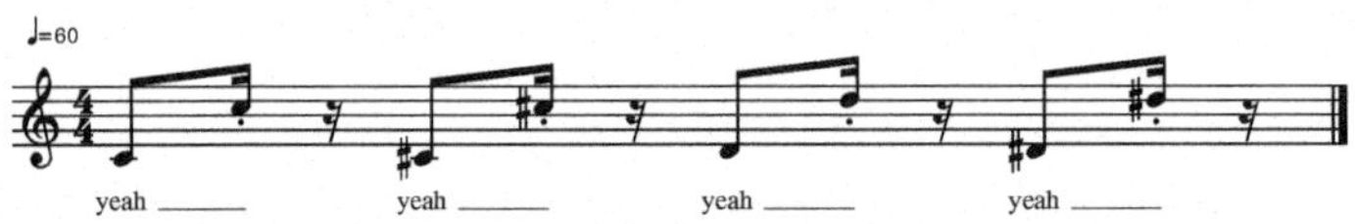

as in previous sessions F3–A5
10. 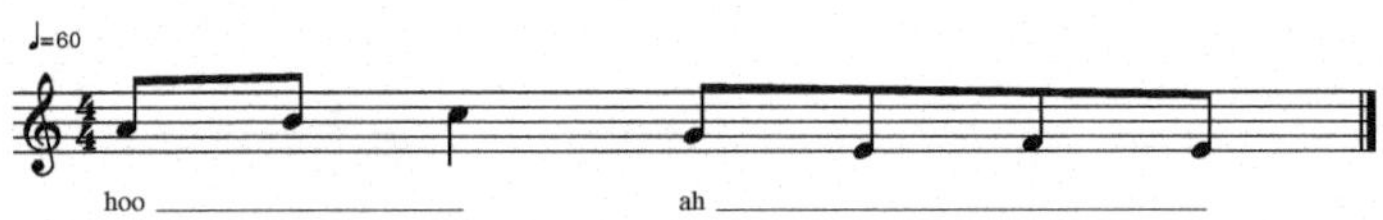

as in previous session B3–D5
11. Worked on applying techniques to songs from set lists
12. Cool-down
13. Speaking voice: Conversational level
Discharged from therapy. Reevaluation with stroboscopy revealed some remaining irregularity and fibrotic changes of vocal fold edges, remaining varix, improved vocal fold vibration, and reduced hyperfunction.
</td></tr>
</table>

Note. *Vocal hygiene, medical management of GERD and seasonal allergies, and vocal pacing were addressed throughout the therapy process but are not included in this chart, which focuses on the evolution of the exercise regimen.*

REFERENCES

Barkmeier-Kraemer, J. (2013). Hiding vocal tremor. In A. Behrman & J. Haskell (Eds.), *Exercises for voice therapy* (2nd ed.). San Diego, CA: Plural.

Behrman, A., & Sulica, L. (2003). Voice rest after microlaryngoscopy: Current opinion and practice. *Laryngoscope, 12*(2), 2182–2186.

Edwards, M. (Ed.). (2014). *So you want to sing rock 'n' roll*. Lanham, MD: Rowman and Littlefield.

Gilman, M. (2014). *Body and voice: Somatic re-education*. San Diego, CA: Plural.

Klimak, M. M. (2003). *Level one course Estill voice craft with compulsory figures for voice: Study guide*. Lexington, MA: Mary McDonald Klimak for EVTS.

LeBorgne, W. D., & Rosenberg, M. (2014). *The vocal athlete*. San Diego, CA: Plural.

LeFevre, C. (2011). Tongue management. *Journal of Singing, 68*(2), 157–162.

LeFevre, C. (2015). Techniques for maintaining low larynx and open throat in classical singing. *Journal of Singing, 71*(4), 459–463.

National Institute of Dental and Craniofacial Research. (2014). Retrieved July 14, 2014, from http://www.nidcr.nih.gov/DataStatistics/

FindDataByTopic/FacialPain/Prevalence TMJD.htm

Rosenberg, M., & LeBorgne, W. D. (2014). *The vocal athlete: Application and technique for the hybrid singer.* San Diego, CA: Plural.

Titze, I. R., & Verdolini Abbott, K. (2012). *Vocology: The science and practice of voice habilitation.* Salt Lake City, UT: National Center for Voice and Speech.

Verdolini Abbott, K., Li, N. Y., Branski, R. C., Rosen, C. A., Grillo, E., Steinhauer, K., & Hebda, P. A. (2012). Vocal exercise may attenuate acute vocal fold inflammation. *Journal of Voice, 26*(6), 814.e1–814.e1B.

CHAPTER 13

Speaking Voice Therapy for Singers

So far, the focus of this book has been on the singing voice. However, we use the same instrument for speaking and singing, and the same convergence of factors that affect the singing voice will also have an impact on the speaking voice. It is very rare (though not unheard of) for one to be affected without the other. Therefore, the speaking voice must be directly addressed as a part of the overall rehabilitation plan. As with the singing voice, the goal of speaking voice rehabilitation is to restore the voice to the best possible quality, restore healthy mucosa and laryngeal function, optimize coordination of voicing subsystems, promote vocal conditioning, and eliminate phonotrauma and maladaptive muscle tension.

WHO PROVIDES SPEAKING VOICE REHABILITATION?

For those of you on the speech-language pathology path, completing a clinical placement in voice disorders as part of your graduate clinical experience is an essential component of your preparation for a career in voice rehabilitation. Once you are out of graduate school, it will be much more difficult to find opportunities for supervised training. There are numerous continuing education courses in voice rehabilitation that can provide excellent opportunities for expanding and deepening your knowledge and resources relative to speaking voice therapy, but without the supervision and mentorship afforded by a hands-on practicum, it is much more difficult to acquire the requisite expertise. If you are coming to voice rehabilitation later in your SLP career and did not have the benefit of a clinical practicum and/or clinical fellowship, I recommend taking appropriate courses but also seeking out observation experience and, if possible, supervised intervention with an expert clinician.

Speaking voice therapy is outside the scope of practice for voice teachers—even those who have advanced training in voice science and who have studied and observed the clinical aspects of voice care. Although many voice teachers have excellent understanding of vocal mechanics and singing voice pedagogy, training the speaking voice is not typically a part of the academic preparation of a voice teacher. Even if the voice teacher has acquired experience in *habilitation* of the speaking voice—perhaps through acting classes or speaking coaches—*rehabilitation* of the speaking voice must be provided by a licensed SLP. If the voice teacher has been working with the singer as a part of the singing voice rehabilitation process (with the appropriate training, as discussed earlier on in this book), it will be essential to have an SLP as a part of the vocal health team who can provide voice therapy for speaking voice. Having said this, it would certainly be beneficial for voice teachers to seek mentoring opportunities with voice-specialized SLPs to expand their understanding and knowledge relative to speaking voice therapy. This collaboration is often a two-way street, as the voice teacher possesses considerable skills and insight relative to shaping voice that can apply to speaking as well.

The ideal scenario is for the singer to work with a provider who is qualified to address both the speaking and singing voice holistically in voice therapy. If a clinical singing voice rehabilitation specialist (SLP with appropriate singing training) is available, the singer is spared the financial and scheduling burden associated with compartmentalizing speaking and singing voice interventions. At the very least, speaking and singing interventions should occur concurrently rather than sequentially (American Speech-Language-Hearing Association [ASHA], 2005).

"SPEAK HIGHER" IS NOT THE GOAL

One of my voice teachers used to say (in dramatic, melodious, Julia Child-esque tones), "Speak like you sing!" I took her at her word, which unfortunately (as a coloratura soprano) led me to talk in my head voice for much of my early teaching and performing career. When I got a review for an operetta performance that spoke favorably of my singing but observed that I "chirped" my dialogue, I began to rethink this advice, and that set me on the path to finding my "true" speaking voice. Since then, I have heard many voice teachers instruct their students to "speak higher" and have heard from many of my singing patients that they were similarly instructed. Unfortunately, this advice is also sometimes doled out by SLPs who are not adequately trained in voice therapy.

Putting aside the risk for garnering negative attention from music critics, speaking at a higher pitch does nothing to improve vocal efficiency. The vocal folds are under greater tension at higher pitch, there are more vocal fold collisions associated with the higher frequency, and maintaining the inappropriate laryngeal posture necessary to speak at an artificially high pitch can lead to maladaptive muscle tension or even painful phonation. And it just plain sounds unnatural! The appropriate laryngeal configuration for speaking employs robust activation of the TA. In other words, the natural register for speaking is chest voice (or perhaps chest-dominant mix for women). Therapy focused on pitch change has generally been discredited and is not believed to improve healthy phonation (Heuer et al., 2006). For an excellent discussion on debunking the "speak higher" myth, see Michael (2012).

SPEAKING VOICE THERAPY APPROACHES

Optimal speaking voice is achieved through coordination of the respiratory, phonatory, and resonance subsystems of voice. Thus, any therapeutic approach should address all three. There are a number of well-established treatment paradigms for voice therapy and abundant resources for learning about them. In-depth exploration is beyond the scope of this text, but brief summaries of some of the most well known and well researched are provided below. For an excellent overview of a variety of therapy approaches illustrated by case studies, see Stemple and Hapner (2014). Another helpful resource is Behrman and Haskell (2013).

Symptomatic Voice Therapy

Symptomatic voice therapy was first introduced by Daniel Boone (1971). The focus of the treatment is direct modification of the specific symptoms exhibited by the patient (e.g., breathy voice, hard glottal onsets, poor projection, etc.). In this approach, the clinician looks for what the patient is doing already that results in better voice and is achieved with little effort and uses this discovery as the starting point for therapy. There is an emphasis on utilization of facilitating techniques —that is, any technique that helps the patient achieve good voice. Facilitating techniques might include "yawn-sigh"; articulatory movement (shifting tongue position, open mouth positions, or use of chewing motion for jaw mobility); respiration training; pitch, loudness, and inflection changes; laryngeal manipulation; ear training; reducing phonotraumatic behaviors; reducing glottal onsets; use of laryngeal massage/manipulation and relaxation techniques; providing education, explanation, and feedback; use of negative practice and voice models; and/or targeted vocal pacing (Stemple, 2014). The approach is highly individualized and invites the clinician to respond directly to each patient's unique presentation.

Physiologic Voice Therapy

Physiologic voice therapy focuses on coordination of the respiratory, phonatory, and resonance subsystems of voice, rather than focusing on a single component (Stemple, 2014). In a sense, this approach starts at the opposite end of the spectrum from symptomatic voice therapy, with the assumption that if the mechanism is appropriately coordinated, the isolated symptoms will resolve. There are a number of physiologic voice therapy treatment paradigms.

Vocal Function Exercises (VFEs)

One of the best-known and most used physiologic approaches to voice therapy is vocal function exercises, which we have already explored in depth in Chapter 11 (see that portion of the text for a review). In Chapter 11, we examined the benefits of VFEs as a part of the singing voice rehabilitation exercise regimen, but the exercises are also highly effective for the speaking voice. I have found these exercises to be especially beneficial when combined with an approach (resonant voice, for example) through which the patient can systematically apply the coordination to increasingly complex linguistic tasks (as will be described below).

Resonant Voice

Clinically defined as voice production that is "both easy to produce and vibrant in the facial tissues" (Titze & Verdolini Abbott 2012, p. 286), resonant voice is a mainstay of voice therapy. It is based on acting voice traditions, specifically the teachings of the great acting teacher Arthur Lessac. Resonant voice allows for a robust and projected voice that is neither pressed nor breathy, with minimal mechanical stress on the vocal folds (Titze & Verdolini Abbott 2012). This is accomplished by optimizing the interaction of source-filter so that the vocal tract actually helps the vocal folds vibrate more efficiently. We have discussed this phenomenon from various perspectives in preceding chapters. The assistance of vocal tract inertance results in low-impact and large-amplitude vibration with vocal folds that are lightly adducted. This lowers phonation threshold pressure (PTP) and reduces laryngeal effort, promoting resolution of traumatic injury and unloading maladaptive muscle tension. This ideal coordination of source-filter also makes this approach an excellent choice for voice habilitation and prevention of injury.

Resonant voice (also sometimes called "forward focus") utilizes semi-occluded vocal tract sounds and exercises to achieve optimal coordination. The patient is encouraged to explore the vibrating sensations in the face and head to use as a sensory reference and target, although the resonance actually takes place in the vocal tract (see Chapter 11 for a detailed description of SOVT and associated benefits).

Lessac-Madsen Resonant Voice Therapy (LMRVT). Lessac-Madsen resonant voice therapy (LMRVT) is a resonant voice therapy program that was designed by Dr. Katherine Verdolini Abbott. This program has its foundation in resonant voice as described above but incorporates specific biomechanical and motor learning principles (see Chapter 9 for more information on motor learning) and strategies to support therapy adherence. To learn more about LMRVT, see Verdolini Abbott (2008). LMRVT courses are also regularly offered in various locations.

Accent Method

The accent method was developed by Svend Smith in the 1930s and was inspired by African drumming (Heuer et al., 2006; Stemple, 2014). This approach has a heavy emphasis on breath support and targets modal voice (TA-dominant register). The patient is taught to use rhythmic abdominal contractions to produce "accents" while sustaining various sounds such as fricatives and closed vowels (SOVT), resulting in musical rhythmic patterns executed in a marcato fashion. The patient starts with unvoiced sounds to isolate breath support without phonation and adds voicing once proficiency is achieved. Complexity is increased by gradually accelerating the pace and by moving on to nonsense words and phrases and finally to meaningful words and phrases. For more information on the accent method, see Kotby (1995).

Flow Phonation

The concept of this approach was developed by Stone and Casteel, and later called "flow phonation" by Gauffin and Sundberg (Stemple & Hapner, 2014). The emphasis is on air flow in a structured hierarchy of tasks. The first three stages are *airflow release, breathy phonation,* and *flow phonation* (maintaining the airflow but removing the breathy component). Each level is first executed in an unarticulated manner (e.g., sustained sounds, first voiceless, then voiced) and then articulated (short phrases of connected speech). Facilitators are used to focus attention on airflow, such as cup-bubble (blowing through a drinking straw that is submerged in a cup of water), gargling, and exhaling with a tissue in front of the mouth for visual confirmation of airflow. Once the skills are acquired, a fourth stage is added that is called *articulatory precision* (deliberate focus on articulatory movement). In this last stage, the patient is encouraged to focus on "speaking clearly" and to explore the sensations associated with the interaction of breath flow and articulation.

PhoRTE: Phonation Resistance Training Exercises

Phonation resistance training exercises are designed primarily for cases of hypofunctional voice (Ziegler, Verdolini Abbott, Johns, Klein, & Hapner, 2014). The method is based on the exercise principle of overload. The goal is to achieve louder phonation through increased expiratory muscle activity, increased TA/LCA activation (to increase subglottic pressure), and use of megaphone mouth shape on /a/ to optimize acoustic energy through interaction of source and filter. Exercises include sustained /a/, pitch glides on /a/, and functional phrases in high and low voice, all at loud phonation (Stemple & Hapner, 2014; Ziegler et al., 2014). The patient progresses through a hierarchy ultimately to conversation. Because of the overload target, increased subglottic pressure with vigorous TA activation, and loud dynamic level, this approach is not indicated in cases of phontrauma but has been demonstrated to be effective for hypofunctional voice (Ziegler et al., 2014), which might include vocal fold paresis, paralysis, atrophy, or neurogenic voice disorders.

Lee Silverman Voice Therapy (LSVT)

Similarly to PhoRTE, LSVT targets loud voice to treat hypofunctional voice, specifically the dysarthria of Parkinson disease (Ramig, Bonitati, Lemkie, & Horii, 1994). However, the treatment protocol is more intensive than PhoRTE. The patient attends four sessions per week for a period of at least a month and must practice exercises multiple times per day. The systematic exercises emphasize phonatory effort and maximum frequency range, and are primarily aimed at prolonged loud phonation (Ramig et al, 1994; Heuer et al., 2006). The patient is cued to "Think loud" and "Think shout." For obvious reasons, this approach is also not appropriate for hyperfunctional voice or phonotraumatic injury. Clinicians must complete a training course and must be LSVT certified to provide the therapy.

Confidential Voice

In confidential voice, the patient is instructed to use a soft, breathy voice (but not a whisper), as if speaking to someone a few feet away or using a "library" voice. The idea is to achieve low effort and low intensity, with the vocal folds barely adducted. Due to the low intensity and lack of projection, confidential voice is not functional for communication. It is typically used briefly when the patient first begins voicing following phonosurgery to avoid mechanical stress that could lead to reinjury or negatively impact healing (Heuer et al., 2006).

Manual Circumlaryngeal Massage

Circumlaryngeal massage can be a very effective intervention for muscle tension dysphonia. The clinician applies systematic kneading using the thumb and index finger in a rotary massage of the entire extralaryngeal area, including over the hyoid bone, along the superior cornu of thyroid cartilage, in the thyrohyoid space, in the suprahyoid region (base of tongue), and the anterior border of the sternocleidomastoid muscles. The massage and manipulation can be utilized with the patient at rest or during phonation. The goal is to release muscle tension, improve circulation, and relieve pain and discomfort (Mathieson et al., 2009; Roy, Ford, & Bless, 1996; Stemple & Hapner, 2014). The clinician needs to be trained in the technique, as it is possible to interrupt circulation of the carotid artery or to cause injury by placing excessive pressure on laryngeal cartilages.

Eclectic Voice Therapy

In describing eclectic voice therapy, Stemple (2014) extols the value of having many resources and using what works for the patient. The idea is to draw from any and all treatment paradigms to customize a rehabilitation plan that best suits the patient. I am a strong advocate of this approach. The more you know about different therapy methodologies, the more tools you will have in your tool box. Mixing and matching can expedite the process, as it ensures a good fit between the treatment protocol and the patient's specific needs. Rigid adherence to one method or another can undermine your effectiveness as a clinician.

HIERARCHY OF TASKS

Whatever treatment approach you decide on, it will be necessary to structure tasks in a hierarchical fashion, starting at a level that the patient can successfully achieve and gradually increasing the complexity so that the patient can ultimately accomplish optimal coordination of respiration, phonation, and resonance at the conversational level. A typical hierarchy is sound, syllable, word, phrase, sentence, paragraph, conversation.

Singers are often already familiar with abdominal breathing, and in many cases you may not need to spend much time teaching this technique. However, it will not be unusual for you to work with singers who have been singing for years without understanding breath support. In these cases, you will need to teach them how to use abdominal breathing. Work on the breath pattern in isolation, and then have the patient practice sustained exhalation without phonation (/s, ʃ, f/, etc.). Ensuring good coordination of respiratory mechanics as a first step will usually save you time when you add voicing.

When the patient is ready to add phonation, start out by exploring different sounds to see if any result in spontaneous improvement in voice. SOVT sounds make great choices, for the reasons previously enumerated. Try not to get stuck on one sound or group of sounds—keep at it until you find what works for the patient, even if it seems counterintuitive. Once you've found the facilitating sound, proceed through the hierarchy utilizing that sound as a "launcher" as the patient ascends the complexity ladder.

For phrases and sentences, you can have the patient repeat a phrase or sentence after you (thus providing a model), have the patient read the sentence (greater cognitive demand, increasing complexity), or respond to questions you have asked (even greater cognitive load with linguistic processing and formulation, further increasing complexity). Once the patient can successfully produce sentences, have him or her compile a list of phrases and sentences used on a daily basis and employ these for practice material. Examples might include how the person typically answers the phone, things said at home ("Kids, dinner's ready, come and eat," "Did you get your homework done?") or at work ("Our specials today are . . . " or "Everyone get out your math books and turn to page . . . "), or even conversational placeholders ("um," "yeah," "ok," "like," etc.). Practicing these everyday utterances until they are perfectly coordinated promotes carryover into real-life speaking situations quickly, and these typical phrases and sentences can act as "recalibrators" throughout the day, reminding the patient to pay attention to how he or she is using the voice.

At the paragraph reading level, avoid materials that are linguistically complex (such as textbooks or technical papers) so that cognitive resources can be allocated to the vocal task. If the patient routinely reads books to children, have him or her bring the favorites into the session to use as practice material. Text or lyrics from songs also make a great choice.

Sometimes patients will demonstrate greater success at higher linguistic levels than at lower ones. For example, they may do better with phrases than with syllables. If this is the case with a given patient, there is no need to work on the less complex steps, since speaking in isolated syllables and words is a somewhat unnatural communication activity and not particularly functional.

Carryover Into Conversation and Real Life

Carryover into conversation is essential and can sometimes be a big hurdle. Provide as much structure as is necessary, such as sticking to a specific topic or role-playing a real-life conversation. Encourage the patient to target a period of 5 to 10 minutes per day when he or she will deliberately focus on applying technique in a real-life conversation. If the "new" voice is markedly different from the voice the patient initially presented with, he or she may feel self-conscious about the change. For some people, it may be easier to try out the new voice when speaking to a stranger. On the other hand, some people find it easier to explore the new voice with a conversational partner whom they feel supported by and are comfortable with. Discuss these options with the patient, and chart a plan of action that is most likely to yield a successful outcome.

Sometimes patients may do very well on structured tasks and even with conversation in the therapy room but have difficulty accessing the new voice in real life. If this happens, have the patient make recordings in a variety of speaking situations, such as when reading to the kids, or speaking to a spouse or friend, or on a telephone conversation at work. This can easily be accomplished with a cell phone voice memo. (Note: when suggesting recording of conversations, it's not a bad idea to remind the patient to consider implications for the confidentiality or privacy of others.) Review the recordings together to see if you can identify what the obstacle is, or have the patient role-play the conversation with you so that you can furnish feedback to shape a better outcome.

PROMOTING ACCURATE SELF-ASSESSMENT

Part of the speaking voice therapy process involves guiding the patient to accurately assess his or her own voice. Most of us have difficulty hearing our own voices accurately due to the way our hearing works. Recording patients at any level of the hierarchy and playing back the recording can be a powerful way to help them train their ears to hear what you hear and note small changes. I find it is most helpful to allow this to happen as organically as possible rather than just telling them what I hear. For example, I might play back the recording for us to listen to together and then say, "What did you hear?" "What do you think of that voice?" or "Were there some words that sounded different than others?" If they seem at a loss, you can lend a little prompting such as, "Did you notice a little bit of a gravelly sound at the end of that phrase?" The more they can learn to self-assess, the more they will be empowered for successful home practice.

As discussed in Chapter 9, negative practice (e.g., having the patient deliberately produce the vocal behavior targeted for reduction) can be very effective for stimulating the patient's awareness and discrimination of the sounds and sensations of efficient versus inefficient vocal production.

THE IMPORTANCE OF NATURALNESS

Depending on how severe the dysphonia is at the start, the patient's voice might change only a little or might change dramatically over the course of therapy. Remember that our voices are central to our identity, and it can take time to adjust to the new voice. It is critical for the new voice to sound natural, both to you and to the patient. Record, playback, and analyze together frequently to make sure you're in agreement, and adjust as needed. Even for patients who really don't like their dysphonic voice, it can be a challenge to fully embrace and embody the new, especially if they are worried that the people around them will notice and make negative comments. For some patients, the transition is easy and they never look back. For others, you may need to develop a strategy for "unveiling" the new voice. As stated earlier, this might mean that the patient starts using the new voice at first only with people he or she feels very comfortable with, or only with strangers.

REDUCING INEFFICIENT VOCAL BEHAVIORS

Glottal Fry/Creaky Voice

Glottal fry is typically a reflection of inadequate breath support: The breath flow stops, and the voice keeps going, necessitating recruitment of the muscles of the larynx, pharynx, and neck to power the voice, which typically exacerbates the dysphonia by adding pressed quality (fry plus pressing equals creaky voice, as noted in Chapter 9). This is a situation in which a flow phonation and/or resonant voice approach can work very well. Explore sensations of breath flow with the patient, and gradually apply these to speaking tasks. If the glottal fry is only occurring intermittently (such as at the end of a phrase), cuing the patient to actively exhale at the end of the utterance can help establish improved coordination in which the breath flow extends slightly past the end of phonation. It is essential for the exhale to emerge directly from the voicing without any pause or silence interrupting the breath flow. Once the speaker successfully maintains airflow past the end of the utterance, you can fade the audible exhalation.

Glottal Onsets

Glottal onsets occur when the vocal fold adduction gesture precedes the airflow.

The vocal folds start in a closed position (as when holding your breath), then breath pressure is applied. Because the vocal folds are already adducted, it takes more subglottic pressure to set them in motion, resulting in increased laryngeal effort and greater collisional force on the vocal fold edges. Glottal onsets are not inherently "bad." In fact, the glottal stroke is phonemic in some languages and it is appropriately used in English for emphasis. However, if this is a habitual phonation pattern, it can place unnecessary stress on the vocal folds and (perhaps more significantly) undermine the coordination of respiration and phonation so that the speaker never achieves good breath support. Elision is a great way to reduce this. Using sentences loaded with vowel-initial words, show the patient visually where the liaison will take place.

Here is an example of a written sentence with elision notated:

Ed‿eats‿eels‿every‿Easter.

When spoken, the sentence should come out as "E deet seel zevry yeaster" or /'ɛdit'sɪəl'zɛvri'jistɚ/. This can be a bit awkward at first, but will improve with practice. Once the patient can achieve elision smoothly, you can start to fade the elision, keeping the breath-initiated onsets the patient has now learned.

"SAFE YELLING"

Although yelling is often discouraged in voice rehabilitation, and while we do want to ensure that unnecessary yelling is reduced, it is possible to yell with good technique, and you will likely encounter some patients who will need to learn how to accomplish this. This comes up often for actors. Acting voice rehabilitation is a specialty unto itself and beyond the scope of this text. However, we will briefly touch on an approach to safe yelling.

Safe yelling is essentially belting. See Chapter 10 for details of the physiology and acoustics of belting. As in belting, safe yelling utilizes a megaphone mouth shape, a vocal tract that is shortened by retracting the lips and slightly elevating the larynx (to keep the first formant elevated), vigorous TA activation to generate second harmonic (H2) energy at the source, and twang resonance to narrow the epilaryx tube. This will result in the same favorable interaction of H2/F1 we find in healthy belting, yielding a loud, well-projected, brassy quality with minimal mechanical stress on the vocal folds. "Hey" and "yeah" make good practice words, as they feature vowels with high F1 frequency.

1. Have the patient explore an exaggeratedly twangy resonance in a TA-dominant register. You can try syllables like /njæ/ or /njaʊ/. Possible cues might include "bratty voice" or "witchy voice."
2. Once the exaggerated twang is established, try it with "yeah" and "hey," dialing back the twang a little if needed to make it more speech-like.
3. Breath support is key, so make sure the patient is expanding the ribs and abdomen on the inhale, and engaging the abdomen to ensure breath flow during phonation.
4. Have the patient start at a low pitch and glide up on "yeah" or "hey." This should be a spoken rather than sung gesture, so the glide will be unstructured but should span an octave or less. The lower pitch should be at medium loudness, and loudness should increase as the pitch ascends. The idea is to anchor the voice in TA-dominant

register and keep TA active and engaged as the pitch goes up. All of this should occur in speaking range.

5. Cue the speaker to access the twang resonance sensation, especially at the top (highest frequency) of the yell.
6. Add an abdominal compression to "punch" the top of the yell. You can also use the epigastric gesture described in Chapter 9 to enlist the diaphragm and abdominal muscles for added power.
7. Once the coordination is reliable on single words, move on to short phrases or sentences and fade the glide. The abdominal and/or epigastric gesture should be used to achieve emphasis wherever it is needed in the phrase. For example, if the target phrase is "I said no!" have the patient experiment with different emphases ("I said *no*!" "I *said* no!" etc.). Make sure the patient is not clenching the abdomen. Abdominal movement should be associated with good airflow.

CASE STUDY

The patient is an engineer who sings in a professional a cappella group. Speaking voice is characterized by pressed quality, pharyngeal tone placement, and intermittent vocal fry. He has to speak a lot at work, giving presentations, leading meetings, and speaking on the phone with clients. He has small children at home and finds that when it is time to read to them at night, his voice is exhausted from speaking all day.

Goal: Improve resonance to reduce laryngeal strain, eliminate pressed quality, and improve breath support, all in the interest of improving vocal stamina and reducing vocal fatigue.

Speaking voice therapy process:

1. We started with respiratory coordination in isolation to establish a low abdominal breathing pattern. He had a tendency to use excessive abdominal clenching when exhaling, so we worked on flow phonation strategies such as exhaling through a drinking straw or exhaling with a tissue held in front of the mouth to promote steady release of air without clenching.
2. For a speaking voice "warm-up," we used the adductory power exercise from vocal function exercises, phonating through a stir straw from C3–G3 to achieve optimal source-filter interaction and establish a reference sensation for resonant voice without pressing. We also used full-range pitch glides, ascending and descending to stretch vocal folds, phonating through the stir straw.
3. We explored SOVT sounds. /z/ proved to be a facilitating launching sound for him. In order to maintain the "buzzy" quality of the fricative, he had to be mindful of maintaining breath flow. The semi-occlusion at the mouth also facilitated reduction of laryngeal effort.
4. We proceeded through the hierarchy from /z/ initial syllables to sentences. We added sentences from his work day and used the books he read to his children to practice at the sentence level as well.
5. We moved on to prepared presentations and simulated meetings to practice working at the conversational level.

By this point, he was demonstrating markedly improved coordination of voicing subsystems very consistently in therapy sessions but still reported that he was fatigued by the end of the day. I had him record himself in different speaking situations throughout the day. When we reviewed the recordings together, it was clear that he was reverting to his old voice when speaking on the phone, especially when on speaker. We practiced role-playing phone calls until he was able to achieve his new voice consistently. He also put a post-it on his phone to remind him to use good vocal technique with every phone call. Solving the phone problem proved to be the final key in resolving his dysphonia. He reported feeling much less fatigued and was able to resume reading to his kids at night.

REFERENCES

American Speech-Language-Hearing Association. (2005). *The role of the speech language pathologist, the teacher of singing, and the speaking voice trainer in voice habilitation* (Technical report). Rockville, MD: American Speech and Hearing Association Ad Hoc Joint Committee with the National Association of Teachers of Singing and the Voice and Speech Trainers Association. Retrieved from http://www.asha.org/members/deskref-journals/deskref/default

Behrman, A., & Haskell, J. (2013). *Exercises for voice therapy* (2nd ed.). San Diego, CA: Plural.

Boone, D. (1971). *The voice and voice therapy.* Englewood Cliffs, NJ: Prentice Hall.

Heuer, R. J., Rulnick, R. K., Horman, M., Perez, K. S., Emerich, K. A., & Sataloff, R. T. (2006). Voice therapy. In R. T. Sataloff (Ed.), *Vocal health and pedagogy advanced assessment and treatment* (2nd ed., pp.227–251). San Diego, CA: Plural.

Kotby, M. N. (1995). *The accent method of voice therapy.* San Diego, CA: Singular.

Mathieson, L., Hirani, S. P., Epstein, R., Baken, R. J., Wood, G., & Rubin, J. S. (2009). Laryngeal manual therapy: A preliminary study to examine its treatment effects in the management of muscle tension dysphonia. *Journal of Voice, 23*(3), 353–366.

Michael, D. (2012). Dispelling vocal myths, Part IV: "Talk higher!" *Journal of Singing, 69*(2), 167–172.

Ramig, L. O., Bonitati, C. M., Lemke, J. H., & Horii, Y. (1994). Voice treatment for patients with Parkinson's disease: Development of an approach and preliminary efficacy data. *Journal of Medical Speech Language Pathology, 2*, 191–209.

Roy, N., Ford, C. N., & Bless, D. M. (1996). Muscle tension dysphonia and spasmodic dysphonia: The role of manual laryngeal tension reduction in diagnosis and management. *Annals of Otology, Rhinology, and Laryngology, 105*(11), 851–856.

Stemple, J. C. (2014). Principles of voice therapy. In J. C. Stemple & E. R. Hapner (Eds.), *Voice therapy clinical case studies* (4th ed., pp. 1–11). San Diego, CA: Plural.

Stemple, J. C., & Hapner, E. R. (Eds.). (2014). *Voice therapy clinical case studies* (4th ed). San Diego, CA: Plural.

Titze, I. R., & Verdolini Abbott, K. (2012). *Vocology: The science and practice of voice habilitation.* Salt Lake City, UT: National Center for Voice and Speech.

Verdolini Abbott, K. (2008). *Lessac-Madsen resonant voice therapy: Clinician manual.* San Diego, CA: Plural.

Ziegler, A., Verdolini Abbott, K., Johns, M., Klein, A., & Hapner, E. R. (2014). Preliminary data on two voice therapy interventions in the treatment of presbyphonia. *Laryngoscope, 124*(8), 1869–1876.

PART IV

Vocal Pacing

CHAPTER 14

Vocal Pacing: Spending the Interest, Not the Principal

Vocal pacing refers to achieving balance in amount, type, and intensity of voice use. As noted previously, vocal pacing is one of the major components of voice rehabilitation —particularly for singers with injuries that may be exacerbated by overuse (or in some cases, even by normal voice use)—and is one of the most important factors you will address as part of the rehabilitation process. For some singers, vocal pacing may not necessarily mean reducing vocal load. For example, singers with vocal fold atrophy may in fact need more vocal exercise, not less. However, in all likelihood, most of the singers you will see will have a degree of voice overuse and will require counseling and strategies for improving the balance of voice use and voice rest.

In many cases, bringing voice use into balance can be the pivotal element in recovering from a vocal injury. It will not be unusual for you to devote a large portion of a session or multiple sessions to addressing vocal pacing. In fact, you may find that you sometimes devote entire sessions to this topic. The singer's occupation, style of singing, singing environments, social habits, and family demands can all impact vocal pacing and should be carefully reviewed to discover opportunities for improvement. This chapter includes guidelines for creating a voice use journal, strategies for prioritizing voice use, planning voice use, and reducing nonessential voice use, as well as recommendations for applying vocal pacing strategies to both speaking and singing.

The specific vocal pacing recommendations furnished in this chapter are also included in the educational handouts in Appendices 14A–P. Because vocal pacing strategies can differ depending on the singer you are working with, the educational handouts encompass not only the broad topics herein but particular populations of singers you will most likely encounter in your practice. Keep in mind that these handouts are merely a starting point to aid you in customizing the vocal pacing plan to each individual singer. Your creativity and growing experience will supply you with even more ideas and strategies.

FOUNDATIONS OF VOCAL PACING

Vocal Pacing Education

There are numerous ways to explain vocal pacing to the singers you are working with. You will undoubtedly arrive at your own methods and analogies, but

I will share a few that I have found to be beneficial with you.

The Vocal Clock: We all have a vocal clock that starts ticking the minute we get up in the morning. We have so many hours and minutes of voice use on the clock that we can expend before we cross the line into overuse. Everyone's clock is different, and different kinds of voice use take up different amounts of time on the clock. For example, speaking at a conversational level (with good vocal technique) takes fewer minutes "off the clock" than speaking with a projected voice (even with good technique). Singing typically involves a higher fundamental frequency than speaking (meaning more vocal fold collisions per second), and often the collisional force of impact during singing is greater than in efficient speaking, and therefore it takes up more minutes on the clock. Certain types of singing take up more minutes than others. Use of extended vocal techniques such as "growl" can be more costly in terms of the vocal clock.

Another way of framing vocal pacing is to think of the voice as a bank account: One wants to spend the *interest* and avoid dipping into the *principal* if at all possible. With this analogy, you can explore the relative expense of differing types and amounts of singing.

It will likely be necessary for you to come back to these basic principles again and again as you guide the singer to better vocal pacing. Having a shared reference and vocabulary surrounding vocal pacing will help to keep this process focused and efficient.

It is imperative that singers understand that vocal pacing goals must encompass both speaking and singing voice activities and that optimizing vocal pacing requires a holistic approach that incorporates strategies for bringing all types of voice use into balance.

When Resistance Arises

Be prepared to meet some resistance on the part of the singer. Singers are usually outgoing and gregarious people, and they sometimes feel that having to monitor their voice use is stifling and burdensome. When you begin working with them, they will probably have a lot on their plates in terms of voice use. They likely would not have taken on an excessive vocal load if they didn't regard all of their vocal activities as high priority for one reason or another. Because of this, they may feel there is no room for reducing voice use. It is up to you to guide them to the realization that something has to give in order for them to get better. The goal is to empower the singer to arrive at a decision regarding what can be unloaded or modified to bring voice use into better balance. Framing this decision as a series of choices can help the singer through the process. For example, if the singer expresses the feeling that it will be impossible to remove any vocal activities from the current load, you can respond by saying, "You absolutely have the option to keep all of these activities on your schedule. However, doing so may have an impact on whether or not you reach your goals for voice recovery. In order for you to meet your goals, we have to find a way to reduce your load so that your injury can heal." This places the power of and responsibility for change in the hands of the singer and may be less likely to lead to feelings that something is being "taken away."

Prioritizing Voice Use

An effective way to empower singers to take control of their vocal pacing is by having them prioritize their voice use. Have the singer make a list of all his or her voice use over the course of days, weeks, or months. Once the singer has compiled the list, review it together with a goal of numbering each activity in ranking order of importance. Initially, the singer may feel that everything on the list is of equal importance, but the act of numbering and ranking activities can be very powerful in revealing the true importance. Singers often discover that there are several vocal activities on the list that aren't necessarily high priority for them; rather, they are high priority for other people in their lives. It can be helpful to make multiple priority lists from different perspectives to gradually arrive at the singer's true priorities.

For example, "Karen," a music educator and professional actor and singer, was asked by a local community theater company to be music director for a musical. She was not going to get paid very much for the engagement but felt compelled to take it on because the director of the show was a good friend. He told her, "There's no one else who can do it, I really need you." She put this engagement on her list of priority activities, but in ranking the list, she realized she was doing it more out of a sense of obligation than for any benefit she would receive. Through this process of prioritization, she was able to explain to her friend that she couldn't take the music directing engagement because she needed to pace her voice to allow her injury to heal. In the end, her friend was very understanding and supportive of her voice rehabilitation, and Karen was able to reduce her vocal load considerably by not taking on this engagement.

This case example brings us to another very important factor in guiding singers to determine vocal priorities and set boundaries for voice use: The *I have to do it because I'm needed* syndrome. Some singers find it difficult to say "no" when asked to share their gifts and as a result, may end up taking on performances they're not really interested in, singing a voice part that isn't appropriate for their range, helping out in a leadership capacity (such as directing a chorus or acting as section leader), or providing an extra coaching session for students. It can be very hard to say "no."

Air travel provides a very powerful analogy for addressing this problem with the well-known phrase: "Put the mask on yourself first." We all hear this when we get on a plane: When the flight crew instructs us on how to use the oxygen mask in case of emergency, they always tell us to put the masks on ourselves first. We all understand the reason for this: We can't help others if we are ourselves incapacitated by lack of oxygen. We know that it is not selfish for us to take care of ourselves first in this situation, yet in other areas of our lives, we often fail to apply the same logic. Singers must understand that if they don't prioritize voice use (e.g., put the mask on themselves first), recovery may be undermined, in which case they may not be able to fulfill their voice obligations anyway. On the other hand, if they take care of themselves, they not only promote their own vocal health but also act as role models for the singers around them, generating an ever-widening circle of healthy voice habits.

Another useful guide in decision making regarding prioritizing voice use is to encourage singers to ask themselves a series of questions about the vocal activity under consideration. The exact questions will vary depending on the individual singer's priorities and goals but might include: "Is this engagement financially appealing? Will it move my career forward significantly? Will it be incredibly fulfilling artistically? Is this a performance or activity that I've dreamed of doing for a long time?" Once the appropriate questions are established, the singer can use them to help decide whether to say yes or no to a given opportunity or request.

Documenting Voice Use

Use of a voice journal can be a powerful tool for optimizing vocal pacing. The format or method for voice journaling should be based on what is most relevant, meaningful, and convenient for the singer, whether using a paper calendar or journal, an electronic journal, a spreadsheet, or mobile device. Some may prefer a table format that allows them to quickly check or fill in boxes or cells (Table 14–1).

Others may wish to do more lengthy writing (see box below).

Example of Handwritten Prose Journal

Wednesday Nov. 7

Had voice therapy at 8:30 AM

Drank about 52 ounces of water

Voice wasn't that sore today

Tried to catch myself talking from the back of my throat

Thursday Nov. 8

Drank 8 cups of water

Did 30 minutes of exercises first thing in the morning

Voice got sore after reading throughout the day, then did laryngeal massage, felt better, then sang lightly a little to the radio and it now feels like I swallowed a pill down the wrong pipe

Friday, Nov. 9

Exercises for 30 minutes first thing. Felt pretty good. Only a little bit of singing but a lot of talking. About 6.5 cups of water

Sunday, Nov. 11

Did 30 minutes of exercises first thing. Didn't talk very much today and throat felt very good. Drank roughly 40 ounces of water.

Tuesday, Nov. 13

30 minutes of exercises. Didn't talk too much so felt pretty good. Had half the water I needed.

Wednesday, Nov. 14

30 minutes of exercises Not too sore. 16 oz water

Thursday, Nov 15

30 minutes of exercises. 7.5 cups. Voice hurt a little when reading at work.

Friday Nov. 16

30 minutes of exercises. 4.5 cups of water

Monday, Nov. 19

Did exercises for 30 minutes, throat was a little dry today and coughed some in rehearsal, sang a little to the radio but nothing extreme, drank roughly 4 cups of water.

Table 14–1. *Example of Table Format for Voice Journal*

	Voice Rating 1–10	*Speaking Voice Use: Amount/Type*	*Singing Voice Use: Amount/Type*	*Practiced Vocal Exercises*	*Voice Rest*	*Vocal Pacing Strategies*	*Hydration*	*Allergy Medicine*	*Daily Vocal Success Story*	*Goal for Tomorrow*
Monday										
Tuesday										
Wednesday										
Thursday										
Friday										
Saturday										
Sunday										

You might start out by having the singer spend the first week just taking observational notes about voice use (Table 14–2).

Talk to the singer to ascertain what will work best for him or her. The more personalized the documentation, the more likely it is that the singer will use it regularly to keep track of voice use. Review the journal each week as part of the rehabilitation session. It can be very difficult to get a true picture of what a typical day of voice use is like for the singer based on your intermittent sessions. The voice journal can help to fill in the blanks and make your intervention more targeted, accurate, and relevant and therefore, more effective.

In addition to voice use, the journal may be used to keep track of vocal hygiene goals (such as hydration or reducing throat clearing), frequency of practice of rehabilitation exercises, a daily voice rating (1–10, 1 being the individual singer's self-perceived worst voice and 10 being the best), taking medications for voice-related medical problems (allergies, GERD, etc.), or any other factor that is part of the voice rehabilitation goals.

Encourage your patients/clients to document their successes. Sometimes this can get overlooked in an effort to focus on what needs to change and improve, but reviewing the positive lifestyle changes that have been incorporated into daily practice can be very potent. Having momentous successes documented in the voice journal is also very encouraging if the singer later experiences a discouraging setback in progress.

Keep in mind that the voice journal will not work for every singer. It is merely one of the many rehabilitation tools at your

Table 14–2. *Example of Observational Notes in Table Format, College Student: Nonvoice Major*

	Voice Use: Week 1
Monday	Personal phone calls: 2 hours; recreational singing: 1.5 hours; talking to friends in sorority house/cafeteria: 2 hours; talking in seminar class: 1 hour; planning meeting for sorority rush: 1 hour; a cappella group rehearsal: 3 hours
Tuesday	Personal phone calls: 2 hours; recreational singing: 1 hour; working in coffee shop: 4 hours; late dinner with friends at loud restaurant: 1.5 hours
Wednesday	Personal phone calls: 20 minutes; recreational singing: 2 hours; directing sorority singing project: 1 hour; talking to friends in quiet room: 1 hour
Thursday	Personal phone calls: 1 hour; argument with boyfriend: 1 hour; recreational singing: 15 minutes; a cappella group sound check and performance: 2 hours; bar with friends after performance: 1.5 hours; talking to roommate: 30 minutes
Friday	Personal phone calls: 2 hours; recreational singing: 1 hour; greeting at sorority rush event: 3 hours; singing at rush: 30 minutes; talking to sorority sisters after rush: 1.5 hours; talking to roommate: 30 minutes
Saturday	Personal phone calls: 2 hours; loud talking/some yelling at football game: 3 hours; party after football game: 2 hours; singing at party: 30 minutes
Sunday	Personal phone calls: 1 hour; talking quietly with friends: 1 hour; a cappella group rehearsal: 3 hours (quiet/studying most of the day)

disposal. As with all other elements of voice therapy, it is important to adapt your intervention to what is most effective for a particular singer rather than trying to fit each singer into a prescribed "one-size-fits-all" mold. If the journal doesn't seem to work for a particular singer, simply abandon it and focus on other strategies and tools.

Enlisting the Support System

Recovering from a voice injury is hard work, and vocal pacing is often the most challenging component for singers. Enlisting the aid of a personal support system—family, friends, colleagues—is an important strategy for ensuring success. Part of your discussion with the singer about vocal pacing should include exploring whether such a support system might be helpful in meeting vocal pacing goals. The singer could start by informing people in his or her circle about the voice injury, letting them know that recovery will involve decreasing voice use at certain times. Use of a letter, e-mail, or social media to communicate this information will allow the singer to avoid having to repeatedly explain why he or she is changing habits and behavior. The singer may enlist a trusted friend or family member to remind him or her to take vocal breaks and to be mindful of amount of voice use or to act as an advocate to "protect" the singer from being drawn into vocally challenging conversations or speaking situations. The possibilities for recruiting others to help with vocal pacing are nearly limitless, and you should encourage the singer to brainstorm about what might work best. Additional suggestions are provided in the handout "Tips for Enlisting Your Support Network for Vocal Pacing Success" in Appendix 14–A.

The Importance of Self-Advocacy

Usually the people the singer interacts with at home, in performance activities, at work, and at school will understand the need for vocal pacing and will be supportive. However, sometimes the singer may encounter pressure to participate in vocal activities or even frank resistance to his or her attempts to reduce the vocal load. If this is the case, you will need to help him or her to be an effective self-advocate.

In some cases, you and your physician colleagues will need to advocate for the singer by speaking or writing to the person who is obstructing the vocal pacing goals, particularly if this person is in a position of authority over the singer. Sometimes the authority figure's inability to understand the need for vocal pacing may result in punitive consequences for the singer. Your professional or clinical perspective and that of your physician colleagues may carry more weight, and you should not hesitate to offer to intervene if needed. This may involve speaking to a conductor, director, supervisor, school principal, spiritual leader, or anyone else who does not seem to be supportive or is in a position to thwart the vocal pacing goals you have set with your patient/student.

It can be advantageous to explain the need for vocal pacing in terms of what will happen if vocal pacing strategies are not implemented. The director of a musical or opera might be resistant to engaging an understudy for a singer in a principal role but may become more open to the idea with the realization that the success of the entire performance depends on finding a way to lighten the vocal load of the singer. A high school principal may be concerned that allowing the chorus teacher to be excused from lunch duty will appear as favoritism but may rethink that position if he or she understands that the teacher may have to go on extended leave or disability if the vocal load is not brought into better balance. A university choral conductor may feel it is urgent for the student singer to participate in rehearsals for an upcoming concert but may understand the need for reducing that singer's load in the ensemble if he or she realizes the impact continued voice overuse may have on the student's academic success and ability to remain in the music program.

When Setbacks Happen

With your guidance and support, the singers you work with should demonstrate regular progress in optimizing vocal pacing. However, setbacks are very common. This will often happen just as the singer is noticing real improvement in vocal quality, range, and stamina, and it can be an extremely discouraging experience to have the voice get worse again, especially if the occurrence is associated with an episode of voice overuse. The

I never fully appreciated the difficulty of vocal pacing until I was in a bicycle accident and sustained a concussion. The primary treatment was complete cognitive rest, which entailed lying in a darkened room with no visual or auditory stimulation—no reading, no computer, no listening to music, no movies or television: nothing. Obviously this meant not going to work as well. I was able to comply with this recommendation for a while, but felt a sense of urgency about returning to work. "My patients need me. My colleagues need me. I'm not pulling my weight. I've got deadlines." Just the sort of arguments I've heard my singing patients make time and time again. I went back to work too soon, and as a result began to have severe headaches. I had another period of extended cognitive rest and again came back to work too soon. The headaches got worse. It took several cycles of this process for me to figure out just the right balance of work and rest. Sometimes I would have a day when I felt really great—back to normal! Usually, this was when I would overdo it and suffer another setback. In the end it took 6 months of lightening my schedule and taking frequent breaks before I felt fully recovered and able to return to my normal workload. It's possible my recovery would have gone more quickly if I had been more careful and rested more at the beginning.

Throughout this difficult process, the physical therapist who treated me was incredibly encouraging. Whenever I would overdo it and have a bad day (or days) as a result, she would always say, "Of course you had a setback. You're figuring out where the line is and sometimes you can't tell until you cross it." Her support and encouragement were so helpful when I was beating myself up for not being smarter in my pacing and lamenting yet another setback.

It's not an experience I would want to repeat, but I am extremely grateful for the lesson I learned about how very difficult it is to be sidelined from one's normal activity level and to feel that one is taking one step back for every two steps forward. It has always been important to me to be supportive and encouraging to the singers I work with, but since my head injury, I feel I can more sincerely express to them that I know how difficult it is to achieve balance for recovery.

singer may feel self-blame, frustration, or defeat. When this happens, it is very important for you to be encouraging and understanding. Part of the process of determining the optimal vocal pacing regimen for any singer is establishing exactly where the overuse line is so that one can avoid crossing it. It is incumbent upon you to strike just the right balance between firmness and flexibility in your interactions with the singer. You must be clear in your recommendations so that the singer will understand how engaging in various vocal activities will affect or has affected healing and recovery, but at the same time you must be supportive and positive when the singer overdoes it by providing reassurance that setbacks are to be expected on the path to recovery and immediately partnering with the singer to get things back on track.

PLANNING VOICE USE

Most singers sing a lot. The amount, type, and intensity of voice use vary quite a bit depending on style, performing schedule, professional status, and training, but most singers—particularly those recovering from a voice injury or disorder—will benefit from being intentional and deliberate in how they allocate their voice use. You can help the singers you work with to achieve this by partnering with them to develop a plan for voice use.

Planning voice use has numerous advantages for singers. It allows them to adjust their voice use in anticipation of changes in demands. By planning voice use in advance, singers can conserve voice in preparation for the times when demands will ramp up, as during an extended performance engagement. If they don't take the long view in pacing and planning, they might find themselves in crisis mode when the performance rolls around, feeling vocally exhausted just at the point when it is too late to decrease the vocal load. Once they have entered the performance zone, the options for vocal pacing are drastically reduced. The key is to implement a vocal pacing plan long before the performance.

Planning voice use also applies to how voice use is allocated during practice time. A strategic approach to practice will ensure that the singer is adequately prepared for the performance and won't have to cram a lot of practicing in at the last minute.

A visual organization scheme can be a powerful tool in optimizing vocal pacing and planning. The exact nature of the organizer will vary depending on each singer's learning style, organizational style, and particular vocal demands. For student singers who have specific and often lengthy requirements for repertoire preparation in a fixed period of time, it might be better to focus on planning practice time first. For working professionals with busy performance schedules, placing the emphasis on long-range planning might be the more immediate objective. The key is to personalize and tailor the planning strategy to each singer's individual needs. A few examples of organizational models are provided herein to get you started. Your job is to partner with the singer to create a planning scheme that will best align with his or her vocal demands.

Long-Range Voice Use Planning

Begin by having the singer write down all the singing voice demands they anticipate for a period of a few weeks or even months. This should include performances, sound checks, recording sessions, rehearsals, individual practice sessions, voice lessons, teaching, directing, and any other singing activities. Significant speaking voice demands (such as presentations, sermons, or extensive teaching) should also be included. Once everything is listed, review each activity to determine whether or not it requires full-intensity singing. Obviously performances and recording will require "full-voice" singing. To get the most out of a voice lesson and individual practice, the singer likely needs to sing full voice for most of the time. These activities should be noted and ranked at the top of the list. Consider numbering or color-coding activities for visual salience. Putting these activities in a calendar or chart will help in identifying when the intensity of singing will be at its greatest.

Next, determine which activities can be accomplished with *marking* or light singing. Staging rehearsals, choreography rehearsals, even scratch tracks for recordings fall into this category. Number and/or color-code these activities and add them to the calendar or chart.

There may be an additional category that is a mixture of full-voice singing and marking or light singing. Varying the level of vocal intensity in this manner could be employed at a run-through rehearsal, in which the singer can plan to sing full voice for part of the rehearsal and mark for the rest based on which parts of the performance need more practice and/or the director's or conductor's preference.

For singers in a band or vocal ensemble, instrumentalists and/or other singers may be somewhat dependent on the lead voice when learning or practicing repertoire. In such cases, the lead singer should sing only the parts of the song that are necessary for cues or entrances instead of the whole song, or at least sing lightly or in a lower octave whenever possible, saving the performance-level singing for a time when all the parts are learned and the song is ready for a run-through.

Once all the activities have been placed on the chart, look for opportunities to schedule voice rest. It's very important to specifically add the voice rest to the calendar. The goal is for the singer to arrive at the performance feeling vocally fresh and rested. See Table 14–3 for an example of a long-range voice use planning chart in a calendar format. This professional musical theater singer used a paper calendar and highlighters to plan in advance the intensity of voice use she would expend over the course of a very vocally demanding month (although in this example, different shading is used in place of different colors).

Another way to organize the voice use planning chart is by priority. This can be especially helpful for singers who have many different vocal demands and who struggle with determining which are most important. Indicating level of priority in a chart can guide them in adjusting voice use according to importance. Table 14–4 provides an example of voice use planning for a college student in an a cappella group. This student struggled with balancing social activities with academic requirements and the very heavy demands of her a cappella group, The Blue Notes. At first, she felt that all of her activities were high priority, but after repeated setbacks in her rehabilitation, she was able to identify her true priorities. She used color-coding to indicate level of priority for vocal activities (although in this example, different levels of priority are indicated by text style). She then decreased or eliminated lower priority activities if her voice started feeling tired or hoarse or in anticipation of a big increase in voice use.

Table 14–3. *Example of completed voice use planning calendar for a professional musical theater singer in a repertory company rehearsing the roles of Lola in* Damn Yankees *("DY") and Cathy in* The Last Five Years *("5") while performing Franca in* The Light in the Piazza *("Light"). In this example, different shading is used rather than color-coding to indicate levels of intensity in voice use.*

Sing full voice Combination marking/full voice Marking Voice Rest

Sunday	*Monday*	*Tuesday*	*Wednesday*	*Thursday*	*Friday*	*Saturday*
			10–1 Blocking *DY* 2–5 Blocking *DY* 7–10 "5" work-thru Cathy	10–1 Blocking *DY* 2–5 "5" Work-thru Jamie **8 *Light* performance**	10–1 Blocking *DY* 2–5 "5" run-thru **8 *Light* performance**	10–1 "5" run-thru **2 *Light* performance** **8 *Light* performance**
2 *Light* performance **8 *Light* performance**	Off	10–1 Blocking *DY* 2–5 "5" tech 7–10 "5" tech	10–1 Blocking *DY* 2–5 "5" Dress **7–10 "5" preview**	10–1 Blocking *DY* 2–5 Dance *DY* **8 "5" opening**	10–1 Blocking *DY* 2–5 Dance *DY* **8 *Light* performance**	10–1 Dance *DY* **2 *Light* performance** **8 "5" performance**
2 *Light* performance **8 *Light* performance**	Off	10–1 *DY* work Act I 2–5 *DY* work Act II **7–10 *DY* Sitzprobe**	10–1 *DY* run Act I 2–5 *DY* run Act II 7–10 *DY* run show	10–1 *DY* tech 2–5 *DY* tech **8 *Light* performance**	10–1 *DY* tech 2–5 *DY* tech **8 *Light* performance**	10–1 *DY* dress **2 *Light* performance** **8 "5" performance**
2 *Light* performance **8 *Light* performance**	Off	**10–1 DY dress** 2–5 *DY* notes **8 Benefit Cabaret**	10–1 *DY* dance as needed **2 *DY* dress** 7–10 *DY* notes	**2 *DY* preview** **8 *Light* performance**	2–5 *DY* notes as needed **8 "5" performance**	**2 *Light* performance** **8 *DY* performance**
2 *Light* performance **8 *Light* performance**	Off	**8 *DY* performance**	**2 *Light* performance** **8 *DY* performance**	**8 *Light* performance**		

Table 14–4. *Example of voice use planning for a college student in an a cappella group based on priority of vocal activity. This student used color-coding to indicate level of priority, although in this example, different text styles are used instead.*

High priority Medium priority *Low priority*

Sunday	Monday	Tuesday	Wednesday	Thursday	Friday	Saturday
					Practice 30 minutes *Party at Cheryl's*	*Football game* **Campus showcase perf-3 songs**
Reh 7–10 PM	**Practice 30 min**	**1 PM voice lesson**	**Practice 30 min**	Bistro with Blue Notes **Reh 7–10 PM**	**Practice 30 min** **Perf at student union 5 songs** *Party at Ed's*	*Watch game at Jamie's* *Party at Beck House*
Reh 7–10 PM	**Practice 30 min**	**1 PM voice lesson** **7–9 PM Blue Note recording**	**Practice 30 min**	**Reh 7–10 PM**	Blue Note beach retreat	Blue Note beach retreat
Blue Note beach retreat	**Practice 30 min** **5 PM practice with accompanist**	**1 PM voice lesson** **8–11 PM Extra reh**	**Practice 30 min** 5 PM Audition for musical **8–10 PM Extra reh**	**4 PM Sing in studio class** **Reh 7–11 PM**	**Practice 30 minutes** Call backs for musical? *Party?*	*Football game* **Blue Notes Fall concert—My solo!** Blue Note party
Reh 7–10 PM 10 PM Bistro with Blue Notes	**Practice 30 minutes** **Presentation for econ class**	**1 PM voice lesson**	**Practice 30 minutes**	**Reh 7–10 PM**	**Practice 30 minutes**	

The group beach retreat presented a challenging decision for her, falling before an important week of auditions and performances. In the end, she decided to attend the retreat, but only for one day.

Planning Practice Time

Planning how to allocate voice use during practice is another vital element in the overall vocal pacing strategy. Singers who have had training should already be in the habit of engaging in regular practice (although one cannot assume this to be the case—always review the practice habits of all the singers you work with). Singers without training (particularly those who sing in contemporary styles) may not routinely set aside time for vocal exercise and work on repertoire. Part of the rehabilitation process will be to ensure that all the singers you work with understand the importance of regular practice and know how to optimize their practice time.

The first part of the practice period should be allocated to warming up. A singer who is regularly engaging in singing activities should be able to warm up his or her voice in 10 to 20 minutes. Some singers engage in long and elaborate vocalization prior to delving into repertoire. Doing so has great advantages for improving vocal technique by isolating various aspects such as agility, legato, precision, control, phrase line, breath support, and so on. However, the singer should realize that it is not necessary to complete such extended vocalization in order to be warmed up, and should understand the difference between *warming up* and *technical practice*. During times when there is a lot of repertoire to learn and master, it is better to streamline the warm-up so that more of the singing time can be devoted to working on music.

When approaching a new piece of music, singers will often learn it by singing it over and over again. Similarly, when it's time to memorize the piece, vocal repetition is a common course of action. The end result may be that by the time the singer is ready to delve into vocal technique on the new piece, the practice time has all been used up and vocal fatigue has begun to set in. How advantageous it would be to start the vocal clock ticking only when the song has been learned! Fortunately, a surprising amount of what is needed to prepare a new piece of music can be accomplished without singing at all. *Mental practice* is an effective strategy and has been demonstrated to generate motor learning (Helding, 2010; Schmidt & Lee, 2014).

Mental Practice

Using mental practice, a singer can learn new music, work on interpretation, and even memorize songs, all without using up any minutes on the vocal clock. It takes discipline to do this, as it is usually more enjoyable and rewarding to sing the song over and over again, but the benefits are tremendous—a singer can allocate hours to mental practice, saving the singing time for working out the technical details of the piece.

How does one learn a song without singing it? Singers who have a solid foundation in musicianship can presumably read music and even mentally sight-read a new piece. They also should have adequate instrumental skills to enable them to play the vocal line on the piano (or other instrument) and thus learn the melody and rhythm to the point that they are able to hear it in their heads. However, many of the singers you work with may not have this skill set. Often CCM singers have little or no musical training and may be unfamiliar with music notation, typically learning the music they perform by rote. The rote learning can also be accomplished mentally simply by listening to a recording of the song without singing it. For songwriters working on their own music, a recording may not exist. In this case, the singer can sing/play the song once while recording it and use the recording to support mental practice. In any case, learning new songs mentally is entirely achievable with your guidance and with practice.

Other Strategies for Nonvocal Practice

Many of the motor aspects of singing can also be accomplished silently. While listening to or thinking through the song, the singer should sit or stand with optimal posture, breathing at appropriate phrase breaks, and articulating the words silently as if singing aloud (note: the vocal folds adduct to varying degrees when whispering and this adduction may undermine voice rest. It is important to ensure that the singer is not whispering in this activity). In this manner, the neuromuscular training relative to body alignment, breath support and articulation are already under way without using the voice. The singer can add another layer of motor training by sustaining an unvoiced phoneme (such as an unvoiced fricative [/s/ or /f/], an unvoiced lip or tongue trill, or unvoiced raspberry) while thinking through or listening to the song. This provides auditory feedback as to how smoothly and steadily the air is being released and further instills the muscle memory for breath support during phonation by simulating glottal resistance at the level of the articulators. Imagining the sensation of resonance or placement can also be incorporated into this routine. Since this kind of practice is a vocal "freebie," the singer can allocate lot of time to practicing without taxing the voice at all.

Systematic Singing Practice

After running through the song mentally a few times, the singer may try singing it aloud, followed by another round of mental run-throughs, and so on. "Listen three times, sing it once" can be a useful rule of thumb. Through this method, the singer can learn the entire song with minimal voice use. Memorization and interpretive work can be accomplished similarly.

Once the music is learned, the singer can move on to working on vocal technique. Again, it is critical that this be done in a systematic and intentional way. Singing through the song on semi-occluded vocal tract sounds (voiced lip trill, tongue trill, raspberry, straw phonation, etc.) can be a useful step for "priming" breath support and resonance using a task that is less cognitively and physiologically complex and more acoustically favorable than singing on the text.

As when learning a new piece, singers will often execute their technical practice by running through a song from beginning to end. A more strategic system is to target only the sections of the piece that need technical work. An excellent way of doing this is to record oneself singing through the entire piece, then review the recording, noting the spots that need work by marking them on the score or lyric sheet, or simply making a list. The subsequent period of practice time can be devoted to technical work only on those sections. This might be followed by another run-through and recording, again taking notes on the areas that need additional technical attention for the next period of practice. This method of focusing practice only on target areas might be called *detailed practice* or *spot practice*.

We now have a number of different approaches to the practice session that can be broken down as follows:

- Learn the song with mental practice
- Listen to the song while practicing unvoiced sustained sounds or mouthing words
- Practice singing the piece on semi-occluded vocal tract (SOVT) sounds
- Run through and record to target sections that need technical work
- Detailed/spot practice of target sections
- Mental practice of interpretation
- Run through and record for use in memorization
- Listen to recording for mental memorization
- Run through full voice from memory

This can be organized visually on a chart or graph (Table 14–5). Using the chart, the singer can plan how to allocate practice over a period of time and can keep track of where he or she is in the overall plan. See Chapter 16, Case Study 2 for an example of a completed vocal practice planning chart.

In this manner, the singer can ensure that all repertoire is thoroughly prepared and that practice time is allocated in such a way that there is time and attention for each piece. Different types of practice may be applied to different pieces on the repertoire list on any given day.

This is only one suggestion for a systematic approach to practice. The specific system should be customized for the particular singer's needs.

The strategies for planning practice time are summarized in the handout "Tips for Planning Vocal Practice" provided in Appendix 14–B.

More on Planning Voice Use

Vocal Pacing in Rehearsals

For performers, rehearsal can represent a large portion of the vocal load and presents numerous opportunities for improving vocal pacing. The timing of the rehearsal can be important, too. If the singer or group typically practices late at night, they will likely already be fatigued (vocally and physically) when the rehearsal starts. You may need to provide education on the potential impact of both timing and duration of rehearsal and encourage adaptation as indicated.

Depending on the type of singing and situations the singer encounters, the following strategies may be helpful:

- Incorporate intermittent short breaks into rehearsals that are designated as silent time.
- Deliberately alternate vocally strenuous activities with those that are less taxing.
- If the rehearsal typically includes time that is allocated to "business" (such as scheduling, planning events, etc.), positioning this activity in the middle of the rehearsal can provide a natural voice break without altering the overall duration or content of the rehearsal (examples of singers to whom this might apply include CCM singers who regularly rehearse with a band or singers in an a cappella group).
- Plan rehearsal time for upcoming performances well in advance to ensure that the singer/group is

Table 14–5. *Vocal Practice Planning Chart Example*

	"Mental" Learning	***Silent Practice***	***Sing Without Text***	***Run Through and Record***	***Listen to Recording, Take Notes for "Spot" Practice***	***"Spot" Practice***	***Mental Practice of Interpretation***	***Run Through and Record for Memorization***	***Mental Memorization (Listening)***	***Run Through Full Voice From Memory***
Song 1										
Song 2										
Song 3										
Song 4										
Song 5										

Note. *Singers can learn the music without singing, indicated in the chart as "mental learning." "Silent practice" can be accomplished by thinking through the song or listening to a recording while silently mouthing the words (not whispering), or while sustaining an unvoiced sound such as /s/, unvoiced lip or tongue trill, exhaling through a straw, and so on. "Singing without text" includes singing on SOVT sounds such as straw phonation, lip or tongue trill, raspberry, or on vowels. Rather than repeatedly running through the song from beginning to end, the singer can be more strategic in his or her practice by only targeting the places that need technical work. Singers can record themselves running through the song from beginning to end, then listen back to this recording to identify the places or "spots" that need more detailed work. Similarly, singers can listen to the recordings they have made of themselves multiple times for memorization. The singer might use check marks or write in the date to keep track of what they have completed, or write dates into the chart in advance to plan practice time into the future. This chart is merely an example: The specific content and organization can be customized for each singer.*

adequately prepared and to avoid overloading at the last minute.

Vocal Pacing in Recording Sessions

Time in the recording studio can be very intense, as much is riding on the process both financially and artistically. You can help the singer to be mindful in considering vocal pacing during recording sessions. Advance planning, including building voice breaks into the schedule, can be very advantageous. The singer should work with the other musicians and producer to prioritize songs, determine the order of recording, and develop a rough idea of the amount of time to be devoted to each song. If possible, the singer should alternate vocal and instrumental tracks.

Vocal Pacing During Performance

For classical and musical theater singers, the options for reducing vocal demands during the performance are, to a degree, constrained by the medium—the vocal range, duration of the performance, timing of breaks, and so on are largely dictated by the repertoire. In recital, singers have a greater degree of control, and vocal pacing should be considered when selecting the content. The singer may benefit from reflecting on vocal demands relative to singing range, intensity, and complexity in designing the program.

In many ways, CCM singers have more opportunities to adjust vocal demands during performance, which can be critical since they typically do not have the cover or understudy options that are often available to classical and musical theater singers. Presenters sometimes prefer continuous performance without breaks (e.g., very long sets) to keep the audience engaged and avoid people leaving during set-breaks. However, this is not a good arrangement for CCM singers, particularly those who are the only or main singer of the group. Singers who encounter this scenario may need your support to practice self-advocacy or your intervention with the presenter to ensure they have adequate breaks during the performance.

Here are some additional recommendations for guiding the CCM singer in adjusting performance load:

- Review typical set lists and keys. You may need to assist the singer in planning set lists so that the most demanding songs are spread out over the duration of the performance, alternating songs that are vocally easier with those that are more taxing.
- The singer may consider transposing songs to a more optimal key. This is particularly applicable to singers in cover bands for whom the original key may or may not be ideally suited to their individual voices.
- If you are working with a lead singer, explore the possibility of having backup singers or other bandmates sing lead occasionally.
- Adding or lengthening instrumental solos or instrumental breaks may also give the singer time for brief rest during the performance.

UNLOADING UNNECESSARY VOICE USE

Delegation and Consolidation

Delegating vocal tasks is a constructive vocal pacing strategy which will be particularly beneficial for choral conductors, vocal music educators, stage music directors, and church music directors, to name just a few.

- Assign students/choristers to act as section leaders and to take on some of the demonstration of parts in rehearsals.
- Designate assistants in rehearsals or classes, as well as for musical theater productions and other extracurricular vocal activities.
- Have students/choristers lead warm-ups.
- Determine which activities require the singer's musical and vocal knowledge and expertise. Anything that does not meet these criteria (such as making announcements or providing repetitive instructions) should be considered for delegation or for communicating in an alternative manner (blogging, website, handouts, visual presentations, etc.).

Another beneficial vocal pacing strategy is consolidating the vocal load at times when rehearsals and performances increase. For example, a voice teacher may modify the traditional once per week individual lesson of 30 to 60 minutes in ways that are beneficial to both the voice teacher and the student. This may entail teaching students who are at a similar skill level in small groups or combining group and individual lessons in such a way that the overall teaching schedule is shortened. Students will benefit from the opportunity to observe their peers working on similar technical goals.

Minimize Modeling and Demonstration

Singers should be conservative in modeling when leading rehearsals or teaching voice lessons. Encourage the singer to explore ways in which technical adjustments may be elicited with verbal cues and/or description rather than demonstration.

Use of Recordings

For conductors, music directors, voice teachers, and others who teach or lead rehearsals, recording vocal parts (either on an instrument or by singing) and using the recordings to drill parts can help reduce the need for demonstration. The conductor/music director/teacher can also send copies of the recordings home with the singers they lead to facilitate home practice. This will not only decrease the need to demonstrate in rehearsals or lessons, but is also more efficient, allowing more time for music making and teaching vocal technique. Making recordings involves an investment of time and planning on the teacher or conductor's part but will save time and vocal wear and tear in the long run. Many music publishers provide recorded examples for solo vocal music or choral sectionals.

For a voice teacher who has students who require a lot of modeling either to learn the music or achieve a better vocal sound, the teacher can record the model and then play back the recording for subsequent demonstration.

Singers in a cappella groups, musical theater, or other performance genres that include staging/choreography can use recordings and lip-synching during choreography rehearsals.

Avoid Singing or Speaking Over the Music

Choral conductors, music directors, and voice teachers frequently give instructions and feedback while their singers are singing. However, anything said when the teacher/conductor can't be heard may represent wasted voice use. Students/choristers will learn better when they are able to hear what the teacher/conductor is saying and are better able to process verbal information if their attention is not divided between singing and listening. Choral conductors should also avoid singing along with the choir if at all possible.

Choral singers may encounter a related scenario: singing loudly in an effort to lead, as when attempting to correct the out-of-tune singer nearby or help the entire section hear the right notes.

VOCAL PACING FOR SPEAKING VOICE USE

As you guide singers in improving vocal pacing, it is essential to emphasize that good vocal technique and strategic vocal pacing are just as important for speaking as for singing. Indeed, speaking voice use is often more out of balance than singing voice use. As you work on vocal pacing goals, be sure to carefully examine and regularly assess progress for both types of voice use.

The first and most important element is to ensure that the singers you work with have excellent vocal technique for speaking voice. Speaking voice should be targeted as part of the rehabilitation process, with a customized exercise regimen and regular review of how well the singer is applying speaking voice technique in everyday conversational interactions, as outlined in Chapter 13.

The handout "Vocal Pacing for Speaking Voice" provided in Appendix 14–C includes tips for cultivating vocal pacing for speaking voice.

Assessing Speaking Voice Use

Have the singer keep track of speaking voice use in the voice journal, or just make a list of typical speaking voice demands. As you review the list together, assess type and duration of speaking voice activities relative to daily communications, social encounters, work environment, family interactions, interviews and other media events, and at rehearsals and performances. Be sure that you understand the singer's priorities relative to speaking voice activities so that you can identify opportunities for bringing speaking voice use into better balance. The goal is to lead singers to a quantity of speaking voice use that provides adequate voice rest but ensures a fulfilling and connected social and professional life.

Performance-Related Speaking Voice Use

For full-time professional singers, speaking will often encompass professional activities and social interactions. In such cases, careful examination of the typical schedule can yield opportunities for decreasing the speaking voice load. Using travel time and hotel time for voice rest allows the voice to recuperate between performances. It is also important to use set-breaks or intermission for voice rest during performances and minimize talking at load-in and sound check, when applicable. Monitoring voice use during rehearsals is equally important. Rehearsal breaks can be used as voice rest time instead of for socializing. For contemporary commercial singers, using the microphone for discussion during rehearsals minimizes the need to speak loudly over amplified instruments.

Contemporary singers often work a merchandise table after the performance, which can involve a lot of speaking as they meet and interact with fans. This activity is extremely important for building and maintaining fan connections and for generating revenue from sales of the artist's merchandise. The environment will likely be noisy due to crowd sounds and background music, which can induce the Lombard effect (the instinctive tendency of humans to increase the volume of their own voice to complete with ambient noise). Try to help the singer develop a tactical plan to incorporate breaks during this type of engagement and encourage him or her to place the table at a location that minimizes competing sound. It's usually better for the table to be located at the end of a long room against a wall rather than in the center of a room with people surrounding it in all directions. If the singer travels with other musicians or crew, see if some of the other members of the team can take over periodically to provide the singer with breaks.

For all types of singers, the performance engagement may include appearances at social events such as after-parties or fundraisers, often in the context of background noise and poor acoustics. If attendance at this type of event is unavoidable, you can help the singer to be intentional about minimizing negative vocal consequences. The singer should identify whether there will be people in attendance with whom it is particularly important for him or her to interact—either for potential career advantages or for the benefit of the presenting organization. This will, of course, include the host of the event but also may include important patrons of the organization, media personalities, directors, conductors, producers, and so on. If the singer plans the timing of his or her arrival to allow for interaction with these people at an early point in the event, he or she may be able to make an early departure, practicing "the art of the brief appearance" to ensure the maximum impact of attendance with the minimum duration. If possible, the singer should try to engage in conversations at a location that is relatively less noisy to minimize the Lombard effect.

Some social activities surrounding performances may not carry this type of professional obligation, and in these cases, it will be essential to help the singer determine how important the event is and whether attending may create a risk of overusing the speaking voice. For example, if the cast of the show is going out to a restaurant for dinner after the performance, it might be better to excuse oneself in the interest of recuperating before the next day's performance or to only make a brief appearance at the gathering.

Media interactions and interviews can represent an additional vocal load. Such interactions may be critical to the singer's success, ensuring time in the limelight. You can help the singer prioritize interactions based on relative importance and examine how much control can realistically be achieved over the timing and duration of these activities. The singer's management (if applicable) may be recruited to help negotiate a schedule that will be support the singer's vocal pacing.

Some singers act as their own managers and promoters, and may have high vocal demands relative to running the business of their singing careers. If this is the case, review typical voice use associated with such activities to see if better pacing may be achieved through planning voice breaks throughout the day, avoiding business work on performance days when possible and optimizing use of nonvocal communication.

Use of nonvocal communication (e.g., e-mail or text) will be beneficial for all singers, particularly those in the habit of speaking on the phone a lot. Shortening phone conversations and avoiding speaking on the phone when there is a lot of background noise (including when driving and when using a speaker phone) will also help to buy more time for voice rest.

Other Work-Related Speaking Voice Use

We have been focusing on pacing speaking voice use for singers who are at a relatively high professional level, but for many of the singers you will work with, singing will not represent their entire work life. Many singers need to support themselves with a "day job." Food service and childcare can be great day jobs for singers as they often allow for the flexibility that is so important for a singer who is trying to schedule auditions and performances. Unfortunately, these jobs are also vocally demanding. In such cases, part of your counseling may involve encouraging the singer to seek a job that will require less voice use. If this is not possible, attaining optimal scheduling and controlling the environment and circumstances when speaking are critical.

For many, singing is an avocational activity enjoyed in addition to a full- or part-time career in another profession. Sometimes nonsinging careers may also be vocally demanding, as is the case for teaching, sales, business, or law. Whether professional or avocational, it is critical to review the demands of the singer's job to identify possibilities for reducing voice use. This may mean scheduling voice breaks during the day, using personal or vacation days surrounding an important performance, or trying to schedule meetings or presentations at a time when singing voice demands will not be high.

Teachers, choral conductors, and music directors should minimize speaking when students or choristers are talking. Encourage the teacher or choral conductor to develop a nonvocal way to indicate when it's time to be quiet, waiting for the room to be silent before trying to speak. This may require a major shift in how classroom/rehearsal behavior is controlled, but with consistent application of meaningful incentives and consequences, it can be a fruitful method for reducing nonessential voice use.

Use of Amplification for Speaking Voice

If the job requires the singer to speak in front of groups—for teaching, training, presentations, meetings, and so on—use of amplification will be immensely beneficial. Singers sometimes have a "macho" attitude about amplification. "I don't need to use an amplifier because I can project my voice." However, even with good technique, projecting exacts a vocal expense that is deleterious and unnecessary. Use of amplification for speaking is especially important for educators and conductors. Amplification not only reduces the vocal load of the teacher/conductor (Gaskill, O'Brian, & Tinter, 2012) but also improves student attention and learning (Sarff, Ray, & Bagwell, 1981).

There are many voice amplifiers available that are portable and unobtrusive and span a wide range of prices. A few examples include IMAGE Loud Portable Voice Amplifier, AliMed Digital Voice

Amplifier, Amplivox BeltBlaster, and the BoomVox Wireless Amplifier and SoniVox Amplifier by Griffin Laboratories. Voice-Amplifier.com offers multiple voice amplifier styles, as do Aker and Luminaud, including the Spokeman Personal Voice Amplifier, pictured in Figure 14–1.

As the singing voice rehabilitation specialist, your recommendation or that of a physician colleague may carry weight in ensuring that the singer is able to obtain and use appropriate equipment at work. Some insurance policies include coverage for voice amplifiers as medical equipment if prescribed by a physician, and it is worthwhile to explore this possibility.

Social Voice Use

Social voice use can represent a significant vocal load. This facet of vocal pacing must be examined with the same diligence as work-related voice use. Sometimes bringing social voice use into balance can be the most challenging aspect of pacing for

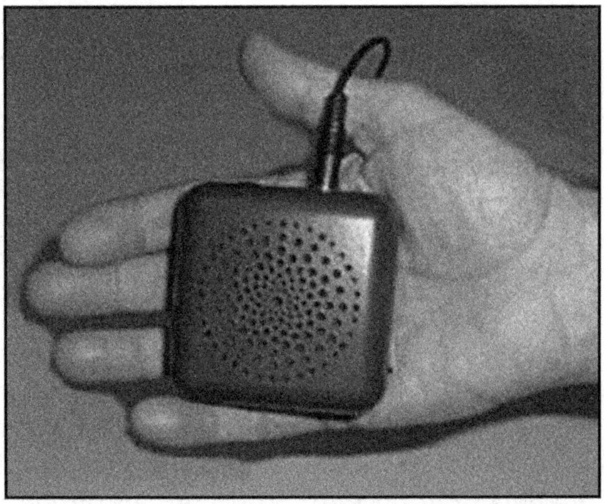

A

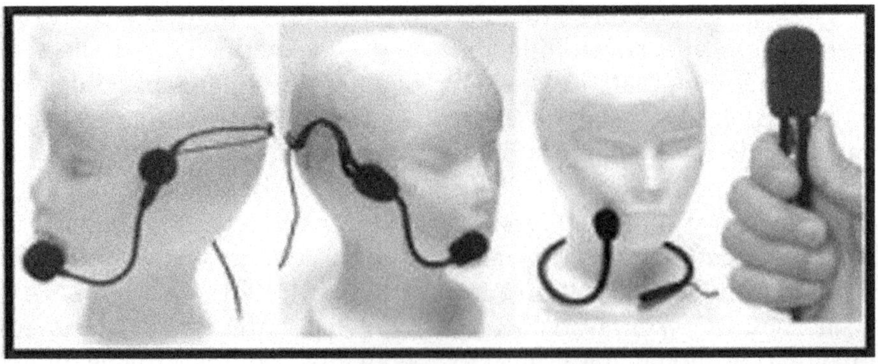

B

Figure 14–1.* A. *Spokesman Personal Voice Amplifier by Luminaud.* B. *Microphone options for Spokeman Voice Amplifier.

speaking voice, as it involves more complex relationships and expectations. The singer may fear being cut off from his or her support system or may feel left out of fun activities and events. Be mindful of this as you counsel the singer. It may take several sessions to understand the nature of the singer's most frequent and vocally demanding interactions. Maintaining a supportive network of friends and family is crucial for the singer's well-being—especially for singers whose careers involve constant travel—and of course it is appropriate to allocate voice use to these relationships. However, regular discussion of social voice use during rehabilitation sessions may reveal social situations that undermine the singer's attempts at vocal pacing.

I once worked with a young jazz singer who was living in New York where she had a wide circle of friends, many of whom were also involved in music. She struggled with pacing her speaking voice use as her friends frequently called her to go out to noisy bars and restaurants. At first she found it hard to resist their calls, but she began to realize that her singing career would be in jeopardy if she didn't achieve better balance, and she became more motivated to avoid these gatherings. She explained to her friends that these noisy get-togethers were having a negative impact on her vocal health. However, her friends were very persistent, often calling or texting her over and over again even after she had already declined. For a long time she succumbed to this pressure, regretting it afterward when her voice was hoarse the next morning. At one point she said, "I don't even enjoy going out that much. I'm really a homebody, but it's really hard to say no." After discussing this struggle in several sessions, she began to realize that the friends who pressured her to go out were perhaps not the best people for her to be around during her recovery. She had other friends who were much more understanding and supportive and who had on many occasions served to remind her about her vocal pacing goals. She started spending more time with these friends. In fact, she ended up sharing an apartment with one of them. Gradually, she was able to be more assertive, avoiding going out to noisy places and instead engaging in activities such as watching movies or quiet dinners at home. She still went out with her partygoer friends, but she was much more judicious about how often, and never when she had an important performance or recording session. I saw this singer intermittently over a period of about 2 years, and it was really only toward the end of our sessions that she felt she had accomplished this balance in her social life. It was hard won, but ultimately she was rewarded by the recovery of her voice and was empowered by her own assertiveness.

Bringing social voice use into balance can be especially challenging when working with high school or college students, for whom social pressure to engage in vocally risky behavior is high. This may involve cheerleading, yelling at spirit activities or athletic events, going to loud parties, fraternity, or sorority activities, and so on. Rather than telling singers not to participate in these activities (which may result in resistance), engage them in prioritizing these pursuits relative to singing. Leading singers to recognize voice use as a series of choices that have consequences may empower them to make responsible decisions and may thus be more effective than telling them to "just say no." Keep in mind that singers in this population are in the process of maturing and it may take a long time

—even years—for them to arrive at the point where they are prepared to put their singing ahead of their social lives. Adolescents and college students often find it particularly difficult to prioritize vocal health over social life through their *actions*, even when they clearly articulate the importance of singing in their lives. Sometimes it is exasperating to observe and interact with this dichotomous behavior, but remember that the brain's abilities relative to judgment and impulse control continue to develop well into the third decade. It can be helpful to set small goals and celebrate and praise the singer when they are achieved. This skill and a little patience can be powerful tools in a successful rehabilitation outcome.

Case Study

"Rachel" was a freshman musical theater major at a prestigious university training program who struggled mightily with bringing social voice use and activities into balance. She recognized that social pursuits were a factor in her vocal health and acknowledged that these activities had a negative impact on her voice. At the same time, she was adamant about her perception that attending two to three parties per week—accompanied by considerable alcohol consumption—was not only desirable but a necessary requirement of her social existence at school.

Not surprisingly, her progress in rehabilitation was initially hindered by her weekend party life. She was often tearful in her therapy sessions, frustrated by her slow vocal progress. Together we drew the line connecting her choices regarding parties and drinking to the vocal consequences they engendered, often yielding a response such as, "But I can't just not go!" or "I'm doing everything I can!" I sometimes found these responses exasperating, but I realized this was a case for very small steps, providing her with choices, and informing her of the likely outcome of her decisions.

I encouraged her to make a contract with herself. Each week she would make a change in her social activities, would maintain that change going forward, and pledge to the next change. I emphasized that the contract was not with me as the therapist but one that she was making with herself, her voice, and her future. After a time, she was able to limit herself to one social event in a noisy environment per week for 1 to 2 hours with minimal drinking. By the time she had completed seven or eight therapy sessions spanning 12 weeks, she stated, "I only go to a party if I really need it for stress reduction." Although her progress was—not surprisingly—slow, she steadily improved and was rewarded by the progress.

Would she have made faster progress in rehabilitation had she been able to more aggressively and rapidly reduce her social activities? Quite possibly so. However, it is my belief (informed by previous experience) that had I taken a more rigid and dogmatic stance with her at the beginning, she would have either fled therapy or attempted to hide her social voice use from me. As a recently liberated young adult, the social pull was just too strong a factor in her self-identity. She couldn't give it up "cold-turkey." Although it was hard for me to watch as she continued to make decisions that were delaying her progress, I had to meet her at the level of her emotional maturity and provide her with a framework for becoming a more responsible and accountable singer, which she ultimately did.

REFERENCES

Gaskill, C., O'Brien, S., & Tinter, S. (2012). The effect of voice amplification on occupational vocal dose in elementary school teachers. *Journal of Voice*, *26*(5), 667.e19–667.e27.

Helding, L. (2010). The mind's mirrors. *Journal of Singing*, *66*(5), 585–589.

Sarff, L., Ray, H., & Bagwell, C. (1981). Why not amplification in every classroom? *Hearing Aid Journal*, *34*(10), 43–52.

Schmidt, R., & Lee, T. (2014). *Motor learning and performance: From principles to application.* Champaign, IL: Human Kinetics.

APPENDIX 14–A

Tips for Enlisting Your Support Network for Vocal Pacing Success

Your friends, family and colleagues can be a big help to you in achieving your vocal pacing goals. The following is a list of ideas for recruiting your support network to help you optimize your vocal pacing. These are only suggestions, and you should only implement the ones that seem useful to you. By enlisting the help of people in your support network, you are empowering them to give you feedback and guidance, and you should consider only those people you know you can trust and who will be supportive and encouraging, rather than nagging, controlling, or bullying.

1. *Let everyone in your circle of friends, family, and colleagues know that you are undergoing voice rehabilitation.* According to your comfort level, let them know what your injury is, what the process for recovery is, and what steps you will have to take in your life to ensure a successful recovery. If you have a wide circle, it might be helpful to share this information in written form (letter, e-mail, social media, blog) so that you do not have to verbally explain what is happening over and over again.
2. *Ask your friends or family to remind you that you need to take voice breaks.* Consider arranging a private signal so that your friend can remind you in public or social situations without drawing unnecessary or unwelcome attention.
3. *Seek social activities that will minimize the risk of overusing your voice.* For example, instead of going out to a noisy restaurant or club, consider a quiet dinner at home where you can control the amount of background noise, or watch a movie together.
4. *Let people at home and at work know that you will periodically be taking voice breaks.* Consider using a signal or sign to let them know when you're "on break," such as wearing a special button or tag, or putting a sign on your office door. These breaks don't need to be very long—10 to 15 minutes several times a day will give your voice a chance to rest and bounce back.
5. *Ask your friends to help you protect your voice.* Sometimes you know you are going to be in a situation in which others may want to draw you into long conversations or involve you in activities that will be unnecessarily vocally demanding. If this type of situation is on the agenda, solicit your friends to advocate on your behalf or help disentangle you from such conversations.

APPENDIX 14–B

Tips for Planning Vocal Practice

Planning how to allocate voice use during practice is a vital element in your overall vocal pacing strategy. Developing a systematic approach to your practice time will help ensure that you are vocally prepared for performances without having to cram at the last minute. This will save wear and tear on your voice and help you be a more polished performer.

1. *Know the difference between "warming up" and "technical practice."* With a good exercise routine, you should be able to warm up in 10 to 20 minutes. Sometimes you might want to spend more time on vocal exercises to work on building your technique. It's important to know the difference. When preparing repertoire or getting ready for a long rehearsal or performance, the short warm-up is best.
2. *Avoid "spending" your voice learning the music.* You can learn new songs with "mental" practice. Think through the song while listening to a recording. You can use an existing recording, or record yourself singing the song. Listen three times, sing it once. Use unvoiced sounds (lip trill, raspberry, tongue trill, sustained "sss," etc.) while thinking through the song to practice breath support and airflow without using your voice. You can spend lots of time mentally practicing without using up your voice. This way, your voice will be fresh and ready to work when it's time to start on your technique.
3. *Use mental practice for memorization and interpretation.* Stand with good singing posture, breathe at appropriate phrase breaks, and mouth the words (silently—don't whisper) while thinking through or listening to a recording of the song. After you have mentally memorized the song, sing through the entire song again from memory, recording and listening back to plan for your next practice section.
4. *Plan your practice time.* Plan what pieces and what portions of pieces will get the most attention in your practice time. When first learning a new piece, it can be helpful to sing it through a few times using semi-occluded vocal tract sounds (voiced lip trills, tongue trills, raspberries, singing through a drinking or stir straw, etc.) Next, record yourself singing the whole song on the words and play it back to take notes about what sections need the most detailed technical work. Focus on those targeted sections for "spot practice" rather than running through the entire song over and over again.
5. *Keep track of your practice schedule and goals.* Make a chart or graph of all the music you need to work on and systematically plan how you will go about meeting your goals. Different types of practice may be applied to different songs on your list on any given day. Try to get a good balance of mental and vocal practice each day.

APPENDIX 14–C

Vocal Pacing for Speaking Voice

Speaking voice use can often be even more vocally taxing than singing voice use. Being strategic in achieving balance in amount and type of speaking voice use is an important part of your overall vocal pacing. The more you can save on speaking, the more you will have to allocate to singing activities.

1. *Make sure you have excellent vocal technique for speaking.* This doesn't mean "speak higher," a common misconception about efficient speaking voice use. Good speaking technique means good breath support, chest or mixed-register, and resonant voice. If you think your speaking voice technique might be contributing to voice problems, consult a qualified speech-language pathologist who specializes in voice care.
2. *When singing voice demands increase, look for opportunities to offload speaking voice use.* Rest your voice before and after a big singing day. Let the people you interact with most often know that you'll be resting your voice during times when singing voice demands are high. Try to minimize scheduling social events during these times.
3. *Avoid socializing in noisy places.* This is especially important when singing voice demands increase, particularly surrounding rehearsals or performances. If you can't avoid the noisy environment, be strategic in using your voice. Try to position yourself close to your conversational partners and avoid speaking over a distance. If you're in a noisy restaurant, sit next to the person you'll be talking to the most. If you're at a party, meeting, or fellowship gathering and want to have a conversation with someone, see if you can move to a quieter place away from the noise and the crowd.
4. *Practice the "art of the brief appearance."* Sometimes a singing engagement will require you to appear at a social function, such as a fundraiser, audience meet-and-greet, or cast party. In such cases, it may be difficult to avoid speaking in a noisy environment. However, you can still be strategic about how you participate in these activities and thereby minimize the vocal consequences. If you can, wait to arrive until the event is in full swing. That way, you minimize having conversations while you're waiting for the arrival of people you need to see. Determine which people you most need to interact with. Make sure you have a conversation with them, but keep it brief. Once you've seen the people you need to see, politely excuse yourself and (if possible) leave the event early. Consider having a "rescue" plan if you think you might be pulled into a long and arduous conversation. Arrange a private signal with a friend so that when you give him or her the signal, your friend can come and politely extract you from the conversation (for example, "I'm so sorry to have to steal Ms. Singer away, but Mr. Patron wishes to speak to her.").

5. *Try to keep media interviews surrounding performances to a minimum.* Obviously, media encounters and events are extremely important for advancing your career and success as a singer, so the idea is not to refuse all interviews, but to be strategic and judicious in scheduling them so that they don't wear you out for the performance. This can be quite challenging. Often radio or television interviews are scheduled in the morning. After being up late the night before for a performance, the morning interview not only adds to your vocal demands but also can undermine adequate rest. If you have a manager, he or she can help by advocating for optimal timing and duration of interviews.
6. *Use amplification if you have to interact with groups frequently.* If you have a day job that requires a lot speaking to groups (meetings, training sessions, presentations, teaching, etc.), or if you frequently direct choral, dance, or theater rehearsals, using amplification can save a lot of vocal wear and tear. Even in small conference rooms, you will benefit from the reduced need to project your voice. There are many options for personal voice amplifiers that are small and unobtrusive. It can take getting used to if you haven't tried it before, but can go a long way toward preserving your voice.
7. *If at all possible, seek a day job that is not vocally demanding.* It may be necessary for singers to have a day job to supplement performing income. Frequently, jobs that offer flexibility and convenience—such as food service or childcare—also come with a heavy vocal load. If at all possible, try to find a job that will require less talking. If that is not possible, apply the recommendations in this section about speaking in noisy environments, and be on the lookout for a better job option to arise.
8. *Be cognizant of how much time you're spending on the phone.* If you talk to people on the phone a lot, consider whether you may be able to accomplish some of your communication by text or e-mail, or at least consider decreasing the duration of your typical phone conversations. Using speakerphone can cause you to unintentionally raise your voice. Be aware that when you are speaking on the phone in the car, you are competing against a lot of noise from the car itself and the road. Try to save your phone conversation for a time when you'll be in a quieter environment.
9. *Do you have to speak a lot to run the business of your performing career?* It's not unusual for singers to act as their own managers and promoters. This can potentially involve a lot of voice use in booking engagements, working with presenters to plan engagements, communication with the other musicians in the group, and so on. If this is true for you, try to see how much of your interaction can be accomplished via written communication, and be mindful of the timing of your exchanges to allow adequate time for rest before and after performances.
10. *Be strategic about voice use at rehearsals and performances.* Try to minimize talking to fans or friends when there's a lot of noise in the background. Use breaks in the rehearsal or performance as voice rest time. If at all possible, have someone help you at the merchandise table so that you can take frequent breaks. Ask for the merchandise table to be set up at the quietest possible location.

11. *Optimize vocal pacing at home and in family interactions.* Let your family members know that you will need to take voice breaks at times. When speaking to people at home, try to arrange it so that you're in the same room, rather than calling to each other from one room to another (or from one end of the house to the other). Keep the background noise to a minimum by turning off or turning down the television, radio, or music if you're having a conversation.

APPENDIX 14–D

Vocal Pacing for Classical and Musical Theater Singers

GENERAL TIPS

1. Always warm up before practice, rehearsal, and performance.
2. Practice excellent vocal hygiene (see Vocal Hygiene handout).
3. Practice excellent pacing relative to your speaking voice use (see Vocal Pacing for Speaking Voice handout). This includes planning speaking voice use during practice, rehearsals, and performances.
4. Whenever possible, advocate for having an understudy or cover. This will give you more opportunities to rest and pace your voice. Should you experience fatigue or illness that affects your voice during the rehearsal period, having an understudy can provide you with the rest and recovery you need to be in good shape for the performance.

PLAN YOUR VOICE USE

1. Be strategic in planning how you will use your voice during your individual practice time. Become an expert at efficient practice (see Tips for Planning Vocal Practice handout).
2. It may be helpful to color-code your schedule, indicating different levels of vocal demands or intensity in various colors. For example, you may indicate marking in one color, combination of marking and full-voice singing in another, and full-voice singing in yet another color. By doing this, you will be able to see at a glance when the demands will increase, and plan accordingly. This will also guide you in planning your voice use surrounding rehearsals and performances. If you have a big audition, rehearsal, or performance coming up, avoid scheduling social activities during that time, adjust your typical practice time, and postpone less important singing activities.
3. Look for opportunities to put more voice time back into your vocal bank account. Start a voice journal and log all of your voice use. Then go through your journal and identify opportunities for offloading voice use. Prioritize vocal demands and say "no" to what is not important.
4. Be judicious in "recreational" singing.
5. Schedule periods for voice rest and write the voice rest time in your planning schedule. This may mean taking short vocal "naps" for 10 or 15 minutes several times per day, or scheduling a voice rest day before or after a big performance.

IN REHEARSALS

1. Plan in advance how much and how intensely you will use your voice throughout the rehearsal. Save your voice for the times when you will focus on the quality of your singing and preparing the performance. Be sure to communicate with the directing

team when you intend to mark so that they know you are practicing good vocal pacing in the interest of the production and not just "slacking off."
2. Staging and choreography rehearsals are a good time to use marking or even lip-synching. Your focus and that of the director/choreographer will be on the movement rather than on your singing, so this can be a time to conserve voice use. Tech rehearsal is another good time to use marking. Again, the focus will not be so much on you and your singing as it will be on the technical aspects of the production.
3. Save your full-voice or performance-level singing for times when the focus will be on the singing, such as in a run-through, orchestra rehearsal, dress rehearsal, or performance.
4. In some situations, it may be beneficial to sing full voice for part of the rehearsal and mark other parts. You might mark the parts that you feel are solidly learned and technically well prepared, and sing full voice for the parts that need more practice. Or, sing full voice at times when you need to check for balance with other singers or the orchestra, and mark during your solo sections.
5. Use rehearsal breaks for voice rest and minimize socializing during breaks.

AT THE AUDITION

1. Prepare your audition music well in advance so that you don't have to cram learning the music at the last minute.
2. Make sure you have a plan for how you will warm up your voice. Often, audition sites don't have designated space for warming up. You may need to warm up at home before going to the audition or in your hotel room. Your voice should easily stay warmed up for an hour or two after completing your routine. Once you get to the audition site, quiet exercises like lip trills or straw phonation can be a good way to stay limber, and can be completed in a quiet corner. Make sure that you don't *over* warm up. Don't leave your money notes in the practice room!
3. Be mindful of minimizing social talking at the audition. Being nervous or excited might put you in a talkative mood, but too much talking might have a negative impact on your performance.

AT THE PERFORMANCE

1. Allow adequate time to warm up, but don't overdo it. Save your voice for the performance.
2. Minimize social talking backstage before *and* after the performance. Dressing rooms can be very noisy places, causing you to speak loudly to be heard. Use your preparation time before the show for quiet time.
3. If you will have a microphone for the performance, work with the sound team if needed to make sure you can hear yourself well in the monitors to avoid over-singing.

ON THE ROAD

1. Use travel and hotel time for voice rest.
2. Minimize "recreational" singing.

IN THE RECORDING SESSION

1. Plan your recording time. Work with the other musicians and producer to prioritize repertoire, determine the order of recording, and develop a rough idea of the amount of time you will devote to each number.
2. Build voice breaks into the recording schedule.
3. Advocate for yourself if you feel the recording schedule is too intense. The producer and other musicians are likely to be supportive if they understand that pushing the duration and intensity of sessions may compromise vocal quality later in the recording process.

APPENDIX 14–E

Vocal Pacing for Contemporary Commercial Music Singers

GENERAL TIPS

1. *It is not normal to be hoarse after rehearsals or performances, and not normal to lose your voice on a regular basis.* If this is happening to you, you may have a voice injury. Repeating the pattern may make the injury worse and could jeopardize your singing future. Don't try to "just push through it." This may result in more severe or even permanent injury. Your long-term vocal health is more important than any given performance.
2. *Always warm up your voice before rehearsals and performances and set aside time for individual vocal practice.* You are a vocal athlete, and as such, you need time to work on your voice and your technique on a regular basis. This can easily be accomplished in 10 to 20 minutes per day. It can be hard to carve out an additional quarter to half hour in a day that is already jam-packed, but regular vocal exercise is essential to your long-term vocal health. If you don't already have a vocal exercise regimen, consider seeking the guidance of a skilled voice teacher or singing voice therapist. It is important that the exercises be customized to your voice, style of singing, and your technical needs. Be deliberate about planning your practice time, especially if you have a lot of music to prepare (see Tips for Planning Vocal Practice handout).
3. *Practice excellent vocal hygiene* (see Vocal Hygiene for Singers handout). This includes not drinking alcohol before and during performances. Smoking (anything) and singing don't mix. If you are a smoker, consider quitting for your vocal health if other health risks haven't motivated you so far. Drug use and singing also don't mix. Any substance that alters your consciousness will have a negative impact on your coordination, as well as your ability to be aware and use good judgment.
4. *Practice excellent pacing relative to your speaking voice use* (see Vocal Pacing for Speaking Voice handout). This includes planning voice use during practice and rehearsals.
5. If you play an instrument while singing, optimizing posture and microphone position can be very beneficial in achieving good vocal efficiency and minimizing risk of injury.

PLAN YOUR VOICE USE

1. *Schedule vocally light tasks and activities for times when other demands increase or in preparation for vocally demanding periods.* It may be helpful to color-code your schedule, indicating different levels of vocal demands or intensity in various colors. By doing this, you will be able to see at a glance when the demands will increase, and plan

accordingly. This will also guide you in planning your voice use surrounding performances. For example, if you have a big concert or show coming up, avoid scheduling social activities during that time, adjust your typical practice time, and prioritize rehearsals.

2. *Look for opportunities to put more voice time back into your vocal bank account.* Start a voice journal and log all of your voice use. Then, go through your journal and identify opportunities for off-loading voice use. Prioritize vocal demands and say "no" to what is not important. Schedule periods for voice rest. This may mean taking short vocal "naps" for 10 or 15 minutes several times per day, or scheduling a voice rest day before or after a big performance.

IN REHEARSALS

1. Plan in advance how much and how intensely you will use your voice throughout the rehearsal and when you are practicing on your own (see Tips for Planning Vocal Practice handout). In rehearsals, save your voice for the times when you will be focusing on the quality of your singing and preparing the performance. At other times, sing lightly or not at all. For example, if you're a singer in a band and you're working out the instrumental parts with the other band members, sing lightly, in a lower octave, or sing only the parts that are necessary for instrumental cues or entrances. Save your "full voice" or performance level singing for when all the instrumental parts are solidly learned and the song is ready for a run-through.
2. Use the microphone to communicate with other performers during rehearsal and sound check rather than trying to project your voice over the music.

AT THE PERFORMANCE

1. Optimize your use of sound engineering. Have the best quality sound equipment you can afford.
2. Advocate for yourself with the presenter, venue, or booking manager to ensure that you have set breaks and that sets are not too long. Continuous performance without breaks is often desirable to the presenter to keep the audience engaged and to avoid having people leave during breaks, but if at all possible, you need to take a break every 45 to 60 minutes.
3. Use set breaks for complete vocal rest time if at all possible. Leave the stage and go to a quiet place during the break rather than interacting with audience members.
4. If you're a lead singer, utilize your backup singers or instrumentalists to create "mini-breaks" for yourself during performances by having them occasionally take the lead.
5. Consider transposing songs to a more optimal pitch range, or at least give yourself the option of singing the song in a more comfortable key on days when you are feeling fatigued or when you have a heavy performing schedule.
6. Arrange your set lists to alternate demanding songs with those that are vocally easier and less taxing. Consider having an alternate or "B-plan"

set list that is less vocally strenuous for days when you are feeling fatigued or during periods when you have a lot of performances.

7. Have a band member who doesn't sing take responsibility for the merchandise table and/or take turns at the merchandise table.
8. Try to keep "meet-and-greets" and audience interactions short and to the point.

ON THE ROAD

1. Use travel and hotel time as voice rest time.
2. Minimize "recreational" singing.
3. Prioritize taking care of yourself, including getting good sleep, adequate nutrition, and exercise.

IN THE RECORDING STUDIO

1. Plan your recording time. Work with the other musicians and producer to prioritize songs, determine the order of recording, and develop a rough idea of the amount of time you will devote to each song.
2. Build voice breaks into the recording schedule. If possible, plan to alternate vocal and instrumental takes.
3. Advocate for yourself if you feel the recording schedule is too intense. The producer and other musicians are likely to be supportive if they understand that pushing the duration and intensity of sessions may compromise vocal quality later in the recording process.

APPENDIX 14–F

Vocal Pacing for Worship Soloists

1. *Your voice is a gift that deserves your care.* If you are a worship musician, your singing and directing activities are intricately intertwined with your spiritual life. You may feel that decreasing your vocal load is selfish, "slacking off," or shirking obligations. The opposite is true. Getting help with a voice injury and bringing your vocal load into a sustainable balance demonstrate your commitment to your spiritual life and creator by cherishing and caring for the vocal gift that has been entrusted to you. By doing so, you also set an example for other singers and worship musicians.
2. *It is not normal to be hoarse after rehearsals or performances, and not normal to lose your voice on a regular basis.* If this is happening to you, you may have a voice injury. Repeating the pattern may make the injury worse and could jeopardize your singing future. Don't try to "just push through it." This may result in more severe or even permanent injury. Your long-term vocal health is more important than any given service or performance.
3. *Always warm up your voice before rehearsals and services and set aside time for individual vocal practice.* You are a vocal athlete, and as such, you need time to work on your voice and your technique on a regular basis. This can easily be accomplished in 10 to 20 minutes per day. It can be hard to carve out an additional quarter to half hour in a day that is already jam-packed, but regular vocal exercise and preparing your voice for rehearsal and services are essential for your long-term vocal health. If you don't already have a vocal exercise regimen, consider seeking the guidance of a skilled voice teacher or singing voice therapist. It is important that the exercises be customized to your voice, style of singing, and your technical needs. Be deliberate about planning your practice time, especially if you have a lot of music to prepare (see Tips for Planning Vocal Practice handout).
4. *Use amplification as much as possible.* If you typically speak a lot during rehearsals or services, using amplification saves unnecessary wear and tear on your voice. It can also be helpful to use amplification when teaching classes or leading activities. If possible, try to find an amplifier that is portable so that you can take it with you to rehearsals in other rooms, auditoriums, places of worship, and so on. If you engage in contemporary worship activities, use of good microphones and monitors is critical to avoid overusing your voice. Work with the sound technicians to ensure optimal equipment and settings. If your singing activities involve working with a band or orchestra, use the microphone when speaking to them in rehearsals.
5. *Make your voice use count.* Make a list of all your voice use and determine which activities require your knowledge and expertise. Anything that

does not meet these criteria should be delegated to others or communicated in an alternative manner (blog, website, handouts, PowerPoint, recording, etc.). Plan in advance how much and how intensely you will use your voice throughout the rehearsal and when you are practicing on your own (see Tips for Planning Vocal Practice handout). In rehearsals, save your voice for the times when you will be focusing on the quality of your singing and preparing the performance. At other times, sing lightly or not at all. For example, if you sing with a chorus, band, or orchestra and you're working out the instrumental/choral parts, sing lightly, in a lower octave, or sing only the parts that are necessary for cues or entrances. Save your "full voice" or performance-level singing for when all the other parts are solidly learned and the song is ready for a run-through.

6. *Plan your voice use in advance.* Schedule vocally light tasks and activities for times when other demands increase or in preparation for vocally demanding periods. Consider making the days before and after intense rehearsal or services vocally light. It may be helpful to color-code your schedule, indicating different levels of vocal demands or intensity in various colors. By doing this, you will be able to see at a glance when the demands will increase, and plan accordingly. This will also guide you in planning your voice use outside the rehearsal room, which is especially important during times in the worship calendar when services and musical occasions increase. If you have a special event or service coming up that requires more voice use in rehearsals, avoid scheduling social activities during that time.
7. *Prioritize vocal demands.* Start a voice journal and log all of your voice use. Go through your journal and rank activities in order of importance and say "no" to what is less important. At first, it may seem impossible to unload anything—it will all seem important. However, with thoughtful review and consideration, you will discover that there are many situations in which your voice is not needed. You may need to practice assertive self-advocacy when discussing the need to lighten your vocal load with colleagues and the leadership at your place of worship, especially if you have always been one to take on extra responsibilities. Your singing activities are important to you, the worship team, and the congregation, and must take priority over other duties.
8. *Minimize using your voice to teach music.* If you typically help the choir, other singers, or instrumentalists learn music, or if you teach music classes, develop alternatives to repetitive singing. Record yourself singing the part and use the recording for teaching, use an instrument to demonstrate the part, or recruit section leaders or choir members to take on some of the demonstrating.
9. *Be mindful of pacing your speaking voice use.* If your worship activities involve a lot of speaking, this area represents an important part of your vocal pacing plan. Include speaking voice demands in your voice journal and look for opportunities to trim. For example, if you typically engage in fellowship time before or after services, you might contemplate shorten-

ing the duration of your participation. Avoid speaking when there is a lot of competing background noise. If you teach classes or direct activities, try scheduling them on days when your singing load will be lighter. If you are consistently fatigued on rehearsal and performance days, you may need to pare down or eliminate some of your speaking demands on the surrounding days. See the Vocal Pacing for Speaking Voice handout for additional tips on bringing speaking voice use into balance.

10. *Look for opportunities to offload voice use.* Be creative in thinking of alternative ways of communicating. What do you say over and over again in the rehearsal? Make a list of these things, and find a way to say them without using your voice. This could be a printed sign, a hand signal, or a gesture. Consider delegating nonessential vocal tasks to other members of the worship team or congregation.
11. *Enlist your community in preserving your voice and in your vocal recovery.* To the degree that you feel comfortable disclosing your voice injury and vocal rehabilitation, communicate with the choir, congregation, and colleagues to let them know you are working on your vocal health so that you can continue to do your best as a worship leader. Sharing this experience with your worship community can be an important lesson for them in vocal health and provides an excellent model. If they know about your voice problem, they will likely be more than willing to help in rehearsals, and they may even serve an important role in reminding you about being consistent in your new vocal habits.
12. *Use your creativity.* Your goal is to maximize the efficiency of your voice use, unload all unnecessary voice use, and look for opportunities to rest your voice. With this goal in mind, you will come up with many ideas for how this can be accomplished in your specific setting. Remember, even God rested on the seventh day!

APPENDIX 14–G

Vocal Pacing for Voice Teachers

1. Practice excellent vocal pacing relative to your speaking voice use, individual practice, and performing activities (see handouts for Vocal Pacing for Speaking Voice, Tips for Planning Vocal Practice, and for appropriate performing and conducting activities).
2. *Warm up before teaching.* You can warm up your voice in 10 to 15 minutes. You don't need to complete an elaborate technical practice session. Save that for when you are ready to focus on your individual practice.
3. Whenever possible, adjust your teaching schedule to be lighter at times when you have a heavier rehearsal and performing schedule.
4. *Be conservative in modeling during the lesson.* Often the easiest way to get the students to produce the sound you want is by giving them a demonstration. However, over the course of a day or week of teaching, this can add up to a lot of voice use that you could be devoting to your own singing endeavors. You may be able to elicit the technical adjustment you are seeking with verbal cues and description alone. If you have students who require a lot of modeling, consider recording yourself giving the model, and use playback for subsequent demonstration.
5. *Avoid giving a lot of instruction or feedback while your students are singing.* They won't be able to hear you well, which will make it less likely that they will implement your instruction. Also, you will likely attempt to project over their sound, which may cause you to overuse your voice.
6. If you have a very heavy teaching schedule, be creative in how you allocate your teaching time. With beginning students, there may be a lot of redundancy in your instruction from one student to the next. Consider teaching students who are at a similar level in small groups. This will benefit you by not having to repeat the same instructions over and over, and by teaching in groups, you may be able to shorten your overall teaching schedule. Your students will also benefit from the opportunity to observe their peers who are working on the same technical goals. You can still give each student some individual time, but perhaps for a shorter period than if you were teaching them all individual lessons.
7. If your pedagogical load includes classroom teaching, use amplification in the classroom. Even in a small room and with good speaking voice technique, speaking in a projected voice for prolonged periods on top of your private instruction creates an unnecessary vocal expense.
8. Optimize the acoustics in your studio, as well as your positioning in the room when teaching (e.g., make sure that your posture is not affected by your position in the room, location of the piano, etc.). Consider using sound-absorbing materials (rugs, wall covers, etc.) if the room acoustics are especially live.

APPENDIX 14–H

Vocal Pacing for Choral Singers

Vocal pacing means achieving a balance of voice use and voice rest. As a choral singer, you are a vocal athlete. Your voice needs regular vocal exercise *and* you need to have good vocal technique for a lifetime of vocal health. If your voice doesn't get regular vocal exercise, your skill might deteriorate over time, and the intense vocal demands of rehearsal and performance might tire you out. If your voice is not getting enough rest, you may be at risk for developing a voice injury or exacerbating an existing injury.

1. *Practice excellent vocal pacing relative to your speaking voice.* See Vocal Pacing for Speaking Voice handout.
2. *If you engage in multiple performing activities or a lot of recreational singing, you may need to decrease your overall vocal load to bring voice use into optimal balance.* See relevant vocal pacing handouts for tips that are customized to your vocal activities (student singers, a cappella group singers, active professionals, worship singers, etc.)
3. *Vocal fitness is essential for lifelong singing health.* If you have never taken voice lessons, consider doing so to develop and enhance your vocal technique. Look for a teacher who is experienced in teaching your style of singing (classical, contemporary, gospel, etc.). Even if you have had vocal training in the past, it can be beneficial to take a refresher now and then. Working with the right voice teacher can help you develop a vocal exercise regimen that is just right for your voice and your singing goals.
4. *Regular practice of vocal exercises is critical for keeping your voice strong and healthy.* Singing with the choir once or twice a week may not be enough to keep your voice in shape. Think of rehearsals and performances as being comparable to running a marathon. Runners make sure to train and prepare for the big race. You should be exercising your voice a little bit throughout the week to be ready for *your* big race.
5. *Practice your choir music outside of rehearsal.* A choir rehearsal is very cognitively demanding. You have to follow the music, watch the conductor, listen to the singers around you, monitor your own singing, and anticipate what's coming up. It can be hard to focus on using good vocal technique. Preparing your part in advance and working on your vocal technique will help you use your voice in the most efficient and skillful way during the rehearsal. Some of your practice can be accomplished "mentally" by thinking through the part in your head or listening to a recording while following along with your music.
6. *Consider keeping a voice journal to track all of your voice use, speaking and singing.* If you notice that your voice is often fatigued, you may be using your voice too much, or you may not be exercising your voice regularly enough. Keeping a voice journal will help you track the peaks and

valleys of voice use, determine how they correspond to how vocally fit you feel, and adjust your vocal load accordingly.

7. *Plan voice use well in advance.* When vocal demands increase—such as before a big concert or event—find ways to offload other voice use. This may include deferring social plans (especially those that require speaking in noisy environments), taking a day or two off from work if your job is vocally demanding, or reducing other taxing vocal activities (such as teaching Sunday school, public speaking and presentations, leading meetings, etc.). Consider making a chart or calendar to keep track of vocal activities to guide planning.

APPENDIX 14–I

Vocal Pacing for Choral Music Educators

1. *If you are experiencing a change in voice or voice problem that last for more than 2 weeks, get it checked out by a vocal health specialist (laryngologist and/or singing voice specialist).* Don't delay getting help. Getting your voice evaluated is taking care of yourself, and it's also taking care of your students. You can't do your best as a teacher with an untreated voice injury. You would be appalled if your instrumental colleagues just kept playing a violin with a broken bridge or a trumpet with a dented bell. Your voice is your instrument and requires constant care and upkeep.
2. *Put the mask on yourself first.* This is what we're told on the airplane prior to takeoff. The reason for this is simple and sensible: Putting the mask on someone else before yourself is indeed noble and selfless, but you're not doing anyone any good if you are unconscious on the floor from lack of oxygen. To really help in an emergency, you have to ensure that you are in condition to be helpful. This does not make you a selfish person. It is actually an act of extreme generosity and wisdom. Your students will learn best if you can give them an excellent vocal model, which you cannot do if you have a voice injury. After years of giving "110%," the thought of dialing back how much one is giving in and out of the classroom can feel very selfish to teachers. It is not. It seems counterintuitive, but your students will actually learn more and become more skillful if they are given more responsibility. By putting the mask on yourself, you give your students an opportunity to become leaders, be more self-aware, and take a greater role in shaping the choir and improving the performance.
3. *Always warm up your voice before teaching.* Warming up with your students in the classroom is not enough. You need some time to work on your voice and your technique on a regular basis before you begin your teaching day. This can easily be accomplished in 15 to 20 minutes per day. It can be hard to carve out an additional quarter hour in a day that is already jam-packed, but preparing your voice for teaching is essential. This must become a nonnegotiable part of your day. If you don't already have a vocal warm-up regimen, consider seeking the guidance of a skilled voice teacher or singing voice therapist. It is important that the exercises be customized to your voice and your technical needs.
4. *Get your classroom into shape to support your best voice function.* Arrange your classroom in such a way that you are able to achieve optimal body alignment: upright ribcage position, head upright, neck elongated, weight in your legs and feet.
   - If you play piano in the classroom, try to position it so that you can face your students while playing rather than turning to the side. With an acoustic piano, this may be challenging but not impossible.

With an electric piano, you may be able to adjust the height so that you can play while standing. An electric piano can also allow you to record the accompaniment or vocalise, and then play it back so that your hands are free to conduct and you can maintain good body alignment. When conducting, make sure you position the music stand so that you can easily see the music without bending your head down, and so that you can maintain eye contact with the students.
- Arrange the chairs in the room so that you can see all the students easily without compromising your posture. Minimize the distance between you and your students so that you can avoid having to project your voice over an unnecessary distance. This may mean rearranging the seating slightly from one class to another, a task that can be assigned to students.
- Consider videotaping yourself in the classroom over the course of a day or multiple days, and then review the recording. By doing this, you may discover a number of situations in which you could achieve better posture and decreased vocal effort.

5. *Always use amplification.* Singers tend to have a "macho" attitude about amplification. "I don't need to use an amplifier because I can project my voice." You may be very accomplished at projecting your voice, but doing this for 6 or more hours per day is wasting your talent and effort. Using an amplifier in the classroom will not only save wear and tear on your voice, but will help your students to learn better. If possible, try to find an amplifier that is portable, so that you can take it with you to rehearsals in other rooms, auditoriums, places of worship, and so on.
6. *Good leaders know how to delegate.* Delegate any vocal task that doesn't require your musical and vocal expertise.
   - Assign section leaders or student assistants in all choirs, as well as student directors for musical theater productions and other extracurricular vocal activities. Delegate as many tasks to them as you can. This could include making daily announcements, leading daily warm-ups, teaching parts, and so on.
   - Delegate speaking demands, such as leading meetings, to other faculty or staff. This takes some of the vocal load off you and helps them develop their leadership skills.
   - Make a list of all your voice use tasks and determine which require your knowledge and expertise. Anything that does not meet these criteria should be delegated to others or communicated in an alternative manner (blog, website, handouts, power point, whiteboard, etc.).
7. *Anything you say/sing when you can't be heard is wasting your voice.* Your students will not be able to take verbal direction from you if you're speaking when they are singing at full voice and with accompaniment. Your students will learn better if they can hear what you're saying. It may feel like you are losing time in the rehearsal by stopping and waiting until it is

quiet to say what it is you have to say. In actuality, your students are more likely to understand what you say and are better able to process the information if their attention is not divided between singing and listening to you. Singing along with your students will not make them sing better and should be used very judiciously. Minimize speaking when students are talking. Develop a nonvocal way of indicating that it's time to be quiet, and wait for the room to be silent before you start speaking.

8. *You don't have to be a cheerleader to be a good teacher.* Your students are not learning because of your enthusiasm level; they're learning because of your wisdom, knowledge, skill, and experience. They will still learn without shouted encouragement or continuous verbal feedback. You will still be able to communicate your passion and enthusiasm through your body language, facial expression, and the words you carefully choose for feedback. Dialing back the intensity level in the classroom can create an environment in which the students are equal partners in being passionate about music and striving for excellence.
9. *Plan your voice use.* Schedule vocally light tasks and activities (such as watching videos, working on projects, testing, etc.) for times when other demands increase or in preparation for vocally demanding periods. It may be helpful to color-code your schedule, indicating different levels of vocal demands or intensity in various colors. By doing this, you will be able to see at a glance when the demands will increase and can plan accordingly. This will also guide you in planning your voice use outside the classroom. For example, if you have a big concert coming up that requires more voice use at school, avoid scheduling social activities during that time, or arrange for a substitute to take the church choir that week.
10. *Look for opportunities to put more voice time back into your vocal bank account.* Start a voice journal and log all of your voice use. Then, go through your journal and identify opportunities for offloading voice use. Prioritize vocal demands and say "no" to what is not important. At first, it may seem impossible to unload anything—it will all seem important. However, with thoughtful review and consideration, you will discover that there are many situations in which your voice is not needed.
    - Be creative in thinking of alternative ways of communicating. What do you say over and over again in the classroom? Make a list of these things, and find a way to say them without using your voice. You could use a printed sign, a hand signal, or a gesture. Alternatively, you could assign certain students to say certain phrases. For example, you might assign Alicia to say, "Put away your cell phones," so that at your cue, she makes the announcement and you don't have to.
    - Use recordings to supplement teaching parts or warm-up exercises. You can make recordings of individual parts and use them for demonstration in the classroom and to help your students with their home practice.
    - Sometimes your classroom warm-up period may be devoted to training vocal and aural skills,

which will require your expertise and necessitate using your voice quite a bit. However, there may be times when you are running through exercises that are already well known to the students simply to get their voices ready for the rehearsal. Consider deliberately alternating this on a regular basis. For example, if you are teaching four choirs per day, you may choose to do more vocal teaching for first and third period choirs on Monday, but just run through warm-ups using student leaders or recordings for second and fourth periods. Then on Tuesday, reverse the pattern, and so on throughout the week.

- When you stop a rehearsal to make a correction, teach your students to take the lead in determining why you stopped (i.e., what needs to change/be better). At first this will be challenging, because it will take them several tries to get it right. However, they will get better at it very quickly as they get into the habit of being better listeners while they're singing. When they see your cutoff, hands should start going up and they should start making suggestions about what needs to be adjusted. In the long run, you will not only be saving your voice, but will also be teaching your students to be better musicians.

11. *Enlist your community in preserving your voice and in your vocal recovery.* To the degree that you feel comfortable disclosing your voice injury and vocal rehabilitation, communicate with the administrators and other faculty at your school to let them know you are working on your vocal health so that you can continue to do your best as a music educator. Sharing this experience with your students can serve as an important lesson in vocal health and provides an excellent model for them. If they know about your voice problem, they will likely be more than willing to help in the classroom, and they may even serve an important role in reminding you about being consistent in your new vocal habits. If you find this difficult to do for yourself, consider it part of the education you are giving your students. You might even post your voice journal as part of a blog your students can read. You may consider letting your students' parents know about it too. Parent volunteers that participate in the classroom or parent support organizations can also be called on when you are delegating nonessential vocal tasks.
12. *Be a leader in vocal health.* Music educators are on the front line of vocal health awareness. Teach your students principles of vocal health and model them. Teach students vocal pacing, especially when their demands increase. Consider collaborating with another teacher on a vocal health project. You might do a segment on voice anatomy and physiology with the science teacher, or collaborate with the health teacher on vocal hygiene, or with the writing teacher on creating a voice journal.
13. *Save some time in your voice budget for joyful singing.* Remember that you got into this profession because you love singing. Continuing to refresh that love in yourself will not only help

you continue to develop your vocal skills but will also recharge you when your battery is low. You may consider continuing your own voice training with a teacher and/or participating in rewarding performing activities.

14. *Use your creativity.* Your goal is to maximize the efficiency of your voice use, unload all unnecessary voice use, and look for opportunities to rest your voice. With this goal in mind, you will come up with many ideas for how this can be accomplished in your specific setting and for your particular students.

APPENDIX 14-J

Vocal Pacing for Choral Conductors

1. *Put the mask on yourself first.* This is what we're told on the airplane prior to takeoff. The reason for this is simple and sensible: Putting the mask on someone else before yourself is indeed noble and selfless, but you're not doing anyone any good if you are unconscious on the floor from lack of oxygen. To really help in an emergency, you have to ensure that you are in condition to be helpful. This does not make you a selfish person. It is actually an act of extreme generosity and wisdom. Your choristers will learn best if you can give them an excellent vocal model, which you cannot do if you have a voice injury. By putting the mask on yourself, you give your choristers an opportunity to become leaders, to be more self-aware, and to take a greater role in shaping the choir and improving the performance.
2. *Your voice is a gift that deserves your care.* If you are a worship musician, your singing and conducting activities are intricately intertwined with your spiritual life. You may feel that decreasing your vocal load is selfish, "slacking off," or shirking obligations. The opposite is true. Getting help with a voice injury and bringing your vocal load into a sustainable balance demonstrate your commitment to your spiritual life and creator by cherishing and caring for the vocal gift that has been entrusted to you, and set an example for other singers and worship musicians.
3. *Always warm up your voice before rehearsals and set aside time for individual vocal practice.* Warming up with your choir in the rehearsal is not enough. You need some time to work on your voice and your technique on a regular basis. This can easily be accomplished in 10 to 20 minutes per day. It can be hard to carve out an additional quarter to half hour in a day that is already jam-packed, but regular vocal exercise and preparing your voice for rehearsal are essential for your long-term vocal health. If you don't already have a vocal exercise regimen, consider seeking the guidance of a skilled voice teacher or singing voice rehabilitation therapist. It is important that the exercises be customized to your voice, style of singing, and your technical needs.
4. *Always use amplification.* Using an amplifier in rehearsals saves unnecessary wear and tear on your voice. If possible, try to find an amplifier that is portable, so that you can take it with you to rehearsals in other rooms, auditoriums, places of worship, and so on.
5. *Good leaders know how to delegate.* Delegate any vocal task that doesn't require your musical and vocal expertise. If possible, assign section leaders in all choirs. Make a list of all your voice use and determine which require your knowledge and expertise. Anything that does not meet these criteria should be delegated to others or communicated in an alternative

manner (blog, website, handouts, PowerPoint, recording, etc.).

6. *Anything you say/sing when you can't be heard is wasting your voice.* Your choir will not be able to take verbal direction from you if you're speaking when they are singing at full voice with accompaniment. Your singers will learn better if they can hear what you're saying. It may feel like you are losing time in the rehearsal by stopping and waiting until it is quiet to say what it is you have to say. In actuality, your singers are more likely to understand what you say and are better able to process the information if their attention is not divided between singing and listening to you. Singing along with the choir will not make them sing better and should be used very judiciously. Minimize speaking when singers are talking. Develop a nonvocal way of indicating that it's time to be quiet, and wait for the room to be silent before you start speaking.
7. *You don't have to be a cheerleader to be a good choral director.* Your choristers are not learning because of your enthusiasm level; they're learning because of your wisdom, knowledge, skill, and experience. They will still learn without shouted encouragement or continuous verbal feedback. You will still be able to communicate your passion and enthusiasm through your body language, facial expression, and the words you carefully choose for feedback. Dialing back the intensity level in the rehearsal can create an environment in which the singers are equal partners in being passionate about music and striving for excellence.
8. *Plan your voice use.* Schedule vocally light tasks and activities for times when other demands increase or in preparation for vocally demanding periods. It may be helpful to color-code your schedule, indicating different levels of vocal demands or intensity in various colors. By doing this, you will be able to see at a glance when the demands will increase, and plan accordingly. This will also guide you in planning your voice use outside of the rehearsal room. This becomes especially important during times in the worship calendar when services and musical occasions increase or when preparing for major concerts. If you have a special performance or service coming up that requires more voice use in rehearsals, avoid scheduling social activities during that time, consider lightening your teaching load, and reallocate any extra rehearsals or obligations.
9. *Prioritize vocal demands.* Start a voice journal and log all of your voice use. Go through your journal and rank activities in order of importance and say "no" to what is not important. At first, it may seem impossible to unload anything—it will all seem important. However, with thoughtful review and consideration, you will discover that there are many situations in which your voice is not needed.
10. *Look for opportunities to offload voice use.* Be creative in thinking of alternative ways of communicating. What do you say over and over again in the rehearsal? Make a list of these things, and find a way to say them without using your voice. You could use a printed sign, a hand signal or a gesture.
11. *Be conservative in using your voice for purposes of teaching parts.* Use recordings to supplement teaching parts or warm-up exercises. These may be

commercial recordings, or you can record yourself or your section leaders singing parts. Use the recordings for demonstration in the rehearsal and to help your choristers with their home practice. This will not only save you vocal wear and tear but will also increase the efficiency of your rehearsals and allow more time to focus on music making and teaching vocal technique.

12. *Avoid using your voice to "fill in" parts.* Regularly singing a voice part that is not your own can be vocally taxing and may contribute to or hinder recovery from a voice injury. Even if you're filling in your own voice part, you're unnecessarily increasing your vocal load by doing so. If you feel you don't have enough strong singers in your choir to underpin a section or to help with demonstrating parts, this may be a sign that you need to recruit more talent from the community or congregation, or advocate for hiring section leaders. This can be very challenging in small groups or congregations with tight budgets, and you may find yourself in somewhat of an uphill battle against "we've always done it this way" thinking. You should be prepared to make your case to the leadership of your organization or place of worship. If having a choir is a priority, it should be reflected in allocation of resources.
13. *Get your rehearsal room into shape to support your best voice function.* Arrange your rehearsal room in such a way that you are able to achieve optimal body alignment. If you play piano in the rehearsal, try to position it so that you can face the choir while playing rather than turning to the side. When conducting, make sure you position the music stand so that you can easily see the music without bending your head down and so that you can maintain eye contact with the singers. Arrange the chairs in the room so that you can see all the singers easily without compromising your posture.
14. *Enlist your community in preserving your voice and in your vocal recovery.* To the degree that you feel comfortable disclosing your voice injury and vocal rehabilitation, communicate with the choir, congregation, and colleagues to let them know you are working on your vocal health so that you can continue to do your best as a music director. Sharing this experience with your choristers can serve as an important lesson in vocal health and provides an excellent model for them. If they know about your voice problem, they will likely be more than willing to help in rehearsals, and they may even serve an important role in reminding you about being consistent in your new vocal habits.
15. *Use your creativity.* Your goal is to maximize the efficiency of your voice use, unload all unnecessary voice use, and look for opportunities to rest your voice. With this goal in mind, you will come up with many ideas for how this can be accomplished in your specific setting and for your particular choristers.

APPENDIX 14–K

Vocal Pacing for Student Singers: General Tips

1. *Vocal pacing will directly affect your success as a singer.* You have chosen to include singing activities in your life and singing is important to you. The vocal pacing choices you make will have a direct impact on your success in these endeavors. Of course we all want to be able to do everything and none of us wants to feel restricted, but the reality is that there is a limit to how much your voice can do.
   - If you are active in singing ventures such as a cappella groups, musical theater, or singing in worship activities, you are making a commitment to fulfilling your role in the group. Unwise vocal pacing decisions may undermine this commitment.
   - If you sing in a school chorus, are a voice or musical theater major or minor, or are taking voice lessons for academic credit, your academic performance will be measured in part by your ability to fulfill the singing requirements of the course or program. Your grade or even your ability to finish your degree may be jeopardized by poor vocal health.

2. *Priorities are the key.* Putting your vocal activities in order from most to least important will help you to make smart decisions and manage your vocal load optimally. Make a list of all your singing and speaking activities and number them in order of how important they are to you. You may need to reduce how much time you spend on the less important activities to keep your voice healthy or to recover from a voice injury. Sometimes you have to think of priorities from multiple perspectives. For example, if you have an academic requirement to sing in choir and are also active in a student-directed a cappella group, the a cappella group may be a priority in terms of fun and fulfillment. However, if your participation threatens your ability to function in choir, your grade or even your ability to continue in the degree program may be in danger. If you want to be successful in your academic program, you may have to make the a cappella group the lower priority.
3. *It is not normal to be hoarse after rehearsals or performances and not normal to lose your voice on a regular basis.* If this is happening to you, you may have a voice injury. Repeating the pattern may make the injury worse and could jeopardize your singing future. Don't try to "just push through it." This may result in more severe or even permanent injury. Your long-term vocal health is more important than any given performance.
4. *Get your voice checked out if you are having frequent voice problems.* Ideally, you should see a laryngologist (voice doctor) and, if possible, a singing voice rehabilitation specialist. In all likelihood, optimizing vocal pacing will be part of the plan for getting your voice back on track. Often voice teachers or

choir directors will notice if a student seems to have chronic or repeated hoarseness and will recommend evaluation. If you are in a student-led group, you have to monitor your own voice and also help monitor the voices of the others in your group.

5. *Always warm up before practice, rehearsal, and performance.* The warm-up should be customized to your voice and your singing style. Choral or group warm-ups may not be adequate to ensure that you get optimal vocal exercise.
6. *For musical theater or opera performances, advocate for having an understudy or cover whenever possible.* This will give you more opportunities to rest and pace your voice. Should you experience fatigue or illness that affects your voice during the rehearsal period, having an understudy can provide you with the rest and recovery you need to be in good shape for the performance.
7. *Practice excellent vocal hygiene* (see Vocal Hygiene handout). This includes drinking at least 64 ounces of water per day. Caffeine is a diuretic and makes your body lose water. If you consume a lot of caffeinated beverages, make sure you balance that consumption with water or other noncaffeinated beverages.
8. *In the long run, a lifestyle of partying and drinking on a regular basis is not compatible with vocal health.* If singing is important to you, consider how the choices you make may impact your voice.
   - Drinking alcohol is dehydrating. More important, alcohol can make you change your behavior in ways that are ultimately unhealthy for your voice. This includes extended speaking or singing in loud environments (bars, parties, athletic events), yelling, and screaming. Alcohol affects your coordination, so if you are singing while intoxicated, it will be much more difficult for you to pay attention to your technique, which may result in voice injury or exacerbating an existing injury.
   - Smoking (anything) and singing don't mix. If you are a smoker, consider quitting for your vocal health if other health risks haven't motivated you so far. Drug use and singing also don't mix. Any substance that alters your consciousness will have a negative impact on your coordination, as well as your ability to be aware and use good judgment.

APPENDIX 14–L

Social Voice Use for Student Singers

1. *Practice excellent pacing relative to your speaking voice use* (see Vocal Pacing for Speaking Voice handout). This includes planning speaking voice use during practice, rehearsals, and performances. Use rehearsal breaks or offstage time for voice rest as much as possible.
2. Social voice use counts as part of your vocal load. In addition to normal social interactions, other situations that may place high vocal demands on your speaking voice are:
   - Yelling and cheering at athletic or spirit events
   - Frequent partying in noisy environments
   - Fraternity/sorority membership with attending social requirements
   - Student leadership organizations
   - Student worship organizations
   - Summer jobs such as camp counseling, coaching, or working in a restaurant

   If you engage in these types of activities regularly, it is critical to be aware of the potential impact on your voice and to take some time to think about your vocal priorities. Singing in and of itself creates a very high vocal load. A large proportion of social voice use on top of that can tip the balance, resulting in vocal injury or hindering recovery from an existing injury.
3. *The first step in bringing social voice use into balance is to prioritize your activities.* It can be hard to say "no" to fun events when all your friends are going, but as a vocal athlete, your success depends on being a "smart socializer." The reward is walking out on stage and doing what you love to do—singing! If singing is important to you, and especially if singing is part of your academic program, it must take the highest priority. That may mean dialing back on the social activities. You don't necessarily need to stop participating altogether. Start by considering which activities you can let go of, and see if you can adjust how much you engage in the social pursuits that are most important to you. For example, if you love going to basketball games, find a nonvocal way to express your spirit during the game. If you just can't say no to parties, try staying for a shorter time, keeping the alcohol consumption in check, and opting out on parties when important vocal performances are coming up.

APPENDIX 14–M

Planning Singing Voice Use for Student Singers

1. *Become an expert at efficient practice* (see Tips for Planning Vocal Practice handout). Be strategic in planning how you will use your voice during your individual practice time. This becomes even more critical at times when you have a lot of music to prepare, such as before recitals, juries, auditions, and opera or musical theater roles. Planning far in advance is the key to ensuring your voice will be in good shape for the performance.
   - If you are taking voice lessons and you're not sure what you're supposed to be doing during your practice time, ask your teacher for guidance.
   - Be diligent in prioritizing individual practice among your vocal demands. This is the time when you will work on your vocal technique with the greatest attention and focus, which is essential for becoming a better singer.
   - Try to avoid scheduling your practice time late at night when you're tired or after you've already been singing in other activities such as choir, coaching, or voice lesson.
2. *Consider creating a color-coded schedule, indicating different levels of vocal demands or intensity in various colors.* For example, you may indicate "marking" in one color, combination of marking and full-voice singing in another, and full-voice singing in yet another color. Be sure to incorporate speaking voice demands as well, including social voice use. By doing this, you will be able to see at a glance when the demands will increase and can plan accordingly. This will also guide you in planning your voice use surrounding rehearsals and performances. For example, if you have a big audition, rehearsal, or performance coming up, avoid scheduling social activities during that time, adjust your typical practice time, and postpone less important singing activities.
3. *Look for opportunities to put more voice time back into your "vocal bank account."* Start a voice journal and log all of your voice use. This should include voice lessons, choir, group rehearsals, individual practice, rehearsals for musicals or opera, rehearsals with your accompanist or coach, performances, "recreational" singing, and speaking voice use. Then, go through your journal and identify opportunities for offloading voice use. Prioritize vocal demands and say "no" to what is not important.
4. *Be judicious with recreational singing.* This is often the most fun and spontaneous singing, but if you have academic voice requirements or have made a commitment to singing in a group, recreational singing may need to be a lower priority and cutting back can create an opportunity for voice rest. You may not need to cut it out

completely. If you're used to singing in the car all the time, try limiting yourself to one or two songs per trip.

5. *Schedule periods for voice rest and write the voice rest time in your planning schedule.* This may mean taking short vocal "naps" for 10 or 15 minutes several times per day or scheduling a voice rest day before or after a big performance.

APPENDIX 14–N

Vocal Pacing for Choral Students

Being in a school or university choir can be very vocally demanding, particularly if the ensemble rehearses multiple times per week, and can represent a relatively large proportion of your singing load. Enrollment in an ensemble is often a requirement for an academic degree in music, so it is essential that you manage the load and prioritize appropriately.

1. *Be sure to balance the demands of choir with your other singing requirements.* If possible, avoid scheduling your voice lesson, coaching, or individual practice right before or after rehearsal.
2. *Make sure you warm up before choir rehearsal.* Choral warm-ups are intended to provide vocal warm-up but also to warm up the balance, intonation, and quality of the choral sound. The exercises may not be adequate to ensure that your individual voice is warmed up. If you find that you don't feel warmed up after the choral exercises, consider completing your own short warm-up prior to the rehearsal.
3. Even if you are singing classical repertoire in chorus and your lessons, solo and ensemble singing technique can be quite different. If you notice that you feel more fatigued or less technically skillful when singing in chorus, ask your chorus director and voice teacher for guidance in differentiating between the two types of singing.
4. A choir rehearsal room can be a noisy place during breaks and before and after the rehearsal, when everyone is talking. Try to minimize talking when it's noisy.

APPENDIX 14–O

Vocal Pacing for Students in A Cappella Groups

If the suggestions outlined here are not already part of your a cappella group's rehearsal habits, you may need to talk with the group's leadership to ensure implementation. This might require some changes in how the group works but ultimately will benefit the vocal health of the entire ensemble, which will result in better and more reliable performances.

1. *Warm up your voice before rehearsals.* Warm-ups should be appropriate for the style of singing the group does and should be customized for your voice. If you are not taking voice lessons or if your vocal training is in a different style (i.e., your training is in classical singing but the group sings contemporary music), consider exploring local resources for obtaining training that is appropriate to your chosen style.
2. *Mix up the rehearsal elements.* Three to 4 hours is a long time to engage in continuous intense vocal activity. If your rehearsals are long, alternate vocally strenuous activities (working or running through songs at full volume) with those that are less taxing (singing lightly or even lip-synching while working on choreography). If you typically take time during rehearsal for group business (working out schedules, planning upcoming events), consider doing this in the middle of the rehearsal to provide a voice break.
3. Take short breaks periodically during the rehearsal, and designate breaks as "silent" time.
4. *When learning new songs, learn parts by listening repeatedly rather than singing repeatedly.* A useful rule of thumb is "listen three times, sing once."
5. *If you are involved in teaching new parts to others in the group, use recordings as much as possible.* If you need to sing the part for them, consider making a recording of yourself singing the part in advance, and use this recording to facilitate teaching. Try to divide the teaching responsibility among the more experienced members of the group.
6. *Plan the group's rehearsal schedule well in advance so that you don't have to cram or add extra rehearsals as the performance approaches.* Increasing the vocal load right before the concert can result in everyone going into the performance more fatigued and at greater risk for injury and may compromise the quality of your performance.
7. *If you lead rehearsals, consider using amplification when you are speaking.* Even in a relatively small rehearsal space, this can save wear and tear on your voice.
8. *Plan and practice good vocal pacing during special events, such as group retreats or tours.* Minimize recreational singing, schedule time for voice breaks (such as during travel time), make sure you get enough sleep, and be mindful of social voice use. Being fatigued or hoarse after such events is an indication that vocal pacing is not optimized and needs more work, especially if this is happening to multiple members of the group.

9. *When recording, plan the session well in advance, alternating vocally intense songs with those that are less taxing.* Avoid scheduling marathon recording sessions, which can result in poor-quality performance as everyone becomes exhausted. Try to schedule multiple shorter sessions. Try to offload other vocal demands (such as social voice use) to conserve voice for the recording session.

10. *If your group uses amplification, maximize the quality of your equipment and sound mixing.* Make sure the microphone arrangement on stage doesn't interfere with good posture, use monitors, and work with the sound engineer to ensure that everyone in the group can hear themselves and the rest of the group in their monitors. Use the best-quality equipment you can afford.

APPENDIX 14–P

Vocal Pacing for Students: Theater and Opera

IN THEATER AND OPERA REHEARSALS

1. Use rehearsal breaks for voice rest, and minimize socializing during breaks.
2. Plan in advance how much and how intensely you will use your voice throughout the rehearsal. Save your voice for the times when you will focus on the quality of your singing and preparing the performance. Be sure to communicate with the directing team when you intend to mark so that they know you are practicing good vocal pacing in the interest of the production and not just "slacking off."
    - Staging and choreography rehearsals are a good time to use marking or even lip-synching. Your focus and that of the director/choreographer will be on the movement rather than on your singing, so this can be a time to conserve voice use. Tech rehearsal is another good time to use marking. Again, the focus will not be so much on you and your singing as it will be on the technical aspects of the production.
    - Save your "full-voice" or performance-level singing for times when the focus will be on the singing, such as in a run-through, orchestra rehearsal, dress rehearsal, or performance.
    - In some situations, it may be beneficial to sing full voice for part of the rehearsal and mark other parts. You might mark the parts that you feel are solidly learned and technically well prepared, and sing full voice for the parts that need more practice. Or, sing full voice at times when you need to check for balance with other singers or the orchestra, and mark during your solo sections.

AT THE PERFORMANCE

1. Allow adequate time to warm up, but don't overdo it. Save your voice for the performance.
2. Minimize social talking backstage before *and* after the performance. Dressing rooms or backstage areas can be very noisy places, causing you to speak loudly to be heard. Use your preparation time before the show for quiet time.
3. If you will have a microphone for the performance, work with the sound team if needed to make sure you can hear yourself well in the monitors to avoid over-singing.

AUDITIONS AND COMPETITIONS

1. Prepare your audition music well in advance so that you don't have to cram learning the music at the last minute.

2. Make sure you have a plan for how you will warm up your voice. Often, audition sites don't have designated space for warming up. You may need to warm up at home before going to the audition or in your hotel room. Your voice should easily stay warmed up for an hour or two after completing your routine. Once you get to the audition site, quiet exercises like lip trills or straw phonation can be a good way to stay limber and can be completed in a quiet corner. Make sure that you don't *over* warm up. Don't leave your money notes in the practice room!
3. Be mindful of minimizing social talking at the audition. Being nervous or excited might put you in a talkative mood, but too much talking might have a negative impact on your performance.

CHAPTER 15

Getting Back on the Horse: When, Where, and How to Return to Performing

In many cases, the singer will be able to continue performing during the rehabilitation process, although perhaps with modifications to the performance schedule. In Chapter 2, we examined considerations for determining whether or not to recommend that the singer temporarily discontinue performing during the rehabilitation process, weighing factors such as severity of injury, risk of further injury, professional status, financial impact, risk of harm to the singer's reputation as a performer, and the degree to which it would be frustrating to the singer to perform below personal standards, among others. For purposes of this chapter, we will assume that a recommendation has been made to suspend or at least significantly reduce performing, and the time has come for the singer to contemplate "getting back on the horse."

Performing is central to the singer's identity, and it is essential that he or she get back to performing as soon as possible during the recovery process. In many cases, the singer's return to a regular performance schedule will occur in a fairly organic manner and may not require detailed attention during the rehabilitation process. In other cases, you may spend several sessions guiding and preparing the singer in planning a safe and successful "comeback." Returning to performing too soon or in the wrong context can have disastrous consequences and may delay recovery. However, postponing the return for too long may present financial difficulties for the singer, foster fear of singing, and promote deconditioning. It is appropriate and desirable for the singer to get back to performing while still undergoing rehabilitation so that both of you can assess and regroup as needed until the singer is safely back on the performance track.

In this chapter, we discuss guidelines for determining when it is appropriate for the singer to resume performing, how to optimize the circumstances surrounding the return, strategies for maximizing success once performance is resumed, and addressing the singer's potential fears and concerns about resuming performing.

THE INJURY OF CONFIDENCE

Singing is the only music-making endeavor in which the human body is the instrument. As such, singing can be a very vulnerable act. It takes a great deal of courage and moxie to walk out on stage and perform with no external instrument between oneself and the audience. When things start to go wrong, this assurance can be undermined. The physiologic vocal injury must heal, but there is also an injury to the singer's confidence, which can persist beyond the physical recovery. Performance needs to be recommenced in a way that will promote resolution of the "injury of confidence."

WHEN TO RESUME PERFORMING

How will you know when it is time for the singer to start performing again? It has been my experience in working with thousands of singers with voice injuries that those reporting about 80% perceived recovery in combination with measurable improvement in the factors enumerated below do well when they return to performing. As you gain experience in working with singers who have vocal injuries, you will refine your ability to predict when the singer will be ready to resume performing with a fair amount of precision.

As has been noted previously, it will be helpful to have an audio and/or video recording of the singer that predates the injury (ideally from a time when he or she felt vocally fit) to serve as a baseline to determine whether the singer's typical function has been restored or approximated. In addition, there are a number of elements that can be assessed to determine whether the time is right, as outlined below.

Evidence of Physiologic Recovery

Videostroboscopic examination of the larynx should occur at appropriate intervals throughout the rehabilitation process. The interval between examinations will vary depending on a number of factors but it is certainly advisable to repeat stroboscopy prior to resuming performance. This will determine whether there has been improvement in vocal fold appearance and function, or whether there is any contraindication to performing.

Pitch Range Has Improved

Remember that, depending on the injury, deficit in range may have occurred at the top or bottom end of the singer's voice or in transitional pitch zones. Depending on the nature and severity of the injury, the singer may or may not experience a complete recovery of preinjury range. The goal will be to maximize range to a level that is adequate for typical performance. If range does not fully recover despite maximal outcome from behavioral, medical, and surgical interventions, the singer may need to consider adjusting voice part and/or making adaptations to repertoire, such as transposing songs to different keys or choosing new repertoire that falls within the singer's postrecovery range.

Vocal Stamina Has Been Optimized

The singer should be able to complete a vocal exercise regimen and period of singing repertoire that approximates what is needed for performance with minimal fatigue, and the voice should be strong enough to do the necessary preparation for the performance (practice, rehearsal). Ideally, an increase in duration of singing will have occurred gradually in an additive manner throughout the rehabilitation process. It is not essential for fatigue to be completely eliminated—what is more important is how quickly the fatigue resolves. If the singer has been off his or her typical singing schedule for a prolonged period, closely monitored overload may be a necessary to maximize stamina (see Chapter 11 for discussion of exercise physiology and overload relative to singing). I have observed both in my own singing and that of my patients that mild fatigue resolving by the next day indicates a sustainable load has been achieved. As noted above relative to recovery of pitch range, preinjury stamina may not completely recover, and adjustments in duration and intensity of performance may continue to be necessary on an ongoing basis.

Vocal Quality Has Improved

The qualitative vocal complaints (hoarseness, roughness, breathiness, strain, voice cracks and breaks, vocal instability, etc.) described by the singer at the initial evaluation should overall be resolved prior to returning to performance, based both on your trained perceptual evaluation and the singer's report. Some dysphonia may be a part of the singer's "vocal signature" and, as long as the singer is satisfied with vocal quality and voice has recovered adequately to meet performance demands, may reflect the singer's baseline.

WHERE TO RESUME PERFORMING

The primary concern regarding location for performance during or after rehabilitation is to ensure a venue that will not pose any obvious risk for exacerbation of injury or reinjury. This means that the size of the venue should be such that the singer will be able to project adequately without straining. For contemporary singers who don't have their own sound equipment, try to ensure that the venue's equipment will support rather than undermine the singer's vocal health (see Chapter 18). The singer should have a place to warm up at the venue or warm up adequately prior to arriving at the venue. If the venue will be particularly loud, the singer will need to plan a vocal pacing strategy to avoid speaking over noise, particularly if the performance will involve interactions with the audience. In the best of all possible worlds, the venue should be one that the performer is familiar with, to minimize surprises related to acoustics, setup, stage entrances and exits, dressing room or green room, and so on. Air quality and temperature may be factors, too. Environments that can trigger laryngeal sensitivity (outdoor venue, dusty or damp venue, etc.) should be avoided if possible for this first venture back into performing.

HOW TO RESUME PERFORMING

Optimize Vocal Pacing

The singer should schedule a performance when there will be plenty of time for vocal voice rest before and after. Scheduling a single performance as a "trial" rather than a tour or run of performances will provide an opportunity to assess and regroup after the performance and adjust the plan as needed. If the first performance goes well, the performance schedule can gradually be ramped up as tolerated.

Seek a Low-Pressure Performance

Scheduling a relatively low-stakes performance for the first time back in the game can help to take the pressure off. Ideally, the situation should allow for the performance to be canceled without adverse consequences if there is a last-minute setback or if the singer is not ready in time. If the singer has a more significant performance coming up, it will be best to try to find an opportunity for a "trial run" that will be less pressured.

Structure the Program for Success

The program should be designed to be a little shorter, a little less intense, and a little less complex than what you and the singer believe is feasible. Thus, songs should be in keys and ranges that are comfortable, the program should be of a duration that is below the singer's current tolerance, and challenging repertoire should be avoided. If there are other performers involved, consider having them share the load. If this performance goes well, you and the singer can consider gradually increasing length, intensity, and complexity for the next performances, as long as the singer is tolerating the increases.

Staging the Return to Performance

Some singers will experience considerable anxiety about returning to performing, particularly if they have had negative or upsetting experiences during a performance as a result of the voice injury. If this is the case, encourage the singer to resume performing in stages. Here's an example:

"Dora" has been a classical church soloist for years. She developed vocal fold lesions, and underwent voice therapy. She made excellent progress and her voice returned to baseline. While still undergoing voice therapy, she was invited to be the soprano soloist for a Christmas cantata, which was several months away. Although she missed performing terribly and wanted to accept the engagement, she was very anxious at the prospect of singing in front of the congregation. We planned the following steps to ease her back into performing:

1. She sang the solos for me during her therapy sessions and we targeted areas for technical practice.
2. She sang the solos with the church organist, who was an old and trusted friend.
3. She sang the solos in the empty sanctuary with the organist playing and with only her husband listening.
4. She sang the solos in the empty sanctuary for a small group of trusted friends.
5. She sang the solos in the empty church for the choir director.
6. She sang the solos during a choir rehearsal.

In this manner, her confidence was gradually restored and she was successfully able to perform the solos in the Christmas cantata, to her great delight.

SETBACKS

Sometimes the singer will return to a normal performance schedule only to have a setback down the road. In this case, repeat stroboscopy may be indicated and depending on results, rehabilitation may need to be briefly restarted. Reassure the singer that this is not an unusual occurrence. Go over the circumstances surrounding the setback to see if you and the singer can identify any contributing factors. These may include changes in vocal hygiene, pacing, type and intensity of singing, or medical factors such as allergies or reflux. Address the contributing factors as needed. It may be necessary to adjust the performance load again and gradually rework the process.

CHAPTER 16

Vocal Pacing Case Studies

This chapter contains a number of case studies illustrating the principles discussed in the preceding chapters and in the vocal pacing educational handouts in Appendices 14A–P. The singers in these cases span a range of age, injury, professional level, singing style, vocal demands, and singing situations. Although all relevant factors were addressed in each case (including vocal coordination and conditioning, emotional factors, medical factors, and vocal hygiene), the emphasis in these examples is on the vocal pacing portion of the rehabilitation plan.

CASE STUDY 1: PERFORMER AND TEACHER OF INDIAN CLASSICAL SINGING WITH FIBROTIC VOCAL FOLD LESIONS

"Bina" was a 55-year-old performer and teacher of Indian classical music whom I evaluated in our clinic. Her vocal diagnosis was bilateral fibrotic vocal fold lesions. Surgical and behavioral options were reviewed, and she opted for voice therapy to begin with. Therapy goals encompassed improving vocal hygiene, medical treatment of allergic rhinitis, improving vocal technique for speaking and singing, and optimizing vocal pacing.

Bina was trained in Indian classical singing, but her training focused much more on musical elements than on vocal technique. She typically warmed up by singing a number of traditional musical scales. She sang these scales using the associated syllables, some of which were not helping her to optimize resonant voice. Using vocal exercises that are based on typical Western scales would have been inappropriate for this singer. Therapeutic singing voice exercises were designed based on the traditional Indian scales but incorporating semi-occluded vocal tract sounds and vowels that facilitated improved resonance, as well as targeting improved breath support.

The biggest contributing factor to her voice injury was presumably her incredibly demanding vocal load. At the time of her evaluation, she taught Indian classical singing to at least 50 students at any given time. She gave them all weekly private lessons 30 to 60 minutes in length. Most of the students were children, but she also taught adults. In addition, she performed four to six times per month, and the performances were usually about 2 hours in length. Bina was a very extroverted and expressive person with a busy social and family life that typically involved a lot of speaking. Her family was fairly vociferous in conversation, with people speaking loudly and sometimes on top of each other. Her parents and some of her extended family lived in India, and she had regular long phone conversations with them.

Bina reported that by the end of the day, her voice usually "gave out" and she often experienced painful phonation. In the past, her voice usually recovered when she had a break from teaching and performing, but at the time of her evaluation, her voice had become hoarse and fatigued, she had lost much of her high range, and she was having difficulty getting through performances.

We began working on vocal pacing by examining her weekly schedule, discovering several areas in which she could potentially reduce voice use. She identified performing and teaching as the highest priorities, but her family and social interactions were very important to her, too. Clearly, her teaching load was the most overwhelming element in terms of sheer quantity of voice use. We came up with the following targets for exploration:

1. Reduce teaching load.
2. Incorporate voice "mini-breaks" during teaching day and at home.
3. Strategically reduce social voice use.
4. Decrease duration and frequency of family phone calls. Consider supplementing with written communication (e-mail).

In examining her teaching load, we first discussed reducing the number of students. She felt she couldn't do this, as she was at the time one of the only people in the community teaching this kind of singing and many families sought her out to train their children. We reviewed the "put the mask on yourself first" principle, and she realized that if she continued with her current load, her voice might not recover, leaving her students without a teacher. She was already finding it very difficult to get through a teaching day and her voice had steadily gotten worse over time.

In probing the lesson structure, it became clear that for her younger students, the content of the lessons was fairly consistent and repetitive, teaching basic principles of the musical tradition. We explored the possibility of grouping these younger students into blocks. We identified at least 30 students who would be appropriate for group lessons. Her studio could accommodate four to six students per group. We established a hierarchical structure with beginning, intermediate, and advanced groups. By teaching in groups, Bina would reduce her teaching time by about 9 hours per week.

Bina felt the students' parents would be resistant to this idea, wanting their children to have Bina's full attention for the duration of the lesson and she did in fact encounter some opposition to the plan when she first began speaking with the parents. It was clear that this was a situation in which Bina would have to practice self-advocacy. Bina crafted a letter to all the parents of her younger students, explaining her voice injury and the need for reducing her vocal load. She indicated in the letter that if she did not reduce her teaching load, she might have to cut back on the number of students she could teach. Faced with the choice between group lessons or no lessons, the parents quickly rallied to the idea and were ultimately very supportive.

Of the remaining students, at least 10 were adults who were experienced and did not necessarily have to have lessons every week. Bina put these students on a bimonthly schedule. In the end, her teaching load went from about 35 hours per week to a much more sustainable load of 15 or 20 hours. She also arranged the schedule so that she would have a 15-minute break after every 2 hours of teaching.

We then turned to the family and social voice use. Bina was afraid that resting her voice at home would interfere with her family interactions. However, she felt she could incorporate a period of voice rest in the evening after teaching and before the family meal. It took her family a little while to adjust to this, but ultimately they were very supportive, and it became part of the routine for Bina to have 15 to 30 minutes of quiet time after her teaching day. Bina tried to explain the need for reducing length and frequency of phone calls to her family in India. Some family members were willing to use e-mail for communication on occasion, but Bina's mother felt hurt and upset by Bina's request for shorter conversations, and she didn't like to use e-mail. With all the other vocal pacing strategies Bina had incorporated, she was able to leave her typical phone call schedule with her mother intact, in the interest of family harmony. She did, however, call on her husband and children to talk briefly with her mother during the conversation so that Bina could take mini-breaks.

At the beginning of therapy, Bina was having so much difficulty getting through performances that we decided she would take a hiatus from performing in the short term. After about 2 months of her new routine of vocal hygiene, vocal exercise, and vocal pacing, she was able to gradually resume performing, and by the end of her course of therapy, she had returned to her typical performance schedule. She arranged her teaching schedule so that she never taught on the day of a performance and usually had a light schedule the day before.

Bina had a few setbacks, including once when she had back-to-back performances at an Indian cultural festival and once after a trip to India to see her mother, with associated increase in voice demands visiting family and friends. However, she was quickly able to get her routine back on track. At her follow-up evaluation, the vocal fold lesions had not completely resolved (as is typical for fibrotic lesions) but they were softer and smaller, and vibration was improved. At that point, she was satisfied with the outcome of her voice therapy and since her voice was fully adequate to meet her vocal demands, she opted not to undergo surgery.

CASE STUDY 2: PLANNING PRACTICE TIME FOR A COLLEGE OPERA SINGER WITH VOCAL NODULES

"Nicolas" was getting ready to start his final semester as an undergraduate voice major with plans for a career as a professional operatic singer when he was seen in our clinic. He had just finished the fall semester during which he came down with an upper respiratory infection at a time when he was facing a number of performances, including a leading role in a university opera production. He saw an otolaryngologist near where he was going to school and was treated with antibiotics and oral steroids. He was able to get through the performance, but his voice did not fully recover. By the time we saw him in December, he had noticed a loss of high range, decreased vocal stamina, and occasional voice breaks occurring on a regular basis. He was very concerned about his voice, especially as he had been cast in the role of Figaro in *Le Nozze di Figaro*, with rehearsals beginning in January.

Videostroboscopy revealed sessile excrescences at the mid-membranous folds bilaterally, consistent with early nodules. He had never experienced any voice problems prior to this incident, and the nodules were likely relatively new, resulting from the combination of the upper respiratory infection and coincident heavy vocal demands. No contributing medical factors requiring treatment were identified.

Nicolas had excellent vocal habits. His hydration was good. He consumed caffeine and alcohol in moderation. He didn't engage in an excessive amount of social voice use, knew to avoid phonotraumatic behaviors such as hard throat clearing and yelling, rarely indulged in recreational singing, and deliberately minimized using his voice in noisy environments. Almost all of his singing activities were in classical style, although he sang in a student a cappella group that performed mostly contemporary music. He had not had any training in CCM singing.

With the exception of occasional vocal fry, speaking voice technique was quite good. Although the symptoms he had described were apparent during the assessment of his singing voice, his classical technique was quite strong. He had brought a recording of his junior recital, which demonstrated vocal technique and ability at a very high level for an undergraduate singer. It was clear that he was getting excellent instruction. Assessment of contemporary technique was postponed in the interest of focusing on the more urgent concerns of getting through the acute stage of his recovery and the upcoming opera performance.

The main problem that had to be addressed was his vocal load. In addition to the upcoming major operatic role and participation in the cappella group, he was enrolled in two choirs at school. He also had a senior recital to prepare, which had to be completed in the spring. Because his vocal stamina was compromised, he was struggling to prepare the role of Figaro before rehearsals started. He was feeling overwhelmed at the prospect of having so much repertoire to learn and prepare at a time when his vocal stamina was at such an ebb.

Fortunately, Nicolas was highly motivated to do whatever it would take to recover from his injury, and—equally important—the faculty in his department were very supportive as well. Although he had initially expressed his desire to continue with the a cappella group if at all possible, he did not hesitate in his decision to drop it once he understood the importance of reducing his vocal demands. Although he had planned to continue singing in two university ensembles during his final semester for his own enjoyment and to help fill a need for strong male voices, he had already fulfilled his ensemble requirement. Since the semester hadn't yet started, he could easily drop the chorus classes without academic repercussions and did so promptly with the support of the director.

This left the opera and the recital. Although rehearsals for the opera began in January, it wouldn't actually open until March. Since he had not been able to practice much, Nicolas needed to be able to devote all of his practice time to working on the role and would not have much time to prepare repertoire for a full recital in April. He was concerned that if he wasn't able to start practicing his recital repertoire until late March, he would not be able to prepare to the level he expected of himself. Nicolas had sung more operatic roles than is typical of an undergraduate student—Figaro would make his third leading role. I asked his voice teacher whether the department would consider waiving his senior recital and allow his operatic roles to fulfill the performance requirement. This is not an unusual practice in academic music programs. Although this particular department had not previously done so for an undergraduate student, the faculty decided to allow it in Nicolas's case. If his voice recovered to a level that would allow increasing his practice time, he would go ahead with the recital, but having the waiver took the academic pressure off and enabled him to focus on recovery for the near future.

Nicolas was daunted by the sheer amount of work he faced in preparing the lengthy role of Figaro. He described his typical approach to learning new repertoire. He usually started singing the piece right away, repeating it until it felt musically secure. Once the piece was learned, he would run through it from beginning to end several times during practice. He was also in the habit of accomplishing memorization through repeated singing. Clearly, given his injury, the sheer amount of repertoire he had to prepare, and the rehearsal schedule, his usual approach would not work.

We developed a strategy together. Nicolas made a list of all Figaro's numbers in the opera, including recitative, arias, and ensembles. We discussed different ways of learning and practicing music. He would use mental practice for learning the music and for memorization (playing the part on the piano, listening to recordings, or simply thinking the music in his head). Another approach would be to focus on singing only the portions of the piece that needed the most technical work ("spot practice"). Another category of practice would be to sing through the piece from beginning to end, recording himself during the run-through. He would then listen to the recording to identify which portions he should target for spot practice.

Together we created a chart, listing all the numbers he had to learn for the role in rows and all the different types of practice in columns (Table 16–1). The goal was to allocate some form of practice to the entire role at least once per week, making sure there was a good balance of singing and nonsinging practice each day and ensuring that each piece got at least some vocal practice each week to promote muscle memory. Nicolas later added a column for "rehearse blocking while listening to recording." He used the rehearsal schedule to guide which pieces would get priority attention and this helped him feel more prepared and secure going into rehearsals throughout the week. Since he had dropped the choirs and a cappella group, he had more time in his daily schedule to allocate to practice. He spent 2 to 4 hours per day "practicing" but only 30 to 60 minutes of actual singing, depending on his singing schedule for the rest of the day.

The school Nicolas attended was over 200 miles from our clinic, making regular voice therapy sessions a challenge. I corresponded with his teacher to provide recommendations for exercises that would help with recovery, which she implemented immediately. She began teaching him two 30-minute lessons per week instead of the usual 60-minute single lesson. She was aware of the practice plan and provided Nicolas with additional guidance on what to target technically.

I saw Nicolas a few weeks into the semester. He reported that he felt his voice was getting stronger, that his practice time was fruitful, and that he was feeling more prepared, although the approach felt radically different from his preinjury routine.

Table 16–1. ***Example of Completed Vocal Planning Chart for Nicolas. Text style indicates intensity of vocalization.***

Bold = Singing *Italic* = Mental practice (nonvocal practice) Regular text = low-intensity voice use.

	Learn (Mental Practice)	**Sing Number Without Text (Lip Trill)**	**Run Through and Record**	*Listen to Recording Make Notes for Spot Practice*	**"Spot" Practice**	Practice Speaking Text	*Memorize (Mental Practice)*
ACT I							
Duet: Cinque, dieci	*Mon, Tues*	**Tues**	**Weds**	*Weds*	**Thur, Fri**	Tues, Weds	*Thur, Fri, Sat*
Recit	*Mon*	**Tues**	**Weds**	*Weds*	**Weds, Fri**	Tues, Weds	*Thur, Fri, Sat*
Duet: Se a caso	*Mon, Tues*	**Tues**	**Weds**	*Weds*	**Thur**	Tues	*Thur, Fri, Sat*
Recit	*Mon*	**Tues**	**Weds**	*Weds*	**Weds, Fri**		*Thur, Fri, Sat*
Aria: Se vuol ballare		**Mon**	**Weds, Fri**	*Thurs, Fri*	**Fri**	Mon, Tues	*Thur, Fri, Sat*
Recit		**Mon**	**Tues**	*Tues*	**Tues, Thur**	Mon	*Thur, Fri, Sat*
Recit		**Mon**	**Tues**	*Tues*	**Tues, Thur**	Mon	*Thur, Fri, Sat*
Non più andrai			**Mon, Sat**	*Mon, Sat*	**Tues**		n/a
ACT II							
Recit	*Tues*		**Fri**		**Sat**		
Finale	*Mon, Tues*	**Weds, Thur**	**Fri**	*Sat*	**Sat**	Mon, Tues, Weds	

	Learn (Mental Practice)	**Sing Number Without Text (Lip Trill)**	**Run Through and Record**	*Listen to Recording Make Notes for Spot Practice*	**"Spot" Practice**	Practice Speaking Text	*Memorize (Mental Practice)*
ACT III							
Recit	*Tues, Weds*		**Thur**	*Thur*		Thur, Fri, Sat	
Recit	*Tues, Weds*		**Thur**	*Thur*		Thur, Fri, Sat	
Sextet	*Tues, Weds*	**Weds**	**Thur**	*Thur*	**Sat**	Thur, Fri	
Recit	*Thur*		**Fri**	*Sat*			
Finale	*Thur*		**Fri**	*Sat*			
ACT IV							
Recit	*Fri*						
Recit	*Fri*						
Recit: Tutto è disposto		**Mon**	**Tues**				
Aria: Aprite un po'		**Mon**	**Tues**	*Tues*	**Sat**	Mon	
Recit	*Fri*		**Sat**	*Sat*		Sat	
Recit	*Fri*		**Sat**	*Sat*		Sat	
Finale	*Mon, Wed*	**Tues**				Tues	

Note. *Nicolas's practice planning chart for the role of* Figaro *for 1 week, including some singing and some "mental" practice every day. Over the course of the week, he did at least some work on every number in the opera.* Non più andrai *was already in his repertoire, so he didn't have to spend as much time preparing it. This stage of preparation took place before rehearsals began. It is clear that in this first week, his strategy was to learn and memorize Act I as much as possible in preparation for staging rehearsals. Nicolas updated the practice plan each week as he made his way through the role, later adding a "rehearse with blocking column" as an additional "mental practice" category.*

We worked briefly on optimizing speaking voice technique, which he quickly assimilated. We discussed the possibility of addressing contemporary singing styles after concluding the semester, but in the end, he decided that it was unlikely that he would have much occasion to engage in that type of singing as he went on to graduate school and his professional career.

At his 3-month follow-up examination, bilateral mid-fold swelling was still evident on stroboscopy but had decreased considerably. The opera was over and he felt it had gone very well, although he felt his stamina had still not fully recovered. He opted not to do a senior recital but did complete auditions for graduate school and was accepted into the program of his choice. We were able to complete a few more sessions of voice therapy with excellent results. Nicolas said that he intended to use his new practice planning protocol on a permanent basis.

CASE STUDY 3: PROFESSIONAL ROCK BAND COLLABORATING ON VOCAL PACING AND VOCAL HEALTH

"Southern Cross" is a folk rock band with four lead singers and two additional instrumentalists. All of the singers play instruments at various times, some more than others. The band was just beginning its career ascent with a major label recording contract and extensive national tour when I met them. They frequently toured for 2 to 3 months at a time, with concerts up to five times per week—sometimes multiple performances on the same day. It wasn't unusual for performances to span several states in the course of a week. The band traveled by van, resulting in long drive time and erratic sleep schedules. They usually stayed at a different hotel every night.

Not surprisingly given this demanding schedule, each of the four singers experienced a voice injury at one point or another and all underwent voice rehabilitation at our clinic. However, this is an exceptionally smart, disciplined, and dedicated group of young musicians, and they ultimately achieved exemplary vocal health habits, including meticulous attention to vocal pacing. As is critical for all singers, the rehabilitation plan targeted vocal pacing for both speaking and singing voice.

I realized just how committed they were to vocal health when I received a phone call from their manager asking me what he could do to support the singers in keeping their voices healthy. I have often spoken to managers, agents, directors, and presenters to advocate for singers in various situations, but this was the first time the manager had initiated the conversation. The singers had each included their manager in the release of medical information, so I was able to speak with him in depth about their specific challenges and goals. From that point forward, the entire production team—singers, instrumental musicians, manager, tour manager, and sound engineer—all participated actively in creating the most vocally supportive environment possible.

Over time, the group implemented a number of strategies into their regular routine. The manager and the band became more strategic about planning the tour schedule. They avoided scheduling more than one performance in a single day and tried to routinely schedule a day off for every 2 to 3 days of performing whenever possible. As they became more and more successful, they were able to optimize their sound equipment with better microphones and monitors and hired their own sound engineer.

None of these singers had received much formal voice training, and therefore the rehabilitation process included quite a bit of singing habilitation. Each singer in the band had a customized warm-up routine, which was executed religiously before performances, rehearsals, and recording sessions. They each had a recording of their warm-up routine, which they sang as they listened to the recording through noise-canceling headphones. This allowed them to complete their warm-up even when they had limited space. Sometimes they all simultaneously sang through their warm-up routines in a tiny backstage space, producing a sort of musical collage that became well-known to the sound engineer and other musicians.

The singers all adopted excellent vocal hygiene habits, optimizing hydration and completely eliminating use of alcohol surrounding performances. Fortunately, the singers were all nonsmokers to start with. Those who needed medication for allergies or reflux were religious about taking them.

All four singers alternated singing lead and backup. This was already part of their songwriting habits and allowed them to share the vocal load over the course of the concert. As their vocal pacing strategy matured, they began to develop "B plan" programs, changing set-lists at the last minute to lighten the load in the event that a singer became sick or vocally fatigued. They also developed tactical plans for the recording studio to avoid over-singing and to ensure adequate voice breaks for all the singers.

One of the most effective ways they optimized their vocal pacing was by being very mindful of their speaking voice use. Each of the singers received training in optimizing speaking voice technique as part of their rehabilitation, targeting breath support, oral resonance, and minimizing laryngeal strain.

When I first met the singers, they were in the habit of doing a lot of talking during their travel time in the van. This had become their time to debrief after the performance, plan, strategize, dream, and sometimes argue. Often they engaged in extended phone conversations during the drive as well as intermittent recreational singing. As we examined their typical voice use, it became clear that the drive time afforded a significant opportunity for voice rest. In time, it became their regular practice for the drive to be almost silent. Each band member would work on his or her own projects or correspondence via computer or listen to music through headphones.

Time in the hotel room was also dedicated to voice rest. They became more deliberate about phone time, using nonvocal means of communication to stay in touch with friends and family whenever possible.

Speaking voice use surrounding performances was identified as a target for better vocal pacing. Historically, there had been quite a bit of talking during the load-in and sound-check before the performance. The band members would often engage with audience members and fans during set-breaks and before and after the performance. They usually all worked the merchandise table after the show as well. In the interest of vocal pacing, they minimized talking during the load-in, became more protective of their break time (going off to a quiet place away from the audience if possible), and took turns spelling each other at the merchandise table. The instrumental musicians also took on more of the speaking load relative to the merchandise table and in audience interactions.

Off stage, they were conscientious in minimizing time spent in noisy environments. This could be challenging as they were often required to make appearances at publicity events, on television and radio, and were involved in frequent media interactions. In these situations, they tried to be as tactical as possible in minimizing the duration of time spent in such environments and sharing the load for interviews. In their social lives, they tried to avoid speaking in noisy environments or for prolonged periods.

All of these changes and habits made them feel their offstage lives were definitely more monastic than they had been earlier in their careers but at the same time were absolutely certain the steps they had taken were critical to their vocal health. Despite their exemplary vocal health habits, they have each had vocal ups and downs due the incredible demands of their musical careers. What has helped them to avoid getting sidelined or having to cancel performances is their calculated attention to vocal health and regular follow-up with their vocal health care team.

CASE STUDY 4: PROFESSIONAL MUSICAL THEATER SINGER WITH A HEMORRHAGIC VOCAL FOLD POLYP

"Danielle" was a 31-year-old actor and singer in the cast of a Broadway touring company. She had a leading role that was very vocally demanding. She was seen in our clinic when the company was performing at a local venue. The company was booked in the area for 3 weeks, but we didn't see Danielle until halfway through the local engagement. She had been experiencing hoarseness, vocal fatigue, loss of high range, and painful phonation for a number of weeks. Then, one night, her voice "locked up" during a performance. She "pushed" through the performance, and her voice was even worse afterward. Her medical history was notable for GERD and allergic rhinitis, both of which were not consistently treated at the time of her evaluation. Her vocal hygiene habits were overall excellent.

At the time of her evaluation, Danielle had been in the company for 10 months, traveling across the country, usually staying in one location for 3 to 4 weeks before moving on to the next engagement. The typical performance schedule was eight shows per week. As a principal singer, she did not have many rehearsals or coachings to attend, typically less than once per month.

Danielle described herself as a "boisterous" talker and spent an hour or more per day speaking on the phone. Her family lived in her native country, and she was in the habit of speaking with them on a daily basis. She reported that she usually engaged in quite a bit of "recreational singing," which included singing along with the radio, singing songs in her dressing room, and with other members of the cast. The cast had a tradition of enacting a prolonged vocal spirit activity before every performance to get "pumped up" for the show. This involved a lot of shouting and loud chanting.

Danielle was diagnosed with a right vocal fold hemorrhagic polyp. Our laryngologist determined that the optimal treatment would be steroids and voice rest for 1 week, to be followed by repeat stroboscopy and consideration of surgical intervention, and 8 to 12 weeks of postoperative voice therapy. However, Danielle was caught in a bit of a Catch-22. In order to have the surgery and recommended time for rehabilitation, she would have to take a leave from the company. As she was not a United States citizen, her leave would result in losing her work visa, so she would not be able to have the surgery in the United States. If she left to have her surgery in her native country, she would lose her engagement with the company and her insurance coverage.

After much discussion with our team, the music directing team, and company management, Danielle decided to defer the surgery until the end of her contract 4 months later. In the meantime, it was imperative to develop a vocal health plan that would allow her to meet the performance expectations of the company without putting her at risk for further injury. She was especially concerned as the company executives would be visiting the show in the coming week, in part to assess singers for consideration for future contracts.

Treatment started with addressing the medical factors contributing to her dysphonia. She was given a steroid injection and steroid dose-pack. Due to the vascular nature of her polyp, avoidance of blood-thinning medications (such as nonsteroidal anti-inflammatories, or NSAIDs) was recommended. Nexium was prescribed for GERD and a nasal steroid and sinus irrigation for her allergic rhinitis. The immediate treatment plan included 5 days of complete voice rest, followed by repeat stroboscopy and intensive voice therapy for as many sessions as her schedule would allow while she was staying locally, which ended up being three. Vocal pacing was immediately established as a goal of voice therapy.

The vocal pacing strategies implemented as part of her voice therapy included having her understudy go on for one show on the days when two shows were scheduled. This reduced Danielle's performance schedule to six shows per week. Eliminating recreational singing entirely was an obvious way to buy back more time for her vocal clock. During the preperformance cheering session, Danielle participated in the physical parts of the routine but was vocally silent. She also minimized backstage talking and phone calls and did not attend cast parties or fundraisers.

Her family communications represented an important lifeline for her, providing emotional support and a sense of connection, which is so critical in the difficult life of a touring artist. Cutting off family phone calls altogether would have presented an emotional hardship. Instead, Danielle used Skype for family calls, typing her side of the conversation while everyone else spoke theirs. Although cumbersome, this practice allowed her to maintain her family connections at a time when she needed their support while meeting her vocal pacing goals.

Danielle did not have much vocal training. She had been recruited for this production for the authenticity and naturalness of her singing. She did, however, have a regular vocal warm-up regimen, which we reviewed together. During the exercises, she demonstrated a combined abdominal/clavicular breathing pattern and TA-dominant registration to C5. She did not know how to mix. In the short time we had together, a crash course in abdominal breathing for belting was initiated, as well as introduction of "twang" resonance to facilitate mixing.

Danielle's typical routine included constructive exercises such as lip trill glides, but many of the exercises were not appropriate for her and were not well executed technically. Some of the less effective exercises included sustained vocal fry with exaggerated articulatory movements; elaborate, extended scalar passages (spanning a 9th and 11th); and five-note scales singing on the syllables "do re mi fa sol fa mi re do." Although there are potential benefits to any of these exercises, the manner in which she executed them at the time undermined any such benefit. As our time together was very limited, we decided to focus on revising her routine in a way that would ensure quick and accurate implementation of improved coordination of the phonation subsystems.

In exploring an existing vocal exercise regimen with a singer, it can be very helpful to focus on revising the existing routine rather than completely starting from scratch. This supports efficiency in the therapy process but also decreases the likelihood that the singer will be left feeling that their exercise routine is "all wrong." In Danielle's case, the lip trill glides were maintained in her new routine and many of the exercise patterns were retained, although with altered phonemic content. Adductory power over a diatonic octave phonating through a small straw was added to ensure ease of phonation and to help her injured vocal folds to vibrate with the support of the vocal tract, promoting healing of her injury. She mentioned that she liked the exaggerated articulatory motion in her vocal fry exercise. As her vocal fry production was fairly pressed, we decided to eliminate it in favor of a five-tone scale exercise on /m/ with chewing motion, a more effective exercise for her that still featured the articulatory movement she found beneficial. The extended and elaborate 9- and 11-tone scales were extremely challenging technically and as her execution was not proficient, the exercises were not doing her much good. Instead, a simple descending five-note scale and 1-3-5-3-1 arpeggio were added on /jae/, emphasizing "twang" resonance to facilitate achieving mixed register in higher range. A cool-down routine was added including descending glides on lip trills, laryngeal massage, and structured speaking voice exercises. Fortunately, there was time to demonstrate how to apply the new techniques to her numbers from the show.

At the end of our three sessions, she was able to execute her new warm-up routine with very good accuracy. One of the music directors had attended the sessions with her and was able to reinforce what was covered in the sessions as they continued on the tour. Danielle had established a high level of professional success without much training because she was an extremely skillful, intuitive singer. She was also savvy, abundantly motivated, a quick study, and diligent in adhering to vocal health recommendations. She later stated that she felt reducing the amount of nonperformance singing and talking was the most helpful strategy in being able to continue the tour. With the additional support of the company in modifying her vocal load, she made it through the rest of the tour without incident and subsequently returned to her home country for surgery and rehabilitation. She was later rehired by the company for a European tour.

CASE STUDY 5: PROFESSIONAL JEWISH CANTOR WITH EVOLVING INJURY

"Andrea" was a Jewish cantor. We first saw her in our clinic when she was 25 years old. At that time, she was preparing to leave town to sing at a funeral and was very concerned about being able to get through the performance. She reported that she had been experiencing increasing vocal fatigue, effortful phonation, loss of high range, and sometimes voice cracks and breaks that had gradually worsened over a period of several years. She noted that it sometimes hurt to speak or sing, and the pain had recently become more frequent and more consistently associated with voice use. She had taken steroids for similar problems in the past. She had found the treatment helpful and was hoping it would again be effective for her upcoming engagement.

Andrea had a bachelor's degree in voice and had continued voice lessons after graduation. Her training was entirely in classical singing. As cantor, she sang in classical style in some services and contemporary/folk style in others. She noted a "disconnect" between the two—she didn't feel technically proficient when singing in contemporary styles. She often played guitar while singing (performances and teaching) and used amplification almost all the time when performing. She typically completed a vocal warm-up, which consisted primarily of singing scales and arpeggios on vowels and syllables, but she had become less consistent in completing warm-ups due to painful phonation. In addition to her performing activities, she also taught music at the temple school.

She consumed at least two liters of water per day and about five servings of caffeinated beverages (coffee and soda). Her medical history was unremarkable, and there was no evidence of reflux or rhinitis on her examination.

Videostroboscopy revealed relatively mild vocal fold edema, with considerable ventricular and supraglottic hyperfunction, particularly when singing and especially with high pitch.

Her vocal problems appeared to be more chronic in nature than acute, and there was concern on the part of our medical team about repeated use of steroids to get through performances. However, our laryngologist gave her a prescription for a steroid dose pack, indicating that he only wanted her to use it if she absolutely needed it. He counseled her regarding risks of frequent steroid treatment and the importance of addressing the underlying muscle tension and vocal habits. We recommended that she come back for voice therapy after her performance.

We did not see Andrea again for almost 5 years. When she came back, quite a bit had changed in her life. She had gotten married and now had a 3-year-old daughter. Her daughter was in day care and had frequent upper respiratory infections. Due to this exposure, Andrea was getting colds several times a year. Sometimes she had to perform and teach while she was sick. During the years since we had seen her, she had continued to experience intermittent hoarseness, vocal fatigue, voice cracks and breaks, and painful phonation. Her symptoms had steadily gotten worse.

Her vocal hygiene habits had changed somewhat. Water consumption was down to one liter per day, and caffeine consumption had ballooned to two liters per day, which she attributed to the changes in her sleeping habits now that she was a mother, and also to the increase in her workload. She was tired all the time and felt she needed caffeine boosts throughout the day.

She was still cantor, and her duties at the temple had gradually increased in the intervening years, particularly related to teaching music at the temple school. Her vocal load was heavy and diverse, with approximately 20 hours per week of singing related to her job. She sang in two services per week as well as for special occasions such as weddings and funerals. She sometimes prepared small choirs for special services. During the week, she taught music in the temple preschool 2 to 3 days per week and Bar and Bat Mitzvah classes two to three times per week. She gave educational presentations at her temple and as a guest speaker in a variety of settings. Her temple was very involved in community action, which included participation in outdoor rallies three to four times per month. Andrea's responsibility at these rallies (which usually lasted for several hours) was primarily leading singing, sometimes without amplification. Although this was a community activity, she felt her participation was an expectation of her job as cantor of the temple. In addition, she intermittently performed in musical theater productions and had vocal demands related to raising her 3-year-old daughter. At the time she started therapy, she was beginning preparations for the High Holy Days, which would involve prolonged singing during extended services. She was very concerned about whether her voice would hold up.

On stroboscopy, the mild vocal fold edema previously noted had developed into small, focal lesions at the midpoint of the vocal folds bilaterally. She also had prominent vascularity that was not previously noted and a small sulcus on the left. Mucosal wave and amplitude were moderately decreased, and small anterior and posterior gaps were noted even at modal pitch. Anterior to posterior compression was noted, and there was still considerable supraglottic pharyngeal compression as well.

Voice therapy goals included bringing water and caffeine consumption into better balance (which she accomplished over a period of several weeks, in part by using a Fitbit monitor to keep track of water consumption), education regarding contemporary singing technique, and designing a vocal exercise regimen that would support resolution of pathology and that was appropriate for the type of singing she typically engaged in. Her exercise regimen would also include massage and stretching exercises to address her chronic laryngeal pain, as well as speaking voice exercises. Optimizing vocal pacing was a big part of the overall rehabilitation plan.

We worked together to develop strategies for bringing her voice use into better balance. The amount of music in Friday services had recently increased. She began to take steps to offload other voice use to accommodate this increase by delegating some teaching tasks to others, decreasing the number and duration of rehearsals, and modifying speaking voice use surrounding services. She decreased the amount of demonstration she was doing in rehearsals and when teaching. She sometimes recorded herself and used recordings to augment demonstration when teaching and directing.

She purchased a personal voice amplifier and began using it consistently for all teaching and also for singing in situations where amplification was not otherwise provided. She practiced better self-advocacy, negotiating a proportional decrease in other responsibilities when asked to take on additional vocal demands. She received supportive responses from the rabbi and school staff. She continued to participate in community rallies but limited her participation to playing guitar without singing, and when she felt the need to convey enthusiasm, she did so through body movement instead of vocalization. When she had to speak at rallies, she used her amplifier.

The High Holy Days were approaching, providing an opportunity to implement advance planning for vocal pacing. Rehearsals would span approximately 4 weeks, during which her vocal load would increase dramatically. She created a calendar that included all rehearsals and services, as well as other vocally demanding activities, color-coding it to indicate priority. If she began to get tired, she would eliminate or reduce some of the lower priority activities. She reduced her tutoring schedule as much as possible and developed nonvocal activities (listening to recordings and adding movement activities) to supplement her preschool teaching. She had been working on a recording project but decided to defer it until after the holidays. She adjusted her social calendar well in advance to allow for adequate voice rest. She made a video recording of herself reading some of her daughter's favorite books. When her singing load became heaviest, she used these recordings during their typical bedtime routine to provide a break from reading aloud.

All the while, Andrea had been practicing her vocal exercises for speaking and singing, and was becoming much more proficient in CCM vocal technique. Gradually, the painful phonation was eliminated, and she found her vocal quality and stamina improving.

In the end, Andrea got through the demanding period of the High Holy Days without vocal incident and stated that her voice felt stronger than ever. On reevaluation, the tiny lesions had resolved, although there was some remaining vascularity and sulcus. She felt her voice was the healthiest it had ever been, and she made her new vocal habits an ongoing practice.

CASE STUDY 6: PRAISE AND WORSHIP LEADER WITH SURGICAL VOCAL FOLD POLYP AND POSTOPERATIVE VOICE REHABILITATION

"Don" was a 48-year-old gospel singer and praise and worship leader at a large church with a congregation of over 5,000. His responsibilities at the church included leading the musical worship for three to four services per week, often preaching as well. The church had a very high-tech worship space with excellent sound production capabilities, multiple sound technicians, and a lighting director. Services often included additional theatrical elements such as stage smoke. Each week, Don was responsible for leading the musical elements of multiple services—each of which was comparable to a 1-hour theatrical or concert production.

There were both a large choir and small vocal ensemble, and a praise band that ranged from 5 to 10 musicians. Don's preparation for services each week encompassed 6 to 8 hours of rehearsal, in addition to his individual practice time preparing his solos. His pastoral responsibilities included counseling, leading meetings, youth activities, and teaching, in addition to preaching about one service per month. He often had professional singing, preaching, and speaking engagements in addition to his church job. He described his preaching style as passionate, emotional, and assertive, with a fair amount of shouting. As we were discussing his vocal load, Don expressed his feeling that cutting back on vocal demands and activities would make him feel he wasn't fully engaged spiritually. He felt he needed to function at full-tilt to demonstrate his commitment and to be receptive to the Holy Spirit.

Don minored in music in college and had over 4 years of vocal training. However, most of his instruction was in classical singing technique. He had never had any training in contemporary singing. He did not consistently complete vocal warm-ups.

When Don came to see us, he had been experiencing hoarseness, vocal fatigue, loss of high range, and effortful phonation for about 6 weeks. He noted that his vocal demands had been very heavy for 4 or 5 months preceding the onset of his symptoms. He didn't hesitate to seek a voice evaluation, as he had a history of voice injury and vocal fold surgery 14 years earlier. He wasn't sure exactly what this previous injury had been or which side had been operated on, but thought the surgery was for "scarring" of the vocal fold. His previous surgery was followed by 8 weeks of voice therapy. He said his voice fully recovered and, until recently, he hadn't had any recurrence of vocal problems. Don's hydration was good, and he had cut out caffeine entirely when he started having voice problems again. He took oral antihistamines for chronic allergies.

Stroboscopy revealed evidence of GERD and allergic rhinitis, vocal fold erythema, and prominent vasculature bilaterally. On the right vocal fold, there was a varix feeding into a large, pedunculated polyp that was very firm. There was a sulcus posterior to the lesion. On the left, there was also a sulcus as well as an area of reactive swelling contralateral to the right lesion. Closure and vibration were significantly impaired.

The laryngologist recommended microflap surgery to excise the right vocal fold lesion, as well as KTP laser ablation of the prominent vasculature (KTP stands for potassium titanyl phosphate. The KTP laser is a device in the blue-green to green spectrum used for hemostasis). He also prescribed a proton-pump inhibitor (PPI) for GERD and a nasal antihistamine spray, and recommended discontinuing the oral antihistamine. Don agreed to proceed with these recommendations.

At the laryngologist's recommendation, Don observed 1 week of complete voice rest following the surgery. At the end of that week, he was seen in the clinic for reevaluation. Stroboscopy revealed that the right vocal fold lesion was gone. Vascularity was still present, as well as vibration impairment, which was expected for the first week after surgery. One week of gradually increasing speaking voice use was recommended, at the end of which voice therapy would commence.

Voice therapy goals included developing a rehabilitation exercise regimen that would gradually increase in duration and intensity over the course of his recovery, estimated at 12 weeks. Vocal pacing would address progressively resuming vocal activities relative to preaching and singing, and achieving a long-term sustainable vocal load in the interest of promoting optimal vocal health and decreasing the risk for reinjury.

For the first 4 weeks after his surgery, Don did not participate in worship activities at all. He attended services, sitting with the congregation, but did not use his voice while he was there. He had resumed speaking for social and work interactions when he was not in church but continued to be completely silent during services. This was very hard for him, as he felt "cut off" from much of his spiritual life. However, he was very committed to optimizing his recovery. Although I had recommended modifying voice use in services rather than complete silence he was afraid he would overdo it if he participated in services at all or started speaking with his parishioners, choir members, or music team.

In the meantime, he was completing his vocal exercises daily. During the first rehabilitation session, exercises assigned included adductory power, narrow interval glides, and scales (mostly on semioccluded vocal tract sounds and in a limited range) and also speaking exercises at the syllable, word, and phrase levels. He was to practice these exercises in a fairly constrained range for 5 to 10 minutes, one to three times per day. Over the ensuing weeks, the range, complexity, and intensity of these exercises as well as the duration of his practice time gradually increased, in the fashion illustrated in Chapter 12.

Don was often discouraged during the initial 4 to 6 weeks of his recovery. He felt his vocal range and stamina were so limited he couldn't see how he would ever be able to resume leading worship. However, as the weeks went by and he continued to demonstrate steady improvement, he started to feel more confident and we began to discuss resuming his participation in services. Jumping back into his full load of preaching and singing was clearly contraindicated. It was going to be important to plan carefully and reintroduce these activities bit by bit. We reviewed several options for the sequencing of his return to worship leading. Would he go back to preaching first? Or working with the choir? Or singing as soloist? He decided that worshiping as soloist was what he missed the most and would be the most meaningful and fulfilling activity to resume first. He struggled with this decision a bit. "It makes it sound like I'm singing for my own glory." However, with further discussion he realized that his solo singing was when he had the most intimate worship experiences, both with the congregation and with his creator, that his singing touched others and enhanced their worship experience, and that he was not being "selfish" by choosing to lead worship as soloist as his first postsurgery worship activity.

Based on the surgical outcome and the trajectory of his recovery, my prognosis was that by 8 weeks after surgery, Don would have adequate stamina to sing two or three songs, but he decided to sing only one song, erring on the side of caution so that he wouldn't be tempted to do too much. We planned what he would sing, choosing a song that was very familiar to him and not especially vocally challenging. We worked on the song in his therapy sessions and he practiced it regularly at home. A week before he was scheduled to sing, he had a rehearsal with the sound engineer and the instrumentalists. He was so overjoyed to be singing again that he was moved to tears and was glad that he had scheduled the rehearsal far enough in advance to prepare himself for the emotional impact of the actual performance. Don was well loved by his congregation and praise team, and his "comeback" performance was eagerly anticipated. Eight weeks after his surgery, surrounded by the support of his worship community, Don sang "Precious Lord, Take My Hand." He told me afterward that he felt like himself for the first time since his voice problem had started. "I felt He truly did take my hand the whole time I was singing."

All the while, we had been developing a plan for Don's new, permanent vocal pacing regimen. As he gradually resumed his solo singing, praise team direction, and preaching, we knew that it would be necessary to make substantial changes in the weekly amount and intensity of voice use to maintain vocal health and avoid reinjury.

The first step Don made toward achieving better balance in his vocal load was to approach the church leadership about hiring an assistant worship leader. Fortunately, the church had the resources and the willingness to do this, realizing that Don's vocal load had contributed to his injury and that resuming the same load put him at risk for recurrence. Having an assistant made a world of difference to Don, as he was able to delegate quite a bit. The assistant took on some of the load for leading rehearsals, directing the band and leading the congregational singing. In addition, during weeks when Don had extra demands (weddings, funerals, special services, speaking engagements, etc.), the assistant could take on a greater role as needed.

Don had access to excellent sound equipment and sound engineers and was already in the habit of using the equipment effectively during performances and rehearsals. His access to excellent sound and recording resources also made it possible for him to prerecord himself and other singers on the praise team and to use these recordings for demonstration purposes when working with instrumentalists, other soloists, and vocal ensembles. He delegated some of the live demonstration duties during rehearsals to other singers on the praise team. When rehearsing with the band, he tried to minimize singing until the instrumentalists had learned their parts. If they felt they needed to hear his part while they were learning theirs, he isolated the section where he was needed and sang lightly, rather than singing through the entire song full voice.

In services, he began to feature other singers more and strategically structured the program each week so that there was more alternation of solo/ensemble/congregational singing. This allowed him to take mini-breaks intermittently throughout the service. Using these strategies, he was able to reduce the amount of time he sang during services from nearly 60 minutes per service to less than 30 minutes. If he was scheduled to preach in the service, he reduced his singing even more, delegating the bulk of the worship leading to his assistant. He kept his speaking voice demands relatively light on the days before and after services. The church secretary was recruited to block times in his schedule on these days so that he could focus on activities that would allow him to rest his voice. The work Don had done on improving the efficiency of his speaking voice helped him avoid taxing his voice during pastoral and social activities, and also helped him achieve his passionate preaching style with greater technical proficiency.

In Don's case, the vocal pacing strategy was twofold: he had to drastically reduce voice use and gradually resume singing and preaching in a safe way during the postoperative recovery period, and also establish lifelong vocal pacing habits that would promote long-term vocal health. He often struggled with the changes he had to make, feeling that he was not fully serving if he cut back on what he was doing, but over time he came to realize that this balance of voice use and voice rest meant that he was being a good steward of his instrument and signified his mindfulness in protecting the gift he had been given.

CASE STUDY 7: HIGH SCHOOL CHOIR DIRECTOR WITH A VOCAL FOLD POLYP

"Jenn" was a vocal music educator in her early 30s. She directed the choral program in a large urban high school. At the time of her initial evaluation, she had been teaching for 10 years and had built a program of award-winning choirs, recognized among the best in the state.

Jenn's vocal demands were very high, with three high school choruses. Each rehearsed for 90 minutes per day. In addition, she taught a number of after-school activities, including preparing students for honors choir, all county choir, and various auditions, conducting a weekly evening rehearsal for her elite singers, and serving as music director for the annual spring musical. She also sang in her church choir and assisted with directing a community children's choir.

Throughout her career, she had noticed that by the end of the teaching year, she experienced voice changes, including loss of range, decreased stamina, and hoarseness. However, her voice always bounced back over the summer and so she wasn't very concerned about the changes, considering them to be just a part of teaching.

She was evaluated in our clinic in the fall of her 10th year of teaching. She had again noticed loss of range, stamina, and quality at the end of the previous school year, but this time her voice didn't recover over the summer. In fact, she had discontinued singing in the church choir as a result of the problem. The school year was well under way, and her voice seemed to be getting worse. She had experienced a loss of nearly one octave from the top of her range. Her voice was tired at the end of every teaching day. She noticed that her singing voice had become breathy and strained, and she found demonstrating in the classroom difficult. She wasn't able to model the sound she wanted the students to produce.

Jenn's stroboscopic examination revealed a right vocal fold polyp that was translucent and relatively smooth with a feeding varix. She had vibration impairment with reduced mucosal wave on the right side. At high pitch, the lesion resulted in an hourglass closure pattern. The lesion and resulting closure and vibration impairment accounted for her loss of range and increased vocal effort, as well as her vocal fatigue and altered vocal quality. Stroboscopy also revealed moderate anterior-posterior and ventricular hyperfunction. She had signs of laryngopharyngeal reflux and allergic rhinitis. Perceptually, her speaking voice was moderately pressed and strained with frequent vocal fry. Vocal hygiene was notable for inadequate hydration at about 16 to 32 ounces of water consumption per day.

The size and vascular nature of Jenn's polyp warranted consideration of surgical intervention. Undergoing surgery immediately would require an extended leave from her teaching job to ensure recovery and avoid reinjury. Jenn did not feel that she could undertake such a drastic adjustment to her work routine during the school year. We proceeded with medical and behavioral management, deferring consideration of surgery until the end of the school year. If her voice was not adequately improved by then, she would have enough time for surgery and recovery over the long summer break.

Contributing medical factors included GERD and allergic rhinitis, which were treated by our laryngologist. Treatment began with daily PPI for GERD and nasal steroid spray for allergic rhinitis. Throughout the course of her treatment, this regimen was adjusted several times. She did not achieve optimal management of allergies with steroid nasal spray alone and was switched to a combination nasal steroid and nasal antihistamine spray. Oral antihistamine was also added to her regimen, but she was still symptomatic. She had allergy testing and began sublingual immunotherapy. This combination ultimately brought her allergy symptoms under control, and she was eventually able to maintain without the oral antihistamine. Reflux treatment was also tweaked over time, and she ultimately achieved good control of symptoms on dexlansoprazole.

Voice therapy was initiated, targeting vocal pacing, vocal hygiene (primarily increasing hydration), and optimizing vocal technique for speaking and singing.

Jenn had already been proactive in vocal pacing. She had student assistants for most of her classes but had historically used them mainly for clerical tasks. She had been using amplification in the classroom routinely for years but admitted to some yelling and forceful talking while teaching. She reported that she felt she needed to use a "commanding" voice in the classroom to establish authority and control behavior.

We began expanding strategies for vocal pacing right away. She decided to prolong her leave of absence from her church choir position. She continued to participate in the community children's choir but limited her role to that of accompanist. These adjustments allowed her to focus her attention on her teaching job and voice recovery.

At school, she identified a number of speaking situations outside the classroom that could be offloaded, such as lunch duty and corralling students for assemblies. Her principal and colleagues were very supportive, redistributing these activities and changing her assignments to those that were less vocally demanding.

Jenn decided early in the process to let her students know about her vocal injury and voice therapy. She did this in the context of a vocal anatomy and health unit for her choirs, turning her own vocal struggles into an avenue for education and prevention for her students. They were devoted to her and quickly rallied to help her in any way they could. Their participation in her vocal recovery ranged from ensuring that she had a full bottle of water before every rehearsal to reminding her to take voice breaks between classes.

Together, we established a goal of limiting singing in classes and rehearsals to situations that required and utilized her musical expertise and vocal skill. The fact that she already had student assistants for most of her classes provided an immediate opportunity to work on this goal. She started using student assistants for all routine and noneducational tasks, such as taking attendance and making announcements. The student assistants were some of her most accomplished singers. She had them lead warm-ups for one class per day, varying which class they led so that she could direct warm-ups herself in the other classes. With this practice, she was able to ensure that she was regularly including instruction in vocal technique for all of her choirs, while reducing her vocal load by about 1 hour per week. She also used student assistants to lead sectional rehearsals and to do some of the demonstration and modeling in the classroom, further diminishing her singing load.

Jenn noted that there were classroom activities that she engaged in with some frequency that required minimal voice use. She regularly tested students on an individual basis to ensure they were progressing as expected relative to learning music, increasing sight-singing skills and developing vocal technique. She began deliberately planning administration of testing to occur at consistent intervals so that she had 1 hour per week that was devoted to this type of activity.

There were times when classes were devoted to district-wide educational endeavors that were delivered in lecture format. The content was the same for all classes. Jenn videotaped herself giving the lectures, recruiting students to participate in the videos as well. This transformed what would have been hours of lecturing over the course of a week to less than 1 hour of voice use during recording, and the students were even more engaged in the lectures as a result of seeing their classmates featured.

Her after-school activities (as enumerated above) were primarily devoted to teaching students parts and providing additional vocal coaching. In analyzing these rehearsals, she realized that she was doing quite a bit of "spoon-feeding" by providing a lot of modeling and rote teaching of parts. She gradually began having her students become more self-directed in rehearsals. Her student assistants prerecorded parts, and she provided the recordings via a website for the students who needed them to supplement self-teaching. The students were able to use these recordings to practice the music on their own. This allowed Jenn to focus her attention on helping students improve vocal technique during rehearsals. Since she didn't have to devote so much rehearsal time to teaching parts, she was able to decrease the total amount of time she allocated to after-school rehearsals, saving herself another hour or more per week.

The school musical involved directing musical rehearsals three to four evenings per week over a period of about 10 weeks. She realized that it took a bit of time to get the students all assembled and quieted so that she could start the rehearsal. She also found that, as in other activities, she was using her voice a lot to teach and drill parts. She designated a student to act as assistant music director. The assistant then called the rehearsal to order and took on the bulk of the rote teaching. As a result, Jenn could focus her attention on higher level teaching. She began using amplification for musical rehearsals, a practice she had already been employing for her choirs.

Jenn's therapy goals included improving vocal technique for speaking and singing. Early in the therapy process, I had her videotape herself teaching a class, and we reviewed the video together. The pressed and strained vocal quality I had noted in her conversational voice was even more pronounced in the classroom. She had been under the impression that this voice conveyed authority, but when she watched and listened to herself on the video, she was dismayed at the rough quality of her voice. Through self-observation and self-assessment she was motivated to improve her technique. She also realized that she could rely on the microphone to do the projecting for her and did not need to speak so loudly.

We systematically worked through a hierarchy of speaking tasks starting at the syllable and word levels. Once she had achieved appropriate oral resonance and breath support at the sentence level, we began incorporating "real-life" speaking activities. She made a list of sentences she said repeatedly when teaching, and we used these as practice material. She even enlisted her students to help inventory typical statements. By systematically practicing the phrases and sentences she said routinely, they began to serve as "recalibrators" during her teaching day and ultimately helped her achieve better vocal efficiency at the conversational/teaching level.

For years, Jenn had been in the habit of warming up her voice with her students during her first period. However, in watching herself complete warm-ups on video, it was evident to her that her focus was on her students, not on her own voice. Furthermore, for her voice to recover, she needed a routine that was customized to promote healing of her injury. She had a first period planning time that she usually used for correspondence and paperwork, but she gradually began to allocate part of this time for warming up so that she could regularly practice singing. She reported that she immediately noted a difference when singing in the classroom, with less strain and improved quality. Over time, she also began to notice increased range and stamina.

Jenn attended weekly voice therapy sessions for about 10 weeks. At the end of that period, vocal pacing strategies were well established, as was regular vocal exercise. She had noted considerable improvement in vocal stamina and range. Although her voice was still not back to normal, she had achieved a level of improvement and independence that allowed her to continue therapy on an as-needed basis. As it turned out, she did not feel the need for additional sessions that school year. When we met for reevaluation at the end of the school year, the right vocal fold polyp had almost completely resolved.

Jenn was initially concerned that disclosing her voice problem and delegating so much would have a negative impact on the effectiveness of her teaching and would set back all the work she had done over the years to build her program. However, in the end, she found that the opposite was true. The improvement in her voice enabled her to more effectively demonstrate for her students and model the sound she wanted them to emulate. Her students even commented on how much better her voice sounded. In addition, her students benefitted from taking on more responsibility and independence in singing activities. In fact, some of her students decided to pursue careers in music education and reported that this decision was influenced by their experience in leadership roles in the classroom.

CASE STUDY 8: HIGH SCHOOL CLASSICAL AND MUSICAL THEATER SINGER WITH RIGHT VOCAL FOLD PARALYSIS

"Amy" was a 16-year-old rising high school senior when she was first evaluated at our clinic in late July. At that time, she had been taking voice lessons for about 2 years. She sang in musical theater legit and belt styles, and also in classical style in her high school chorus. She reported that her teacher worked with her on both classical and belt technique. She was active in the music program at her church, singing in a contemporary youth ensemble. In addition, she regularly played a leadership role as a counselor and activities leader at church camps. She was planning to sing in a vocal quartet (a cappella group) at her school after summer break, and she reported quite a bit of recreational singing. In short, she had a very vocally busy life.

Amy had started to notice changes in her voice about 3 weeks prior to her initial evaluation at our clinic. She had experienced mild upper respiratory tract symptoms around that time, including nasal congestion and scratchy throat, although she didn't feel she was sick. Shortly after onset of her symptoms, she went to a musical theater camp out of state that required intense and prolonged singing. Her voice quickly deteriorated to the point that she lost it completely and had to leave the camp before the end of the program. She also began to choke intermittently when swallowing liquids. Understandably, she was very alarmed by these symptoms, as was her mother, who accompanied her to the evaluation.

Vocal hygiene habits were overall adequate. Perceptually, her speaking voice was moderately to severely hoarse, breathy, and strained, with intermittent diplophonia, poor projection, and short phrasing. She was unable to produce a normal cough or throat clear. Singing voice was even more impaired, with a pitch range of about seven semitones, severely breathy and strained quality and intermittent phonation breaks. Amy had brought a video recording of a performance from earlier in the year, before the onset of dysphonia. The contrast was considerable. This was not the same voice at all.

Videostroboscopy revealed a right vocal fold paralysis. The right fold had a bowed appearance. Moderate anterior-posterior and ventricular hyperfunction were noted, greater on the left side. The results clearly explained the precipitous deterioration of her voice as well as the dysphagia. Once this diagnosis was made, the next step was to try to determine the etiology of the paralysis. The laryngologist ordered a computed tomography (CT) scan of the neck and chest. We recommended discontinuing singing for the time being and using a voice amplifier for the short term to facilitate communication and minimize hyperfunction.

The CT scan did not reveal any masses or abnormalities, and it was assumed that the paralysis was idiopathic. The laryngologist reviewed surgical options to address the problem, including temporizing injection and permanent options of medialization laryngoplasty or laryngeal reinnervation, although given the recent onset of her symptoms and presumed coincidence of the paralysis, it was deemed too soon to consider permanent procedures. The option of laryngeal EMG to prognosticate whether the vocal fold was likely to regain function was presented to the patient, with the caveat that it is not a perfect test. Amy and her family decided to go ahead with the temporary Cymetra injection.

After the Cymetra injection, Amy noted that her voice was stronger, although she still fatigued very easily and singing was very effortful. At her follow-up evaluation 1 month after the injection, improved glottal closure and vibration were noted and hyperfunction had decreased somewhat. Most important, some movement of the right vocal fold was observed, suggesting that the paralysis was beginning to resolve spontaneously.

Voice therapy began, with goals including optimizing coordination of phonation subsystems for speaking and singing and achieving appropriate vocal pacing during recovery to avoid traumatic vocal fold injury and/or maladaptive compensatory muscle tension.

By this time it was mid-September. School had started, and Amy was enrolled in the chorus. She had been attending choir but had not been singing. She had also suspended voice lessons during the month since her injection. At her first voice therapy session, Amy reported that she had been doing some recreational singing for short periods without fatigue but noted increased hoarseness after cheering at a volleyball game a few days before. Principles of vocal pacing were introduced. It would be critically important to make sure that Amy was getting adequate vocal exercise while avoiding excessive voice use, which could slow down her recovery and put her at risk for traumatic injury or habitual hyperfunction. A vocal exercise regimen was established with 10 to 15 minutes of structured exercises, primarily using semi-occluded vocal tract sounds. When I vocalized her during the first session, improved pitch range was noted, having increased to two octaves. Amy was elated by this improvement. Even so, vocal quality was still breathy, compensatory strain was evident, and she tired fairly quickly.

Improvement was maintained over the following weeks and we decided that Amy could try singing in choir a little bit. She attended a choir retreat and sang intermittently throughout the day without fatigue. She had been practicing her vocal exercises regularly. She still had some difficulty modulating voice use in social situations, as during a trip to the state fair. We reviewed the importance of establishing a tolerable balance of voice use and voice rest and being more mindful of voice use in social settings. She agreed to start a voice journal to document voice use in the coming weeks.

During the entire time Amy had been a patient at our clinic, both the laryngologist and I had been corresponding with Amy's voice teacher and high school chorus director (at Amy's and her mother's request) to keep them apprised of her progress and our recommendations for vocal pacing. In one of these conversations, Amy's choir director expressed concern that Amy might be singing too much. At her next therapy session, Amy admitted that she had been singing for the entire 90-minute rehearsal every day, even though she felt fatigued, strained, and hoarse afterward. Further probing revealed that she was so excited to be singing again she didn't want to feel left out of participation. She felt frustrated that she had been sidelined for so long. However, she realized that overdoing it was slowing down her recovery. Up until this point, we had recommended that she use vocal fatigue and strain as a guide for when to stop singing. We decided to set a more structured protocol. She would start out singing only for the first 15 minutes or so of the rehearsal, stopping at that point even if she didn't feel fatigued. If she tolerated 15 minutes without fatigue or strain, she would increase the duration of singing in each rehearsal by 5 or 10 minutes. With this plan in place, she was gradually able to increase participation in rehearsals to about 75% without fatigue.

Amy had a few setbacks during the following month, associated with excessive speaking at a noisy wedding reception and speaking and singing while she had a cold. Use of the voice journal was very beneficial in helping her recognize and understand the factors that contributed to the ups and downs she was experiencing with her voice.

Since singing in chorus at school was an academic requirement, it was the top vocal priority for Amy. Once vocal pacing was well balanced in that setting, we began to explore adding back other types of voice use. Her self-identified priorities were (in order) increasing recreational singing, resuming voice lessons, and auditioning for the school musical. From her previous experiences, she knew that unlimited recreational singing would negatively impact her goals for resuming voice lessons and singing in the musical, and she set a limit for herself of 15 to 20 minutes of recreational singing per day, which she tolerated without incident. By Thanksgiving, she was ready to go back to her voice lessons.

At her reevaluation in mid-December, videostroboscopy revealed full and symmetrical arytenoid mobility. The paralysis had resolved, although there was still some mild decrease in mucosal wave on the right and phase asymmetry, suggesting there might still be an underlying mild paresis. She had resumed voice lessons and was able to participate in choir rehearsals for the full duration and without a break. A comparison of a preinjury recording and present-day performance of the same song demonstrated a return to baseline, and she was discharged from therapy.

Amy continued to be diligent in vocal pacing. She said that her experience in voice rehabilitation had made her realize that she had overused her voice in the past and declared that she would use what she had learned in voice therapy as a guide in making choices about voice use in the future. Amy went on to perform in the school musical that spring but decided not to pursue the a cappella group, and she postponed resuming her singing activities at church until after the musical was over.

PART V

More Tools for the Toolbox

CHAPTER 17

Aging Voice and the Singer

Chad Whited, Jarrod Keeler, Leda Scearce, and Seth M. Cohen

Our youthful skin, energy, and voice all succumb to the inevitable effects of time. Importantly, in the performer's voice, vocal aging may lead to early termination of a career or interruption of a joyful activity. That being said, we now better understand these changes both histologically and functionally. There continues to be scientific advancement in nonsurgical and surgical therapeutic options to slow the functional decline resulting from the aging process.

PREVALENCE

As the baby boomers make their way into retirement, there is a growing interest in geriatric medicine, not only for increasing the days of our lives but the quality of our lives. Otolaryngologists, speech-language pathologists, and singing voice rehabilitation specialists have our own unique roles to play in this growing field. Voice disorders among the elderly are quite common and have been estimated between 20% and 29% (Cohen & Turley, 2009; Golub, Chen, Otto, Hapner, & Johns, 2006; Roy, Stemple, Merrill, & Thomas, 2007). These studies define their populations of elderly as those over 65 years of age.

One fifth to nearly one third of the populace have voice disorders, but what effect does this have on their day-to-day lives? Large-scale studies have evaluated voice-related quality of life (V-RQOL) showing decreased V-RQOL scores in association with increasing age (Behlau, Hogikyan, & Gasparini, 2007; Golub et al., 2006). Similar studies have shown V-RQOL and Voice Handicap Index (VHI) correlate with each other and are significantly reduced in patients with presbyphonia (Portone, Hapner, McGregor, Otto, & Johns, 2007; Romak, Orbelo, Maragos, & Ekbom, 2014). Fortunately, recent small-scale studies show improvement in voice-related quality of life and overall quality of life with voice therapy exercises such as vocal function exercises (VFE) or phonation resistance training exercise (PhoRTE) therapy (Ziegler et al., 2014).

Although the primary diagnoses of these patients are inconsistent, presbyphonia and presbylarynges are often major underlying factors. Presbylarynges is defined as the age-related changes on the larynx, and presbyphonia is defined as age-related changes to the voice. These two diagnoses are seen with varying frequency within the population of the elderly (Hagen, Lyons, & Nuss, 1996; Kandogan, Olgun, & Gultekin, 2003; Woo, Casper, Colton, & Brewer, 1992). The specific vocal characteristics of presbyphonia are discussed in a later section.

ANATOMY AND PRESBYLARYNGES

As we age, our anatomy changes, and this is especially true in the larynx. The physical exam findings of presbylarynges stem from underlying tissue atrophy and include concavity of the medial edge of the vocal fold or "bowing," prominence of the vocal process, and persistent glottic gap with phonation. These findings can be subtle on flexible laryngoscopy and often require videostroboscopy to fully assess.

Histopathology

The extracellular makeup of the larynx is of paramount importance to laryngeal function as voice production is dependent upon the interaction between the layers of the true vocal folds. Below the epithelial surface are the superficial, intermediate, and deep lamina propria. The superficial layer has wide distribution of hyaluronic acid, which contributes to the viscoelastic properties of the vocal fold (Gray, Titze, Chan, & Hammond, 1999). The intermediate layer is made up of mostly type III collagen fibers and is interwoven with the deep layer consisting of the thyroarytenoid muscle. This cover-body relationship allows movement between the superficial lamina propria/epithelium and the intermediate/deep layer, resulting in the propagation of a mucosal wave and voice production (Madruga de Melo et al., 2003).

Changes from aging result in a relative loss of hyaluronic acid, an increase in collagen, and a decrease in the collagen organization. The critical interaction between the superficial and intermediate/deep layer of the lamina propria is affected with a change in the viscoelasticity (Sato & Hirano, 1997; Sato, Hirano, & Nakashima, 2002).

Atrophy

One of the characteristic findings of presbylarynges is atrophy or decrease in vocal fold mass (Figures 17–1 and 17–2). This is due to atrophy of the intrinsic laryngeal musculature as well as thinning of the

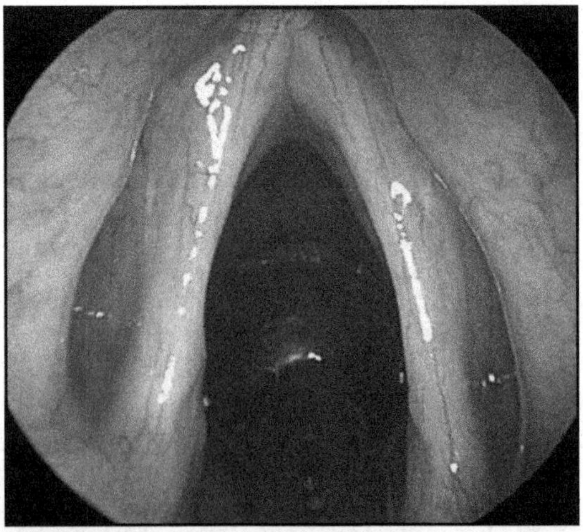

***Figure 17–1.** This is an endoscopic view using a zero-degree scope of presbylarynges. Note how thin the folds are, the concavity of the medial true vocal fold edges, and the exaggerated laryngeal ventricles bilaterally.*

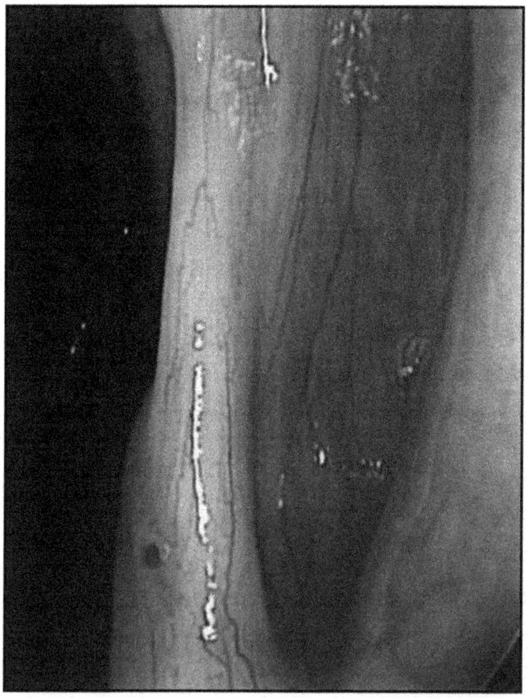

Figure 17–2. ***This is a magnified view of the right true vocal fold of an elderly patient. Note the significant atrophy of the thyroarytenoid muscle, creating an enlarged trough at the junction of the superior surface of the fold and the laryngeal ventricle. Also note the thin leading vibratory edge representing a loss of vertical mass.***

overlying lamina propria. Atrophy can create a concavity of the vocal folds, deepened laryngeal ventricles, reduction in the vertical height of the vocal fold body, persistent spindle-shaped closure, or what is commonly described as "bowing." Generalized muscle atrophy is well known in aging but has proven difficult to quantify (Cooper et al., 2013; Cruz-Jentoft et al., 2010). Muscle atrophy can be as great as 20% to 40% in some muscle groups with the loss of type II muscle fibers (Lexell, Henriksson-Larsen, Winblad, & Sjostrom, 1983; Thomas, Harrison, & Stemple, 2008). This has been described as sarcopenic change, which is physiologic age-related degeneration of skeletal muscle mass, quality, and strength. It is seen beginning anywhere from ages 25 to 40 years. Thomas et al. (2008) performed a comparison of the changes in skeletal muscle noting that cellular, neurologic, hormonal, and metabolic changes lead to sarcopenic change in the thyroarytenoid muscle similar to losses seen in other skeletal muscle.

With muscular atrophy and decreased organization of the extracellular matrix, an overall decrease in the volume of the vocal fold occurs. As the anterior and posterior points are fixed at the anterior commissure and vocal process, the volume lost is visualized most clearly at the midportion of the vocal fold. The concavity of the medial edge and incomplete spindle-shaped closure pattern with phonation are two of the key features on laryngoscopic evaluation of the aging voice. This gap is important as increased breathiness due to air loss increases the listener's impression of vocal age (Winkler & Sendlmeier, 2006). Although study numbers were limited Sato and Hirano (1997) and Sato, Hirano, and Nakashima (2002) demonstrated that males appear to be more affected by atrophic vocal fold changes, perhaps attributing to the increased fundamental frequency of the aging male voice.

Edema

Edema is a commonly found characteristic and, although nonspecific, is frequently seen in the aging voice. As a result of hormonal changes during menopause, the vocal folds of women are believed to have a greater increase in their vocal mass, as has been confirmed with laryngoscopic evaluation (Close & Woodson,

1989). As many as 74% of female and 56% of male larynges demonstrate edema and an increase in the mucosal wave under laryngoscopic evaluation (Honjo & Isshiki, 1980). Hormonal changes associated with menopause cause an increase in vocal fold mass, leading to a decrease in the fundamental frequency and subsequently a lower-pitched voice. Although edema is sometimes a feature of the male aging voice, the atrophy and extracellular matrix changes are thought to be more dominant in men, resulting in an overall increase in fundamental frequency.

Breath Support/ Breath Management

Breath support should not be underestimated in the evaluation of the aging voice. The atrophy of the vocal fold and subsequent persistent incomplete closure pattern result in a leaky valve (Iwarsson, Thomasson, & Sundberg, 1998). As the engine behind the vocal machine, the respiratory system must compensate for this inefficient escape of airflow. The sarcopenic changes and thyroarytenoid muscle loss noted above are present for all skeletal muscle and can decrease the force of the lung bellows. This is worsened by a decrease in elastic recoil of the lungs, resulting in a decrease in loudness and maximum phonation time in older adults (Huber, 2008). Finally and most notably, comorbid lung disease (i.e., chronic obstructive pulmonary disease, malignancy, pneumonia) is more common with age and is an independent risk factor associated with dysphonia and poorer response to therapy (Huber, 2008; Mau, Jacobson, & Garrett, 2010; Pontes, Brasolotto, & Behlau, 2005).

Poor Compensations

Maladaptive compensation frequently exacerbates the underlying problem. As the atrophy of the vocal fold worsens, patients frequently begin to use supraglottic hyperfunction in an attempt to compensate and close the gap. This resulting muscle tension dysphonia is one of the most frequent diagnoses within all of voice pathology and is seen in 10% to 73% of aging voice patients (Bloch & Behrman, 2001; Gregory, Chandran, Lurie, & Sataloff, 2012; Kandogan et al., 2003).

Secretions

Mucus and its effects on voice are well known. Between 83% and 100% of patients with voice dysfunction were found to have thickened, ineffective mucus aggregations on the vocal folds (Bonilha, White, Kuckhahn, Gerlach, & Deliyski, 2012; Hsiao, Liu, & Lin, 2002). Mucous glands decrease in both quantity and quality as we age, leading to less lubricated, drier vocal folds. Also, many medications that are taken by those over 65 years of age have anticholinergic, diuretic, or normal flora altering properties resulting in inspissated secretions. In a pilot study from Copenhagen, 10 patients treated with medical therapy directed to improve micro-organic conditions showed improved overall voice quality-of-life scores compared to standard vocal hygiene (Pedersen, Beranova, & Moller, 2004).

Menopause

Hormonal changes are well known to have effects on the voice. Women experience drastic shifts in their estrogen and progesterone in the peri- and postmenopausal time frame. Vocal harmonics are significantly affected by these hormone changes. Abitbol, Abitbol, and Abitbol (1999) evaluated 17 menopausal women, demonstrating menopausal vocal syndrome with resultant decreased vocal intensity, increased vocal fatigue, a loss of the higher frequencies, and a decrease in overall vocal quality. Raj, Gupta, Chowdhury, and Chadha (2010) demonstrated changes to the frequency range and decreases in the maximum phonation time that were statistically significant compared to premenopausal women. These changes are attributed to both atrophy and edema of the vocal fold mucosa (D'Haeseleer et al., 2011). Specifically for elite vocal performers, 77% experienced vocal changes around menopause. They reported reduced vocal flexibility, loss of highest notes, changes in timbre, reduced stability, and huskiness (Boulet & Oddens, 1996).

CHARACTERISTICS OF THE AGING VOICE

These age-related changes in anatomy and physiology contribute to characteristic changes in the aging voice. Some of these changes are universal and others are sex-specific changes that affect both the speaking and singing voice. Some of the measures that correlate most closely with vocal age include jitter and intensity (Benjamin, 1981; Gregory et al., 2012; Wilcox & Horii, 1980). Specifically, increased pitch variation and decreased loudness were demonstrated as some of the strongest cues for perceived older vocal age (Prakup, 2012).

Speaking rate has been demonstrated to slow as we age, representing a generalized slowing of our motor functions (Harnsberger, Shrivastav, Brown, Rothman, & Hollien, 2008). Formant frequencies have also been shown to become lower, reflecting an increase in vocal tract volume with age (Xue & Hao, 2003). There is an increase in fundamental frequency perturbation in both elderly men and women, although whether the extent of change is equal between both sexes is unclear (Benjamin, 1981).

Throat clearing was also noted to be a complaint among aging vocalists resulting from the change in mucous glands and thickened laryngeal secretions (Gregory et al., 2012). Other characteristics of the aging voice include increased roughness, shimmer, and breathiness (Benjamin, 1981; Gama, Alves, Cerceau, & Teixeira, 2009; Ramig & Ringel, 1983).

Men often experience vocal changes around age 60. Men's voices will deepen from puberty into their 40s and 50s. However, into their seventh decade of life, the fundamental frequency for males begins to increase (Hollien & Shipp, 1972; Honjo & Isshiki, 1980). Women, however, often have a lower or stable fundamental frequency as they age.

For singers, acoustic measures in older singers were significantly better than older nonsingers for jitter and intensity, with singers having less jitter and greater intensity (Prakup, 2012). Perceived age based on voice was dependent on jitter for all subjects except female nonsingers, for whom the perception correlated most closely with intensity. As singers age, they frequently report reduction in their voice range. However, vocal training (which we describe later) has been demonstrated to help delay this deterioration (Martins, Gonsalvez, Pessin, & Branco, 2014).

IMPACT ON THE ELDERLY

As one ages, many aspects of quality of life are affected: independence, mobility, cognition, social interactions, physical strength, and communication skills. These communicative declines are commonly attributed to hearing deficits, overlooking the importance and multifaceted impact of dysphonia within the elderly.

Dysphonia affects approximately 20% of the elderly population. Half of this dysphonic population has a significantly decreased quality of life resulting from their dysphonia that is not generalized (Golub et al., 2006) and a worse V-RQOL score (Ramig & Ringel, 1983). The elderly experience an increased self-consciousness due to voice instability, voice discomfort, and excessive effort. Ultimately, this can lead to the avoidance of social gatherings and frustration from needing to repeat oneself (Roy et al., 2007; Verdonck-de Leeuw & Mahieu, 2004). Voice disorders can also affect the psychiatric health of the elderly. Depression and anxiety are more prevalent in the aging population when there is an associated dysphonia, especially when combined with hearing loss (Cohen & Turley, 2009; Mirza, Ruiz, Baum, & Staab, 2003).

There is also the aesthetic or cosmetic component of the aging voice. People will invest significant energy into working out, maintaining a cardiopulmonary and muscular fitness level. They will spend a lifetime making health-conscious choices, choosing well-balanced meals and refraining from unhealthy habits. Some aging adults will even undergo the risks of anesthesia and expend financial resources for surgical cosmetic procedures to conceal the effects of aging. Yet, as soon as they open their mouths, their numerical age is revealed with a rough, effortful, breathy, unstable voice. There have been procedures described to minimize these changes and restore voice capabilities as much as possible (Valeo, 2010).

SYSTEMIC COMORBIDITIES AFFECTING VOICE

It is important to keep in mind that presbyphonia is a diagnosis of exclusion. Multiple studies have investigated the etiology of dysphonia in the elderly and concluded that typical findings of bowing and atrophy were the cause in approximately 19% of dysphonic patients (Lundy, Silva, Casiano, Lu, & Xue, 1998). Other common etiologies were unilateral vocal fold immobility (19%), benign lesions (12%), tremor (9%), spasmodic dysphonia (8%), and malignancy (4%). Although the exact incidence of comorbid disease presenting as dysphonia within the elderly is unknown, between 80% and 96% of those studied had diagnoses that were not presbyphonia (Calhoun & Eibling, 2006; Cohen & Turley, 2009; Golub et al., 2006; Hagen et al., 1996; Kandogan et al., 2003; Roy et al., 2007; Woo et al., 1992). It is crucial that comorbidities be evaluated during the initial presentation, including neurologic, pulmonary, gastrointestinal, neoplastic, and medication side effects.

Neurologic

Numerous neurologic comorbidities can both affect the voice and present as primary vocal concerns within the aging population (Calhoun & Eibling, 2006). Stroke, amyotrophic lateral sclerosis (ALS), and myasthenia gravis (MG) can present as affectations of the voice. Strokes most often present as dysarthria, although breathing, phonation, articulation, resonance, and prosody are frequently affected (Godoy, Brasolotto, Berretin-Felix, & Fernandes, 2014). ALS produces bulbar symptoms, resulting in dysphagia and dysarthria. One of the earliest presenting symptoms of bulbar involvement in ALS is vocal dysfunction. This dysfunction is characterized by breathy, wet, possibly hypernasal voice with frequent tremor and fluctuation in intensity (Strand, Buder, Yorkston, & Ramig, 1994). Vocal perturbations can even be the presenting signs of myasthenia gravis (Nemr, Simoes-Zenari, Ferreira, Fernandes, & Mansur, 2013).

Essential tremor can present as vocal tremor and result in rhythmic voice breaks or pulsations. Tremor is usually consistent across phonatory tasks and most pronounced during sustained phonation on vowels.

Parkinson disease (PD) is one of the most well-known and well-studied neurologic conditions to affect the voice in the aging population (Canter, 1963). The voice is characterized by low loudness, breathy quality, and decreased prosodic variation. Several speech and language therapies have been developed to assist these patients (Deane, Whurr, Playford, Ben-Shlomo, & Clarke, 2001).

Pulmonary

Pulmonary and tracheal diseases have obvious effects on the voice. As discussed above, breath support is of paramount importance and pulmonary impairment can lead to significant dysphonia. Primary lung cancer can have devastating effects on the voice due to destruction of critical laryngeal structures or vocal fold paralysis. Iatrogenic surgical, cardiac pathology, or primary thoracic malignancy are other common etiologies of vocal fold paralysis, causing nearly 30% of all vocal fold paralyses (Spataro, Grindler, & Paniello, 2014).

Gastrointestinal

Gastrointestinal complaints are frequent causes of dysphonia, with gastroesophageal/laryngopharyngeal reflux representing between 17% and 70% of all aging voice patients (Gregory et al., 2012; Kandogan et al., 2003; Zeitels et al., 2002). Due to the proximity of the upper esophageal sphincter, any refluxate passing through has a direct impact on the glottis resulting in edema, thickened mucus, and/or benign lesions (Hopkins, Yousaf, & Pedersen, 2006; Kotby, Hassan, El-Makhzangy, Farahat, & Milad, 2010; Morrison & Gore-Hickman, 1986; Tobey et al., 2001).

Dysphagia of any type, including Zenker's diverticulum, achalasia, cricopharyngeal dysphagia, or oropharyngeal dysphagia, can result in chemical injury to the larynx or a wet-sounding voice from poor clearing of secretions (Hopkins et al., 2006).

Cancer/Leukoplakia

Laryngeal cancer is one of the most frequent concerns of aging voice patients and otolaryngologists but is not the most frequent diagnosis, representing only17% to 27% of diagnoses in elderly patients (Morrison & Gore-Hickman, 1986). Laryngeal cancer represents approximately 21% of all head and neck cancers (Hoffman, Karnell, Funk, Robinson, & Menck, 1998). Hence, the American Academy of Otolaryngology-Head and Neck Surgery practice guideline makes a strong recommendation for laryngoscopy for the evaluation of any dysphonia, but especially in elderly dysphonic patients (Schwartz et al., 2009).

Paralysis/Paresis

A significant proportion of those presenting for evaluation of the aging voice will have paralysis or paresis, (4% and 75% for complete paralysis and any paresis, respectively) (Gregory et al., 2012; Kandogan et al., 2003; Kendall, 2007). The paretic cord represents a significant cause for dysphonia with well-documented airflow changes, muscle tone discrepancy, and vocal dysfunction (Zeitels et al., 2002).

AGE-RELATED VOICE CHANGES AND THE SINGER

The physiologic changes that occur with aging can have a dramatic impact on the singing voice (Sataloff, Rosen, Hawkshaw, & Spiegel, 1997). Reported symptoms may include changes in vocal range, increased effort with phonation, unreliable or unstable voice, voice breaks and cracks, difficulty negotiating register transitions, reduced projection, difficulty with breath support, decreased phrase duration, unsteady vibrato, and changes in vocal quality (Sataloff et al., 1997). Quality changes may include huskiness, a perceived hollow quality, breathiness, hoarseness, or strain (Anderson, Anderson, & Sataloff, 2006).

Many singers feel they have to give up singing as their voices become more unreliable. This can have an impact on income for some, and self-image or self-esteem for others. Singing may play a significant role in the singer's spiritual life and worship activities. For many avocational singers, singing is a significant element of their quality of life, and giving up singing represents a devastating loss not only of musical enjoyment but also social interaction, as well as physical and mental activity. However, with appropriate medical intervention, neuromuscular retraining, and expectation management, the joy in singing can continue for many years.

An important factor for preserving vocal longevity for singers is regular vocal exercise. Some singers may be in the habit of sporadic or intermittent vocal exercise, often determined by upcoming singing engagements. They may have previously been able to get away with singing only at choir practice and services. They may typically increase practice time when preparing for a specific performance and may practice less frequently when they have no pending engagements. Singers who do not have vocal training (as is often the case with choral singers or contemporary singers) may never have acquired a vocal exercise regimen that is customized for their voices and vocal needs. It is critical that the singer develop the habit of regular vocal exercise, ideally 4 to 5 days per week. Even relatively short periods (15–20 minutes per day) of the right kind of exercise can have enormous benefit in extending vocal longevity when completed regularly (see Chapter 11 for discussion of exercise physiology and singing).

Retirees may experience significant decline in the amount of speaking voice use overall. This should be considered in the approach to vocal pacing for social voice in this population. Those who frequently experience days when speaking voice is at a minimum may find that when there is an uptake in speaking demands —perhaps surrounding rehearsals or performances, family gatherings, or holidays—they are quickly fatigued. Recommending decreasing or avoiding participation on such occasions (as you might with singers whose vocal load is on the excessive side) may be contraindicated for older singers, both from the perspective of achieving balance in overall voice use *and* maintaining quality of life and social connection. Rather, work with the singer to increase vocal exercise globally and balance voice use, including exercises for speaking voice as needed.

For singers with extensive experience and training, it may be necessary to seek retraining from a qualified voice teacher, as vocal technique may require adjustment to adapt to changes in anatomy and physiology. The technique that worked for the younger voice may not fit as the voice matures. It is essential that the singer seek training from a voice teacher with expertise in teaching the singer's style, whether classical or contemporary.

It is also critical for singers to address any medical problems that may be affecting the voice. This may include pulmonary, cardiac, or thyroid disease, as well as seasonal allergies, gastroesophageal reflux, and hearing loss. For singers who experience hearing loss requiring hearing aids, the hearing aid fitting must encompass optimizing programming for singing as well as environmental variables.

Singers should be counseled and educated on optimal vocal hygiene, particularly relative to hydration. This becomes even more essential with the drying of mucous membranes and thickening of mucus that can occur with aging. General fitness can also have an impact on the voice. For example, pulmonary function has an effect on breath support, posture and body alignment may be affected by the skeletal changes associated with aging, and vocal endurance and resilience may be dictated by global fitness. Singers should be encouraged to optimize their physical fitness and to understand the impact of overall fitness on their vocal health.

Vocal Fold Atrophy

As noted above, vocal fold atrophy occurs when the muscular layer of the vocal fold loses bulk and becomes thinner. This can decrease the vertical dimension of the vocal folds on adduction so that there is less area of contact between the vocal folds and decreased ability to square up the vertical edge of the fold during phonation. According to Titze and Verdolini Abbott (2012), this squared-up vertical edge of the vocal folds is very important for optimizing the balance of activation of the thyroarytenoid (TA) and cricothyroid (CT) muscles to achieve appropriate laryngeal configuration for chest voice (or TA dominant) registration. In addition, achieving appropriate vocal registration depends on the ability to make fine motor adjustments in activation of TA and CT muscles, which can be undermined by loss of TA bulk. Vocal fold atrophy can also cause glottal gapping, resulting in difficulty generating sufficient subglottic pressure to achieve clear, projected tone. This gapping also causes air leakage during phonation, which has a direct impact on breath management, as the singer will deplete the supply of air in the lungs more quickly. Singers may note that they have less ability to sustain phonation for long phrases. All of these factors—decreased ability to balance TA/CT ratio, decreased glottal closure, decreased ability to sustain phonation—can result in maladaptive muscle tension as the singer attempts to compensate for the underlying problems.

The resulting muscle tension can then become a contributing factor in and of itself that must be addressed in the rehabilitation process (see Chapter 12 for resources for addressing muscle tension).

Male and female singers may experience a loss of low range associated with vocal fold atrophy. As the vocal folds shorten to produce lower pitch, tension on the vocal folds is reduced and glottal gapping will be more pronounced. Vocal fold atrophy is more likely to affect male singers than females, as women often have an overlay of laryngeal edema resulting from the hormonal changes associated with menopause. This can create its own set of challenges for the female singer (to be discussed below) but may decrease the likelihood of frank glottal gapping and decreased glottal resistance.

The most conservative approach to addressing vocal fold atrophy is behavioral singing voice rehabilitation. If the atrophy is relatively minor, appropriate vocal exercise may enable singers to effectively compensate for the laryngeal changes, allowing them to continue to participate in their chosen singing activities.

Rehabilitation Targets and Approaches

Exercises should focus on optimizing glottic closure, TA/CT ratio, coordination of respiration and phonation, and vocal tract inertance. The utility of semi-occluded vocal tract (SOVT) exercises in achieving all of these goals has been well documented, as outlined in previous chapters. A semi-occluded vocal tract is achieved with phonation through a small-diameter straw, lip and tongue trills, raspberries (labio/lingual trills), voiced fricatives (like /v, z/), Lessac "Y" buzz, kazoo buzz, and nasal consonants. SOVT exercises not only result in improved respiratory/laryngeal/vocal tract mechanics, but they also provide immediate auditory and sensory feedback to the singer, as it is nearly impossible to achieve phonation with these sounds without achieving correct coordination. The pitch and rhythmic complexity of the exercise should be adjusted to meet the singer's current ability, ranging from sustaining one note at a time (as in Stemple's Adductory Power Exercise; Stemple, Lee, D'Amico, & Pickup, 1994), to more elaborate scalar and arpeggiated patterns. Messa di voce (crescendo and decrescendo on a single note) is an excellent exercise for improving vocal coordination in cases of vocal fold atrophy, promoting minute, highly controlled adjustments in TA/CT ratio, airflow, and resistance. Messa di voce combined with SOVT (e.g., executed while phonating through a small straw) provides maximal neuromuscular retraining and optimal coordination.

In developing an appropriate exercise regimen, it is crucial to adapt the exercise to the singer's current level of ability and gradually increase the complexity. For example, some singers may not be able to sustain phonation through a stir straw but may be able to start by phonating through a drinking straw, gradually increasing the occlusion by gently squeezing the straw and eventually moving on to phonation through the smaller straw.

SOVT exercises have the added advantage of allowing singers to use oral airflow resistance to approximate an appropriate degree of laryngeal resistance. Once the singer has achieved the appropriate degree of resistance at the mouth (via any of the SOVT sounds listed above), a sensory reference relative to breath support can be established, which can then be translated to phonation on sustained vowels and ultimately to repertoire. Having the singer alternate SOVT phonation with sustained vowel phonation, with cues to match the respiratory mechanics, can be highly effective in adapting breath support technique to the altered anatomy of the aging larynx.

Exercise should also focus on optimizing TA/CT ratio through the lower register transition or passaggio, particularly for female classical singers who tend do more singing in mixed or head voice (CT dominant) registration. This can be accomplished by starting on a note in the passaggio range and pivoting a minor second above and below to make gradual changes in TA/CT ratio. As the singer progresses, the exercise can expand chromatically above and below the starting pitch over a wider range (as illustrated in Chapter 12, Case Study 2).

If the atrophy is more advanced, exercise alone may not be enough to address the problem, and the surgical interventions that we discuss later in this chapter should be explored. Some singers may wish to proceed with vocal fold augmentation or medialization immediately. In such cases, singing voice rehabilitation is often still indicated following the surgery to minimize the impact of maladaptive muscle tension (which may persist after surgery due to muscle memory) and to guide the singer in adapting to the altered sensation and responses of their postsurgery laryngeal configuration.

Changes in Elasticity of Vocal Folds

As noted earlier, age-related physiologic changes can include alteration of the cellular structure of the vocal folds, which can result in thickening and loss of elasticity. When this happens, the vibratory characteristics of the vocal folds change as well, often yielding decreased mucosal wave. In some cases (often associated with menopause or thyroid disease), the vocal folds become hyperdynamic. In either situation, the singer may note a change in the amount of effort it takes to initiate and sustain phonation and in the flexibility and agility of the voice. This is particularly distressing to singers whose singing style requires a great deal of agility (e.g., the coloratura soprano).

Rehabilitation Targets and Approaches

Again, SOVT exercises can be invaluable in retraining muscle memory to adapt to these changes effectively, as detailed above. Staccato exercise is also helpful in increasing precise coordination of airflow, intrinsic laryngeal musculature activation, and optimal vocal tract configuration. Exercises should also focus on gradually increasing the complexity of the pitch pattern as well as the tempo of the exercise to facilitate recovery of agility (see case studies in Chapter 12 for examples). Use of a metronome can be very helpful in this type of exercise.

Unstable Vibrato

Unsteady or unstable vibrato is a common symptom of the aging voice. Acceptable vibrato frequency and extent is 4.5 to 6.5 Hz in frequency and 0% ± 3% in extent (Titze et al., 2000). Typically, both men and women may find that their vibrato becomes slower in rate and wider in extent, resulting in a wobbling quality. This is largely due to changes in vocal fold tissue, decreased fine motor control of intrinsic laryngeal musculature, and changes in respiratory mechanics and laryngeal valving, and may also be impacted by ossification of laryngeal cartilages and decreased elasticity of the vocal tract. All of the exercise strategies above can help stabilize vibrato and return to a more desirable rate and frequency variation. Improvements in body alignment and torso anchoring can also facilitate improved vibrato, as detailed in Chapter 12.

Body Alignment and Anchoring

Skeletal changes associated with aging can have a marked effect on body alignment, which in turn affects singing. Curvature of the spine can make it more difficult to maintain the necessary rib cage elevation and expansion that is so essential for achieving optimal breath support for singing. Body morphology changes may result in decreased core strength, which makes it difficult to appropriately stabilize and anchor the torso during phonation. Arthritis can affect the entire skeletal system, including the arytenoid joints. As discussed in Chapter 12, the fine motor movements of the larynx during phonation require anchoring gestures, ideally allocated to the lower body, including the muscles of the lower back, lower abdomen, pelvic floor, and lower limbs. Changes in body alignment, joint flexibility, and core strength may result in the singer unconsciously anchoring the larynx in a maladaptive manner, resulting in muscle tension in the neck, shoulders, tongue, jaw, and so on. Singing voice rehabilitation will likely require addressing stability issues.

Appropriate bracing or anchoring of the larynx can be retrained through a variety of strategies and techniques (see Chapter 12). Practicing vocal exercises or repertoire while seated on a fitness ball automatically engages core strength for posture and maintains torso alignment over the pelvic floor. This can be an effective method for reducing maladaptive muscle tension and improving vocal stability. Other strategies include gently pushing back with the feet while in a seated position, standing with the back against the wall (with head support), or slow knee bends during singing exercises. For all techniques, the singing voice rehabilitation specialist must provide regular feedback to ensure that the singer is maintaining optimal alignment from the feet to the top of the head.

Menopause and the Singer

The impact of the hormonal changes associated with menopause is discussed in detail earlier in this chapter and in Chapter 4. These changes can have a dramatic and devastating effect on the female singing voice. The thickening of the vocal folds increases their mass, lowering fundamental frequency. Singers often experience a loss of high range and an increase in low range. This can be particularly problematic for sopranos, whose singing activities depend on higher range. However, all female singers are potentially at risk for significant voice changes associated with menopause. For any singer, the gradual loss or unreliability of high notes can be extremely distressing.

Because the female voice can be so altered during and after menopause, female singers should be counseled regarding the potential for voice changes prior to menopause. The initiation of hormonal therapy may be beneficial and women for whom singing is a high priority relative to income and/or quality of life should be given the opportunity to make an informed decision (Anderson et al., 2006). Research has indicated that hormonal therapy may be able to reverse the effects of menopause on the vocal tract (D'Haeseleer, Depypere, Claeys, Van Borsel, & Van Lierde, 2009). Estrogen therapy has been shown to reduce the amount of vocal decline, including changes in fundamental frequency (Lindholm, Vilkman, Raudaskoski, Suvanto-Luukkonen, & Kauppila, 1997). One study demonstrated an increase in this effect when the application of estrogen is intranasal (Firat et al., 2009). However, the risks associated with hormone replacement therapy include increased risk of cancer, embolism, and heart disease. The decision regarding whether or not to undergo hormone replacement therapy must be carefully weighed against these risks in conjunction with a multispecialty team.

For women who are menopausal or postmenopausal, it may be necessary to make adaptations in repertoire, focusing on that which is appropriate for their altered singing range. This discussion must be handled with sensitivity, as the singer's vocal identity may be intrinsically tied to the voice part she has identified with for all her singing life.

Vocal exercise is essential for longevity of singing life for women during and after menopause. Exercises should focus in optimizing vocal quality, stability, flexibility, and control, including the methods and techniques outlined above.

Changing Expectations

The age-related anatomical and physiologic changes to the voice are magnified in singing, which is a highly athletic vocal activity. Just as other athletes may have to adjust their performance expectations as their bodies change, singers may need to adjust their expectations relative to their voices. This doesn't mean having to settle for a voice that is unrewarding and unsatisfying to them. Rather, they may need to consider adapting repertoire, duration, type of performances, and possibly even voice part or fach. The singing voice rehabilitation provider should always be honest in conveying the prognosis relative to maintaining or improving singing, but ultimately singers must make their own decisions about whether they are satisfied with their vocal performance and whether to continue participating in singing activities. Some singers may decide not to continue performing if they are not able to do so at a level that is fulfilling to them. However, if singing is an important part of life, and if the singer is motivated to do the work that is necessary to maintain or improve vocal function, singing voice providers—laryngologists, speech-language pathologists, singing voice rehabilitation specialists, and voice teachers—should make every effort to support and encourage the singer, providing appropriate medical, surgical, therapeutic, and educational care.

SURGICAL THERAPY

It is worth reviewing the options afforded to the patient and surgeon should the physiologic changes of the aging voice be too great for or refractory to voice rehabilitation.

There is much debate over whether injection medialization or type I thyroplasty is the best approach for patients with symptomatic glottal insufficiency (Cohen, 2010; Rosen & Statham, 2010). To date, there is no ideal head-to-head study comparing the two. In addition, there are little if any data looking at surgical treatments directed solely at presbyphonia/presbylarynges. However, there are benefits and risks worth considering with each, which should be reviewed with the singer. The impact of vocal fold injection (or any kind of medialization) on the singing voice can be highly unpredictable at best. Fortunately, the effect usually dissipates after a period of time as the injectable is reabsorbed, depending on what substance is used. There has been a lot of attention to and practice of injection and medialization for the speaking voice. However, because of the intricate and complex vocal function required for singing (especially with a classical aesthetic), the outcome from injection or thyroplasty may cost the singer more than is gained. The jury is still out on this, and the decision should be carefully reviewed with the singer and laryngologist.

There have been many advances in injection medialization over the past decade with more procedures being performed in office without general anesthesia and more options for injectable materials. Proponents of injection for glottal incompetence cite the flexibility to perform the procedure in the office or in the operating room. There are many different biocompatible materials to choose from, including fat, hyaluronic acid, acellular dermis, and calcium hydroxyapatite. Each has its own strength, whether being autologous, allowing for a medialization trial period, or offering a more extended therapeutic duration. Also, injection medialization allows for relatively fast access to both vocal folds to treat bilateral atrophy. Repeat injections are available to address further aging and atrophy changes. Disadvantages cited against injection are the inconsistent and often temporary results (Laccourreye et al., 2003; McCulloch et al., 2002).

Medialization laryngoplasty, or type 1 thyroplasty, is advocated as a permanent solution to patients with large to small glottal gaps not resolved with voice therapy. Acoustic and perceptual results were equal to or better than injection after medialization laryngoplasty even with treating a larger glottic gap (Dursun, Boynukalin, Ozgursoy, & Coruh, 2008). Advocates also remark on the intraoperative precision allowed during implantation as well as the ability to remove the implant at a later time if needed. Risks include up to a 30% revision rate with migration or further anatomical aging changes (Anderson, Spiegel, & Sataloff, 2003). With the placement of a foreign body, there is always the risk of extrusion or reaction. There clearly is opportunity in the literature for long-term outcomes research in the surgical treatment of the aging voice.

Hirano, Tateya, Kishimoto, Kanemaru, and Ito (2012) have been researching basic fibroblast growth factor (bFGF). They demonstrated that bFGF stimulates fibroblast production of hyaluronic acid and reduces collagen synthesis. Via intracordal injections, a group of 10 patients with a mean age of 70 years improved their maximum phonation time, noise-to-harmonic ratios, mean flow rate, and pitch and amplitude perturbation, and had improved glottal closure on videostroboscopy. Although further and larger study is needed, they concluded that bFGF has a strong regenerative effect on age-related atrophy of the vocal fold.

CASE STUDY

"Sandy" had just turned 80 when she came to our clinic. She was a highly trained singer with multiple degrees in voice and had been a voice teacher in a private studio for many years before retiring from teaching in her 60s. She formerly had a career as a classical soprano soloist, primarily in concert and recital, and as a paid soloist in church choirs. At the time of her initial evaluation, her vocal activities had tapered off quite a bit, but she was still engaged as a paid section leader and occasional soloist at her church. The choir rehearsed once per week for 2 hours and sang in services every Sunday, with intermittent services for special occasions. The choir typically took a hiatus in the summer for about 8 weeks. It was shortly after this hiatus that Sandy came to see us. She found that she was struggling to get through rehearsals and left feeling exhausted at the end. This decrease in vocal stamina was accompanied by increased vocal effort, particularly in her high range; unsteady vibrato; and intermittent voice breaks and cracks. She found it harder to sustain long phrases. "My breath support just gives out." She also noted a constant sensation of mucus and need to clear her throat. She was very alarmed by these symptoms, having never had any problems with her voice other than the occasional brief laryngitis associated with upper respiratory infections. At 80, singing was still central to her life, well-being, and self-image, and she was devastated by what had happened to her voice.

Videostroboscopy revealed remarkably healthy appearing vocal folds—certainly not the bowed and atrophic folds one might expect of a person of her age. It is likely that her long life of singing had helped keep presbylarynges at bay. However, there was a small amount of bilateral atrophy and sulcus vocalis resulting in intermittent tiny anterior glottic gapping and mild reduction in amplitude and extent of mucosal wave. Although subtle, this finding was certainly consistent with the changes she had noted. There was quite a bit of viscous mucus persistently clinging to her vocal folds, but no evidence of GERD.

In reviewing vocal hygiene history, Sandy admitted that she did not drink very much water and had about 16 ounces of caffeinated soda or coffee per day. The thick mucus and sensation of needing to clear her throat were likely related in part to poor hydration. However, she had overactive bladder and found it challenging to tolerate large volumes of fluid intake. During her rehabilitation therapy, we worked on increasing hydration very gradually and minimizing caffeine consumption to find a tolerable level of hydration for her. This ended up being about 24 to 32 ounces per day. We also targeted behavioral reduction of the chronic throat clearing. Over time, she reported that the sensation of mucus in her throat decreased.

Sandy had not been in the habit of exercising her voice much between rehearsals or over the summer hiatus—she had never found it necessary in the past as her voice had always been very reliable, even after taking extended vocal breaks. However, the slow attenuation of her singing activity had finally taken its toll.

The primary focus of intervention was reestablishing a daily vocal practice regimen for her. She said that it had been years since she had one. She typically ran through a few brief exercises prior to rehearsal and services but mostly warmed up with the choir. I asked her to recall the exercises she had done previously. Many were quite intricate agility exercises that spanned a fairly wide range. She noted that she found it difficult to execute these exercises fluidly and accurately now. We added a number of more structured exercises to the routine, including adductory power with messa di voce, glides, and less complex scales and arpeggios. We retained some of the more complex exercises—she liked them and they were very familiar to her, although they were now challenging. We worked on these more elaborate exercises using SOVT sounds such as lip trills and straw phonation to facilitate respiratory-phonatory motor coordination and help optimize vocal tract configuration. Exercises employing dotted rhythms and staccato (as described in Chapter 12 case studies) were incorporated to recalibrate and retrain agility. Rehabilitation exercises also targeted optimizing laryngeal stabilization through torso anchoring, specifically to steady vibrato.

We set an initial goal of 15 to 20 minutes of practice daily. She was highly motivated to improve her voice, but she said it was hard to be consistent in completing the exercises. This was in part a result of feeling frustrated and discouraged by her vocal quality. "I sound like a screechy old woman." She also said that she had always found vocalises somewhat tedious. Even in her prime, she had gravitated toward repertoire work in her practice time rather than exercises. It was necessary to repeatedly circle back to the connection between her goal of continuing to participate in singing activities, her expectation for high quality of singing, and commitment to the practice regimen. We continued to adapt the routine so that the rehabilitation exercises—which were essential for rebuilding vocal technique—were interspersed with brief periods of working on repertoire. We extracted phrases of familiar repertoire to use as vocalises singing them in various keys using SOVT sounds or vowels. Together, we arrived at a routine that both accomplished the rehabilitation goals and engaged her interest and commitment. She ultimately was able to consistently complete a routine 20 to 30 minutes in duration 4 to 5 days per week, in addition to her rehearsals and services.

In the meantime, we tackled the fatigue issue that was occurring after rehearsals and services. She typically engaged in quite a bit of social speaking surrounding these occasions. In fact, choir rehearsals and church services had, over the years, become one of her primary social environments and represented a significant portion of her social interactions. Aside from her church activities, there were sometimes days when she spoke very little.

To simply eliminate or even drastically reduce speaking in the context of her church choir could have had a negative impact on her quality of life and sense of social connection. Instead, we concentrated on establishing an exercise regimen for speaking voice and optimizing the speaking environment at church. We added a few minutes of structured resonant speaking exercises to her daily singing routine. In addition, on days when her social speaking would be minimal, she would engage in 10 to 15 minutes of reading aloud following her singing exercise. Much of the fatigue she experienced when speaking at church appeared to be related to the amount of competing background noise. She worked on minimizing the acoustic competition by making sure she was positioned close to her speaking partner at all times and by moving away from the crowd for longer conversations. If there was a social activity planned immediately after rehearsal or services, she took a short 5- to 10-minute voice break beforehand.

Sandy's had been a case of strategically reducing or modifying voice use in some situations, but increasing at other times to bring the overall picture of voice use into better balance. Although it took a while to establish this new routine, after about 4 months, she was feeling much better about her voice. She no longer felt fatigued in choir rehearsals and services and felt more confident. When the choir went on hiatus over the summer, the music director asked Sandy to participate in a series of afternoon concerts. This was an ideal development, as it provided motivation to continue her exercise routine and regular singing during the break. She also put together a program of music to perform at retirement communities. At 80, she had a level of vocal fitness that singers decades younger would envy.

REFERENCES

Abitbol, J., Abitbol, P., & Abitbol, B. (1999). Sex hormones and the female voice. *Journal of Voice, 13*, 424–446.

Anderson, T. D., Anderson, D. D., & Sataloff, R. T. (2006). Endocrine dysfunction. In R. T. Sataloff (Ed.), *Vocal health and pedagogy: Advanced assessment and treatment* (2nd ed.). San Diego, CA: Plural.

Anderson, T. D., Spiegel, J. R., & Sataloff, R. T. (2003). Thyroplasty revisions: Frequency and predictive factors. *Journal of Voice, 3*, 442–448.

Behlau, M., Hogikyan, N. D., & Gasparini, G. (2007). Quality of life and voice: Study of a Brazilian population using the voice-related quality of life measure. *Folia Phoniatrica et Logopaedica, 59*(6), 286–296.

Benjamin, B. J. (1981). Frequency in the aged voice. *Journal of Gerontology, 36*(6), 722–726.

Bloch, I., & Behrman, A. (2001). Quantitative analysis of videostroboscopic images in presbylarynges. *Laryngoscope, 111*, 2022–2027.

Bonilha, H. S., White, L., Kuckhahn, K., Gerlach, T. T., & Deliyski, D. D. (2012). Vocal fold mucus aggregation in persons with voice disorders. *Journal of Communication Disorders, 45*(4), 304–311.

Boulet, M. J., & Oddens, B. J. (1996). Female voice changes around and after the menopause—an initial investigation. *Maturitas, 23*(1), 15–21.

Calhoun, K. H., & Eibling, D. E. (2006). *Geriatric otolaryngology*. New York, NY: Taylor & Francis.

Canter, G. J. (1963). Speech characteristics of patients with Parkinson's disease: I. Intensity, pitch, and duration. *Journal of Speech and Hearing Disorders, 28*, 221–229.

Close, L. G., & Woodson, G. E. (1989). Common upper airway disorders in the elderly and their management. *Geriatrics, 44*, 67–68, 71–72.

Cohen, S. M. (2010). Vocal fold injection as a treatment for glottic insufficiency: Con. *Archives of Otolaryngology-Head and Neck Surgery, 136*(8), 827–828.

Cohen, S. M., & Turley, R. (2009). Coprevalence and impact of dysphonia and hearing loss in the elderly. *Laryngoscope, 119*, 1870–1873.

Cooper, C., Fielding, R., Visser, M., van Loon, J., Rolland, Y., Orwoll, E., . . . Kanis, J. A. (2013). Tools in the assessment of sarcopenia. *Calcified Tissue International, 93*(3), 201–210.

Cruz-Jentoft, A. J., Baeyens, J. P., Bauer, J. M., Boirie, Y., Cederholm, T., Landi, F., . . . Zamboni, M. (2010). Sarcopenia: European consensus on definition and diagnosis: Report of the European Working Group on Sarcopenia in Older People. *Age and Ageing, 39*, 412–423.

Deane, K. H., Whurr, R., Playford, E. D., Ben-Shlomo, Y., & Clarke, C. E. (2001). A comparison of speech and language therapy techniques for dysarthria in Parkinson's disease. *Cochrane Database of Systematic Reviews, 2*, CD002814.

D'Haeseleer, E., Depypere, H., Claeys, S., Van Borsel, J., & Van Lierde, K. (2009). The menopause and the female larynx, clinical aspects and therapeutic options: A literature review. *Maturitas, 64*(1), 27–32.

D'Haeseleer, E., Depypere, H., Claeys, S., Wuyts, F. L., De Ley, S., & Van Lierde, K. M. (2011). The impact of menopause on vocal quality. *Menopause, 18*, 267–272.

Dursun, G., Boynukalin, S., Ozgursoy, O. B., & Coruh, I. (2008). Long-term results of different treatment modalities for glottic insufficiency. *American Journal of Otolaryngology, 29*(1), 7–12.

Firat, Y., Engin-Ustun,Y., Kizilay, A., Ustun, Y., Akarcay, M., Selimoglu, E., & Kafkasli, A. (2009). Effect of intranasal estrogen on vocal quality. *Journal of Voice, 23*(6), 716–720.

Gama, A. C., Alves, C. F., Cerceau, J. S. B., & Teixeira, L. C. (2009). Correlation between acoustic-perceptual data and voice-related quality of life in elderly women. *Prò Fono, 21*(2), 125–130.

Godoy, J. F., Brasolotto, A. G., Berretin-Felix, G., & Fernandes, A. Y. (2014). Neuroradiology and voice findings in stroke. *CoDAS, 26*, 168–174.

Golub, J. S., Chen, P. H., Otto, K. J., Hapner, E., & Johns, M. M., III. (2006). Prevalence of perceived dysphonia in a geriatric population. *Journal of the American Geriatrics Society, 54*, 1736–1739.

Gray, S. D., Titze, I. R., Chan, R., & Hammond, T. H. (1999).Vocal fold proteoglycans and their influence on biomechanics. *Laryngoscope, 109*(6), 845–854.

Gregory, N. D., Chandran, S., Lurie, D., & Sataloff, R. T. (2012). Voice disorders in the elderly. *Journal of Voice, 26*, 254–258.

Hagen, P., Lyons, G. D., & Nuss, D. W. (1996). Dysphonia in the elderly: Diagnosis and management of age-related voice changes. *Southern Medical Journal, 89*(2), 204–207.

Harnsberger, J. D., Shrivastav, R., Brown, W. S., Jr., Rothman, H., & Hollien, H. (2008). Speaking rate and fundamental frequency as speech cues to perceived age. *Journal of Voice, 22*(1), 58–69.

Hirano, S., Tateya, I., Kishimoto, Y., Kanemaru, S., & Ito, J. (2012). Clinical trial of regeneration of aged vocal folds with growth factor therapy. *Laryngoscope, 122*(2), 327–331.

Hoffman, H. T., Karnell, L. H., Funk, G. F., Robinson, R. A., & Menck, H. R. (1998). The National Cancer Data Base report on cancer of the head and neck. *Archives of Otolaryngology-Head and Neck Surgery, 124*(9), 951–962.

Hollien, H., & Shipp, T. (1972). Speaking fundamental frequency and chronologic age in males. *Journal of Speech, Language, and Hearing Research, 15*(1), 155–159.

Honjo, I., & Isshiki, N. (1980). Laryngoscopic and voice characteristics of aged persons. *Archives of Otolaryngology-Head and Neck Surgery, 106*, 149–150.

Hopkins, C., Yousaf, U., & Pedersen, M. (2006). Acid reflux treatment for hoarseness. *Cochrane Database of Systematic Reviews*, 1, CD005054.

Hsiao, T. Y., Liu, C. M., & Lin, K N. (2002). Videostrobolaryngoscopy of mucus layer during vocal fold vibration in patients with laryngeal tension-fatigue syndrome. *Annals of Otololaryngology, Rhinology, and Laryngology, 111*(6), 537–541.

Huber, J. E. (2008). Effects of utterance length and vocal loudness on speech breathing in older adults. *Respiratory Physiology & Neurobiology, 164*(3), 323–330.

Iwarsson, J., Thomasson, M., & Sundberg, J. (1998). Effects of lung volume on the glottal voice source. *Journal of Voice, 12*, 424–433.

Kandogan, T., Olgun, L., & Gultekin, G. (2003). Causes of dysphonia in patients above 60 years of age. *Kulak Burun Bogaz Ihtis Derg, 11*(5), 139–143.

Kendall, K. (2007). Presbyphonia: A review. *Current Opinion in Otolaryngology & Head and Neck Surgery, 15*(3), 137–140.

Kotby, M. N., Hassan, O., El-Makhzangy, A. M., Farahat, M., & Milad, P. (2010). Gastroesophageal reflux/laryngopharyngeal reflux disease: A critical analysis of the literature. *European Archives of Oto-Rhino-Laryngology, 267*(2), 171–179.

Laccourreye, O., Papon, J. F., Kania, R., Crevier-Buchman, L., Brasnu, D., & Hans, S. (2003). Intracordal injection of autologous fat in patients with unilateral laryngeal nerve paralysis: Long-term results from the patient's perspective. *Laryngoscope, 113*(3), 541–545.

Lexell, J., Henriksson-Larsen, K., Winblad, B., & Sjostrom, M. (1983). Distribution of different fiber types in human skeletal muscles: Effects of aging studied in whole muscle cross sections. *Muscle & Nerve, 6*, 588–595.

Lindholm, P., Vilkman, E., Raudaskoski, T., Suvanto-Luukkonen, E., & Kauppila, A. (1997). The effect of postmenopause and postmenopausal HRT on measured voice values and vocal symptoms. *Maturitas, 28*(1), 47–53.

Lundy, D. S., Silva, C., Casiano, R. R., Lu, F. L., & Xue, J. W. (1998). Cause of hoarseness in elderly patients. *Otolaryngology-Head and Neck Surgery, 118*(4), 481–485.

Madruga de Melo, E. C., Lemos, M., Aragao Ximenes Filho, J., Sennes, L. U., Nascimento Saldiva, P. H., & Tsuji, D. H. (2003). Distribution of collagen in the lamina propria of the human vocal fold. *Laryngoscope, 113*, 2187–2191.

Martins, R. H., Gonzalvez, T. M., Pessin, A. B., & Branco, A. (2014). Aging voice: Presbyphonia. *Aging Clinical and Experimental Research, 26*(1), 1–5.

Mau, T., Jacobson, B. H., & Garrett, C. G. (2010). Factors associated with voice therapy outcomes in the treatment of presbyphonia. *Laryngoscope, 120*, 1181–1187.

McCulloch, T. M., Andrews, B. T., Hoffman, H. T., Graham, S. M., Karnell, M. P., & Minnick, C. (2002). Long-term follow-up of fat injection laryngoplasty for unilateral vocal cord paralysis. *Laryngoscope, 112*(7, Pt. 1), 1235–1238.

Mirza, N., Ruiz, C., Baum, E. D., & Staab, J. P. (2003). The prevalence of major psychiatric pathologies in patients with voice disorders. *Ear, Nose, & Throat Journal, 82*(10), 808–810.

Morrison, M. D., & Gore-Hickman, P. (1986). Voice disorders in the elderly. *Journal of Otolaryngology, 15*, 231–234.

Nemr, N. K., Simoes-Zenari, M., Ferreira, T. S., Fernandes, H. R., & Mansur, L. L. (2013). Dysphonia as the primary complaint in a case of myasthenia gravis: Diagnosis and speech therapy. *CoDAS, 25*, 297–300.

Pedersen, M., Beranova, A., & Moller, S. (2004). Dysphonia: medical treatment and a medical voice hygiene advice approach: A prospective randomised pilot study. *European Archives of Oto-Rhino-Laryngology*, 261(6), 312–315.

Portone, C. R., Hapner, E. R., McGregor, L., Otto, K., & Johns, M. M., III. (2007). Correlation of the Voice Handicap Index (VHI) and the Voice-Related Quality of Life Measure (V-RQOL). *Journal of Voice, 21*(6), 723–727.

Pontes, P., Brasolotto, A., & Behlau, M. (2005). Glottic characteristics and voice complaint in the elderly. *Journal of Voice, 19*, 84–94.

Prakup, B. (2012). Acoustic measures of the voices of older singers and nonsingers. *Journal of Voice, 26*(3), 341–350.

Raj, A., Gupta, B., Chowdhury, A., & Chadha, S. (2010). A study of voice changes in various phases of menstrual cycle and in postmenopausal women. *Journal of Voice, 24*, 363–368.

Ramig, L. A., & Ringel, R. L. (1983). Effects of physiological aging on selected acoustic characteristics of voice. *Journal of Speech, Language, and Hearing Research, 26*(1), 22–30.

Romak, J. J., Orbelo, D. M., Maragos, N. E., & Ekbom, D. C. (2014). Correlation of the Voice Handicap Index-10 (VHI-10) and Voice-Related Quality of Life (V-RQOL) in patients with dysphonia. *Journal of Voice, 28*(2), 237–240.

Rosen, C. A., & Statham, M. M. (2010). Vocal fold injection as a treatment for glottic insufficiency: Pro. *Archives of Otolaryngology-Head and Neck Surgery, 136*(8), 825–827.

Roy, N., Stemple, J., Merrill, R. M., & Thomas, L. (2007). Epidemiology of voice disorders in the elderly: Preliminary findings. *Laryngoscope, 117*, 628–633.

Sataloff, R. T., Rosen, D. C., Hawkshaw, M., & Spiegel, J. R. (1997). The aging adult voice. *Journal of Voice, 11*(2), 156–160.

Sato, K., & Hirano, M. (1997). Age-related changes of elastic fibers in the superficial layer of the lamina propria of vocal folds. *Annals of Otolaryngology, Rhinology, and Laryngology, 106*, 44–48.

Sato, K., Hirano, M., & Nakashima, T. (2002). Age-related changes of collagenous fibers in the human vocal fold mucosa. *Annals of Otolaryngology, Rhinology, and Laryngology, 111*(1), 15–20.

Schwartz, S. R., Cohen, S. M., Dailey, S. H., Rosenfeld, R. M., Deutsch, E. S., Gillespie, M. B., . . . Patel, M. M. (2009). Clinical practice guideline: Hoarseness (dysphonia). *Otolaryngology-Head and Neck Surgery, 141*(3, Suppl. 2), S1–S31.

Spataro, E. A., Grindler, D. J., & Paniello, R. C. (2014). Etiology and time to presentation of unilateral vocal fold paralysis. *Otolaryngology-Head and Neck Surgery, 151*(2), 286–293.

Stemple, J. C., Lee, L., D'Amico, B., & Pickup, B. (1994). Efficacy of vocal function exercises as a method of improving voice production. *Journal of Voice, 8*(3), 271–278.

Strand, E. A., Buder, E. H., Yorkston, K. M., & Ramig, L. O. (1994). Differential phonatory characteristics of four women with amyotrophic lateral sclerosis. *Journal of Voice, 8*, 327–339.

Thomas, L. B., Harrison, A. L., & Stemple, J. C. (2008). Aging thyroarytenoid and limb skeletal muscle: Lessons in contrast. *Journal of Voice, 22*, 430–450.

Titze, I. R., Story, B. H., Burnett, G. C., Holzrichter, J. F., Ng, L. C., & Lea, W. A. (2000). Comparison between electroglottography and electromagnetic glottography. *Journal of the Acoustical Society of America, 107*(1), 581–588.

Titze, I., & Verdolini Abbott, K. (2012). *Vocology: The science and practice of voice habilitation.* Salt Lake City, UT: National Center for Voice and Speech.

Tobey, N. A., Hosseini, S. S., Caymaz-Bor, C., Wyatt, H. R., Orlando, G. S., & Orlando, R. C. (2001). The role of pepsin in acid injury to esophageal epithelium. *American Journal of Gastroenterology, 96*(11), 3062–3070.

Valeo, T. (2010). The voice lift: Should vocal fold surgery be considered a cosmetic procedure? *ENT Today*. Retrieved March 30, 2015, from http://www.enttoday.org/article/the-voice-lift-should-vocal-fold-surgery-be-considered-a-cosmetic-procedure/

Verdonck-de Leeuw, I. M., & Mahieu, H. F. (2004). Vocal aging and the impact on daily life: A longitudinal study. *Journal of Voice*, *18*(2), 193–202.

Wilcox, K. A., & Horii, Y. (1980). Age and changes in vocal jitter. *Journal of Gerontology*, *35*(2), 194–198.

Winkler, R., & Sendlmeier, W. (2006). EGG open quotient in aging voices—changes with increasing chronological age and its perception. *Logopedics Phoniatrics Vocology*, *31*, 51–56.

Woo, P., Casper, J., Colton, R., & Brewer, D. (1992). Dysphonia in the aging: Physiology versus disease. *Laryngoscope*, *102*, 139–144.

Xue, S. A., & Hao, G. J. (2003). Changes in the human vocal tract due to aging and the acoustic correlates of speech production: A pilot study. *Journal of Speech, Language, and Hearing Research*, *46*(3), 689–701.

Zeitels, S. M., Casiano, R. R., Gardner, G. M., Hogikyan, N. D., Koufman, J. A., & Rosen, C. A. (2002). Management of common voice problems: Committee report. *Otolaryngology-Head and Neck Surgery*, *126*, 333–348.

Ziegler, A., Verdolini Abbott, K., Johns, M., Klein, A., & Hapner, E. R. (2014). Preliminary data on two voice therapy interventions in the treatment of presbyphonia. *Laryngoscope*, *124*(8), 1869–1876.

CHAPTER 18

What the Singing Voice Rehabilitation Specialist Should Know About Sound Equipment

Matthew Edwards

Contemporary commercial music (CCM) relies heavily on audio technology. Athletic styles of singing, including CCM, are often associated with vocal pathology but that does not necessarily need to be the case. Because of our constant exposure to amplified singing, many performers attempt to reproduce electronically created qualities with their acoustic voice. Attempting to do so places singers at greater risk for vocal injury. This chapter will help you understand the basics of audio enhancement, how audio equipment can alter the audio spectrum of a singer's voice, how the equipment can be used to protect the health of singers, and how to use audio technology in singing voice rehabilitation. In order to understand how to manipulate the audio spectrum of a singer's voice, you should first review a few basics of sound.

THE FUNDAMENTALS OF SOUND

Frequency

Sound travels in waves of compression and rarefaction within a medium, which for our purposes is air (Figure 18–1). The waves travel through the air around us, into our inner ears via the ear canal, and are converted to nerve impulses that are transmitted to the brain and interpreted as sound. The number of waves per second is measured in hertz (Hz), which is a measurement of the frequency of sound that we perceive as pitch. For example, we hear 440 Hz (440 vibrations per second) as the pitch A above middle C (McCoy, 2004).

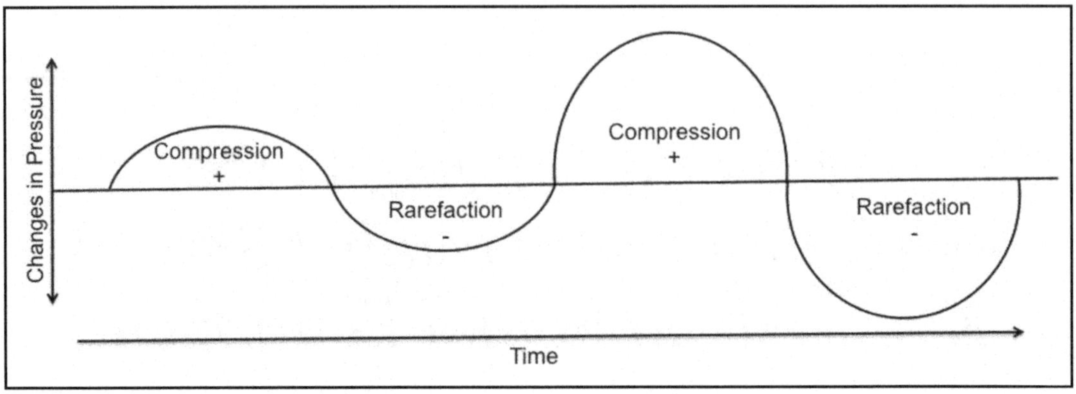

***Figure 18–1.** Waves of compression and rarefaction are pictured above. The further the wave travels from the center line, the louder the sound will be.*

Amplitude

The magnitude of the waves of compression and rarefaction from the centerline (silence) determines the amplitude of sound that we hear as volume (see Figure 18–1), measured in decibels (dB). The larger the waves of compression and rarefaction, the louder we perceive a sound to be (McCoy, 2004).

Harmonics

As mentioned above, in order to create the pitch A above middle C, we must create 440 vibrations per second in the air surrounding us. If an instrument produced a note with the fundamental frequency alone, the sound would be strident and mechanical like the emergency alert signal used on television. Musical sounds and most sounds found in nature consist of multiple simultaneous frequencies. While producing the fundamental, the vibrating mechanism simultaneously produces a series of frequencies above the fundamental called overtones. For our purposes, the overtones we are interested in are called harmonics. Harmonics are whole-number multiples of the fundamental frequency. For example, if the fundamental is 220 Hz, the harmonic overtone series would be 220 Hz, 440 Hz (fundamental frequency times two), 660 Hz (fundamental frequency times three), 880 Hz (fundamental frequency times four), and so on. Every musical note contains both the fundamental frequency and a predictable series of harmonic overtones, each of which can be measured and identified as a particular frequency. This series of frequencies then travels through a resonator; for a singer, the throat and mouth (McCoy, 2004; Nair, 1999).

Resonance

As the harmonics created by the vocal folds travel through the vocal tract, some are amplified and some are attenuated depending on the vocal tract's shape. The alterations that occur to the harmonics as they pass through the vocal tract enable us to distinguish vowel sounds and timbre. We can analyze these changes with a tool called a spectral analyzer as seen in Figure 18–2 (McCoy, 2004; Nair, 1999).

The display produced by the spectral analyzer shows us what is called the spectral envelope. The peaks and valleys from left to right indicate amplitude variations (vertical axis) of the corresponding overtones (horizontal axis). The difference in spectral envelope between instruments is what enables us to aurally distinguish the difference between a violin and a trumpet playing the same note. Differences in spectral envelope also account for two different singers sounding recognizably different when they are singing the same pitch (McCoy, 2004) (Figure 18–3).

In acoustic singing, the throat and mouth act as the resonating tube, and by changing their shape, the singer is able to make adjustments to timbre. In electronically amplified singing, the sound engineer can make electronic adjustments to amplify or reduce specific frequency ranges, thus altering a performer's timbre. To better understand how audio engineers can enhance a singer's voice, let us take a look at the components of the signal chain.

SIGNAL CHAIN

The signal chain or signal path is the course an audio signal travels from the input to the output of a sound system.

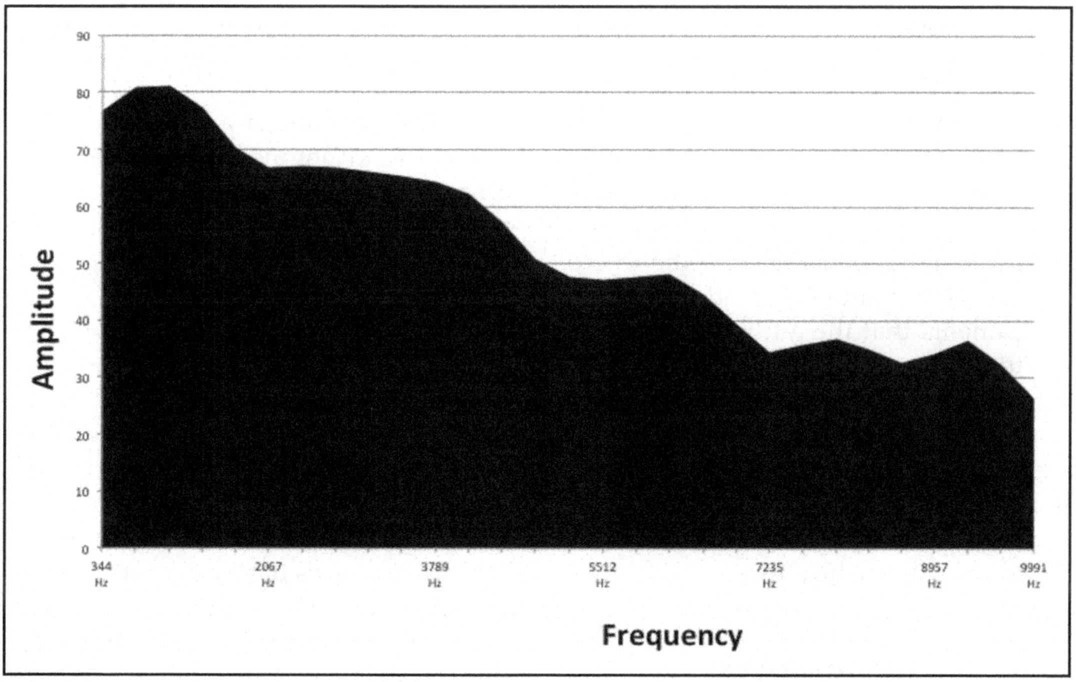

Figure 18–2. *The figure above shows the output of a spectral analyzer. This type of display is called a power spectrum.*

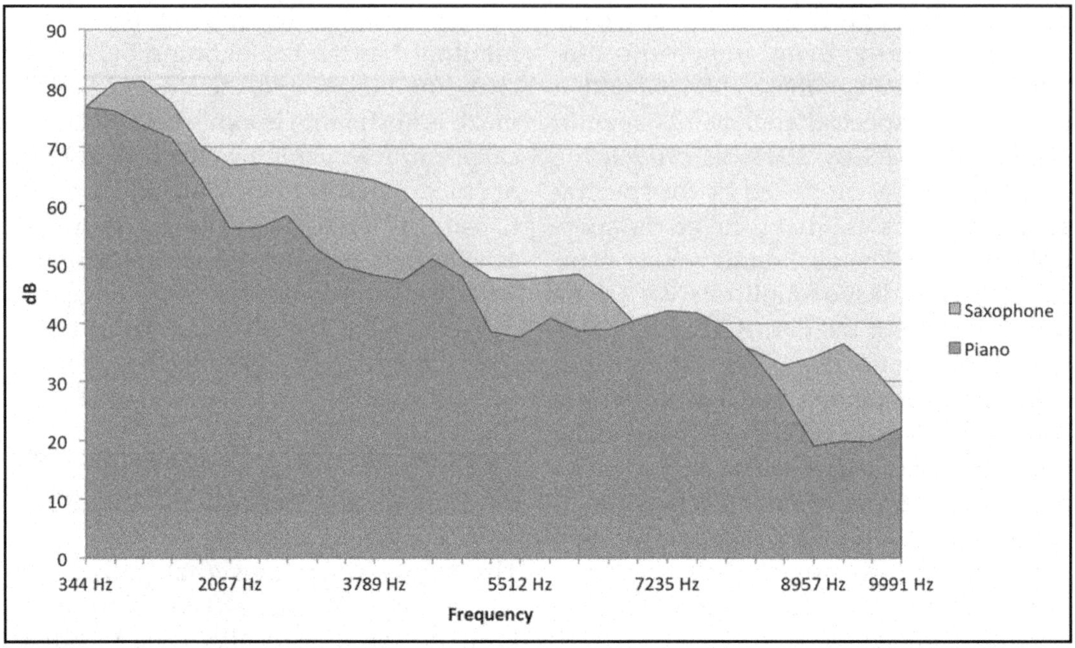

***Figure 18–3.** The figure above shows two instruments playing the same pitch. The peak at the far left is the fundamental frequency and the peaks to the right are harmonics that have been amplified and attenuated by the instruments' resonator resulting in a specific timbre.*

A voice enters the signal chain through the input (the microphone), which transforms the acoustic energy of the voice into a corresponding electrical signal. The electrical signal generated by the microphone is transmitted through a series of components that the audio engineer can use to enhance and/or modify the signal before the speakers transform it back into acoustic energy. Although some engineers strive to replicate the original sound source as accurately as possible, others use the capabilities of the system to alter the sound for artistic effect.

Microphones

Microphones transform the acoustic sound waves of the voice into electrical impulses that can be enhanced and/or amplified by the sound engineer. The three most common microphone types singers will encounter are dynamic, condenser, and electret condenser.

Dynamic

Dynamic microphones consist of a dome-shaped Mylar diaphragm attached to a free-moving copper wire coil that is positioned between two poles of a magnet (Campbell & Greated, 1987). The Mylar diaphragm moves in response to air pressure changes caused by sound waves. When the diaphragm moves, the magnetic coil that is attached to it also moves. As the magnetic coil moves up and down between the magnetic poles, it produces an electrical current that corresponds to the sound waves produced by the singer's voice. That signal is then sent to the soundboard via the microphone cable (Figure 18–4).

Condenser

Condenser microphones are constructed with two parallel plates: a rigid posterior plate and a thin flexible anterior plate. The anterior plate is constructed of either a thin sheet of metal or a piece of Mylar that is coated with a conductive metal. The plates are separated by air, which acts as a layer of insulation. In order to use a condenser microphone, it must be connected to a soundboard that supplies "phantom power" (Figure 18–5). A component of the soundboard, phantom power sends a 48-volt power supply through the microphone cable to the microphone's plates. When the plates are charged by the phantom power, they form a capacitor. As acoustic vibrations send the anterior plate into motion, the distance between the two plates varies, which causes the capacitor to release a small electric current. This current, which corresponds with the acoustic signal of the voice, travels through the microphone cable to the soundboard where it can be enhanced and amplified (Benson, 1988; Campbell & Greated, 1987; Turner & Gibilisco, 1985) (see Figure 18–5).

Electret Condenser

Electret condenser microphones are similar to condenser microphones, but they are designed to work without phantom power. The anterior plate of an electret microphone is made of a plastic film coated with a conductive metal that is electrically charged before being set into place opposite the posterior plate. The charge applied to the anterior plate will

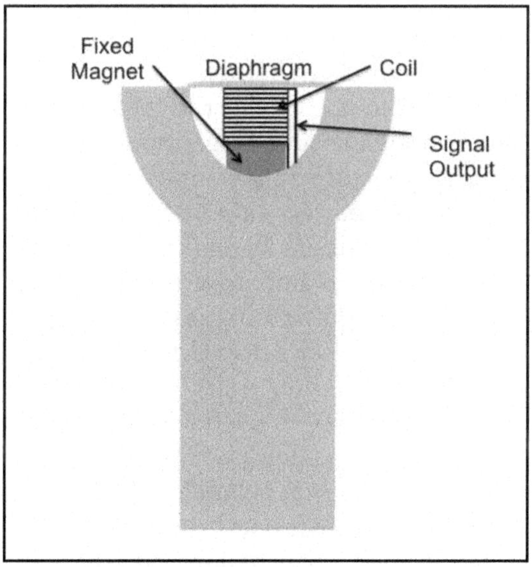

***Figure 18–4.** The basic design of a dynamic microphone.*

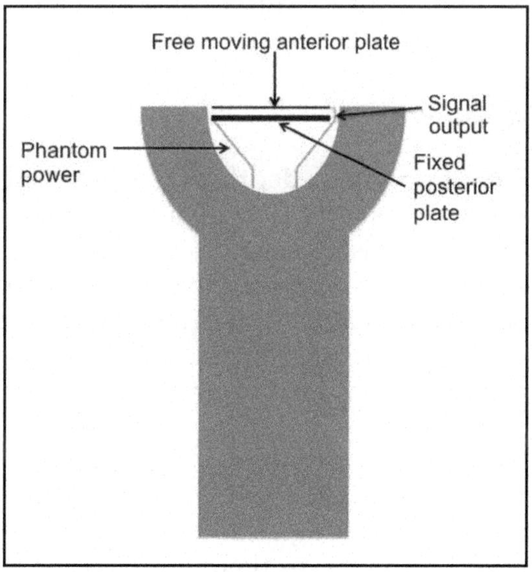

***Figure 18–5.** The basic design of a condenser microphone.*

last for 10 or more years and therefore eliminates the need for an exterior power source (Benson, 1988). Electret condenser microphones are often used in head-mounted and lapel microphones, laptop computers, and smartphones.

Dynamic Versus Condenser

Dynamic microphones are most commonly used in live performance because their lower sensitivity rejects excess stage noise. Recording engineers often prefer using condenser microphones for recording applications due to their high level of sensitivity. You will occasionally find condenser microphones in some live performance venues for genres that do not have excessive stage noise—for example, handheld microphones used by jazz and folk artists and head-mounted microphones used in musical theater.

Although diaphragm type should be your first consideration, there are several other factors you need to consider when selecting a microphone, including sensitivity, polar pattern, and frequency response.

Sensitivity

Providing an in-depth explanation of sensitivity is difficult without going into additional discussions of electricity and electrical terminology. However, a simplified explanation should suffice for our purposes. In the simplest terms, sensitivity describes how responsive a microphone is to the amplitude of the source. For instance, compare a dog's ears to a child's ears. A dog can hear a squirrel running through the back yard while a child cannot. We therefore describe a dog's ears as more sensitive than a child's. Microphones with higher sensitivity can be placed farther from the sound source without adding excessive noise to the signal. Microphones with lower sensitivity will need to be placed closer to the sound source in order to keep excess noise at a minimum. When shopping for a microphone, you should audition several options plugged into the same soundboard with the same volume level settings. As you sing on each microphone, you will notice that some microphones replicate your voice louder than others do. This change in output level is due to differences in each microphone's sensitivity. If your voice is naturally loud, you may prefer a microphone with lower sensitivity (one that requires more acoustic energy to respond). If you have a lighter voice, you may prefer a microphone with higher sensitivity (one that responds well to softer signals).

Amplitude Response

The amplitude response of a microphone describes how sensitive it is to sound arriving from various angles. The amplitude response will vary depending on the angle at which the singer is positioned in relation to the axis of the microphone. Microphone manufacturers publish polar pattern diagrams (also sometimes called a directional pattern or a pickup pattern), to help consumers visualize the amplitude response of a microphone at various angles. Polar pattern diagrams consist of six concentric circles divided into 12 equal sections. The center point of the microphone's diaphragm is labeled "0°" and is referred to as "on-axis" while the opposite side of the diagram is labeled "180°" and is described as "off-axis."

Although polar pattern diagrams are printed in two dimensions (Figure 18–6), they actually represent a three-dimensional response to acoustic energy. Think of a

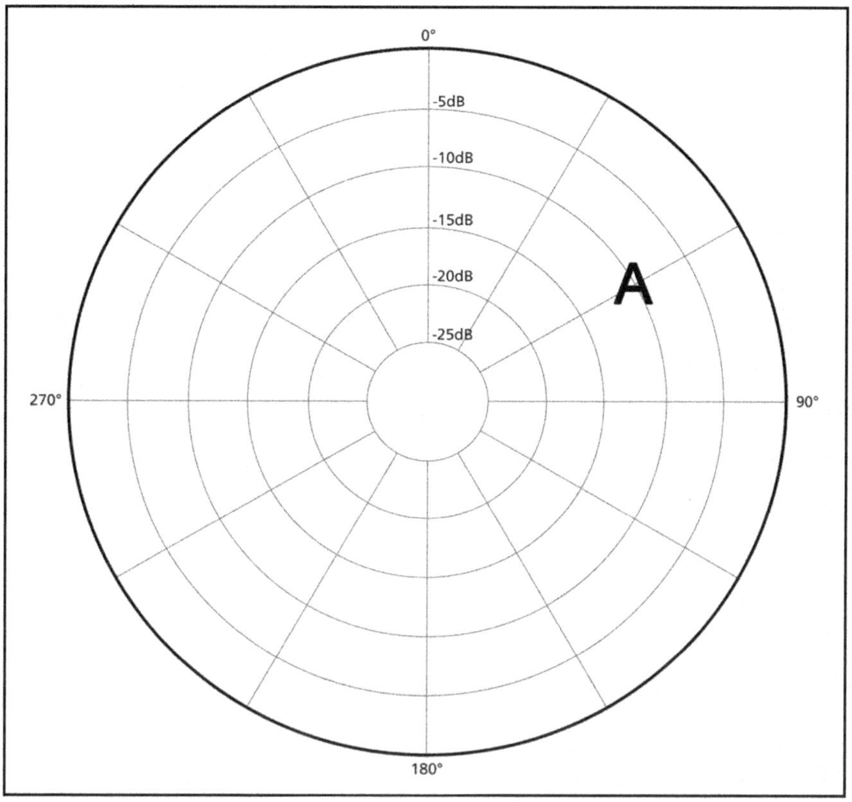

***Figure 18–6.** An example of a microphone polar pattern diagram. Reproduced under Creative Commons, © Galak76. https://en.wikipedia.org/wiki/Microphone#/media/File:Polar_pattern_omnidirectional.png*

round balloon as a real-life polar pattern diagram. Position the tied end away from your mouth and the inflated end directly in front of your lips. In this position, you are singing on-axis at 0° with the tied end of the balloon being 180°, or off-axis. If you were to split the balloon in half vertically and horizontally (in relationship to your lips), the point at which those lines intersect would be the center point of the balloon. That imaginary center represents the diaphragm of the microphone. If you were to extend a 45° angle in any direction from the imaginary center and then drew a circle around the inside of the balloon following that angle, you would have a visualization of the three-dimensional application of the two-dimensional polar pattern drawing.

The outermost circle of the diagram indicates that the amplitude of the instrument or voice is transferred without any amplitude reduction, indicated in decibels (dB). Each of the inner circles represents a −5-dB reduction in the amplitude of the signal up to −25 dB. For example, look at Figure 18–6. If the microphone's response curve crossed point A on this diagram, we would know that the strength of the signal received by the microphone at that point would be reduced by 10 dB. The following examples (Figures 18–7, 18–8, and 18–9) show the most common polar patterns that you will encounter.

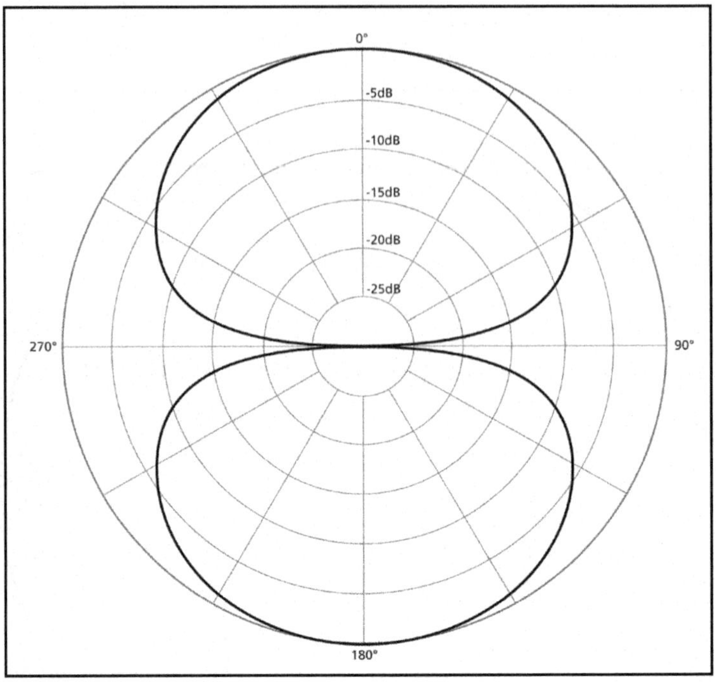

A

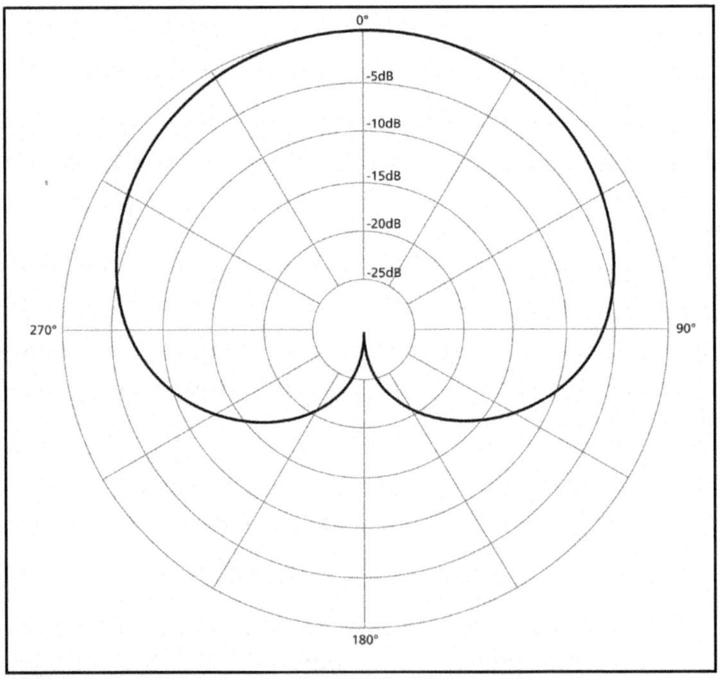

B

Figure 18–7. *A. Represents a bidirectional pattern. B. Represents a cardioid pattern. Reproduced under Creative Commons, © Galak76. https://en.wikipedia.org/wiki/Microphone#/media/File:Polar_pattern_figure_eight.png and https://en.wikipedia.org/wiki/Microphone#/media/File:Polar_pattern_cardioid.png*

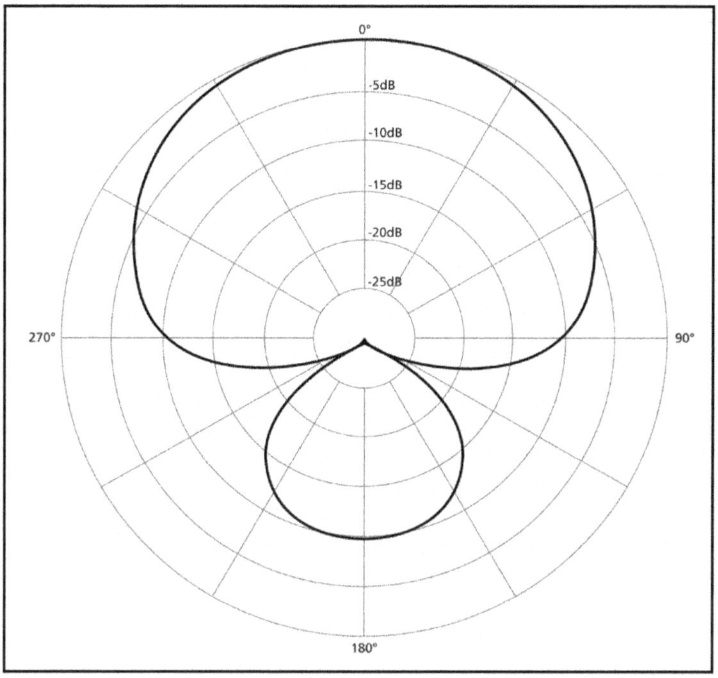

A

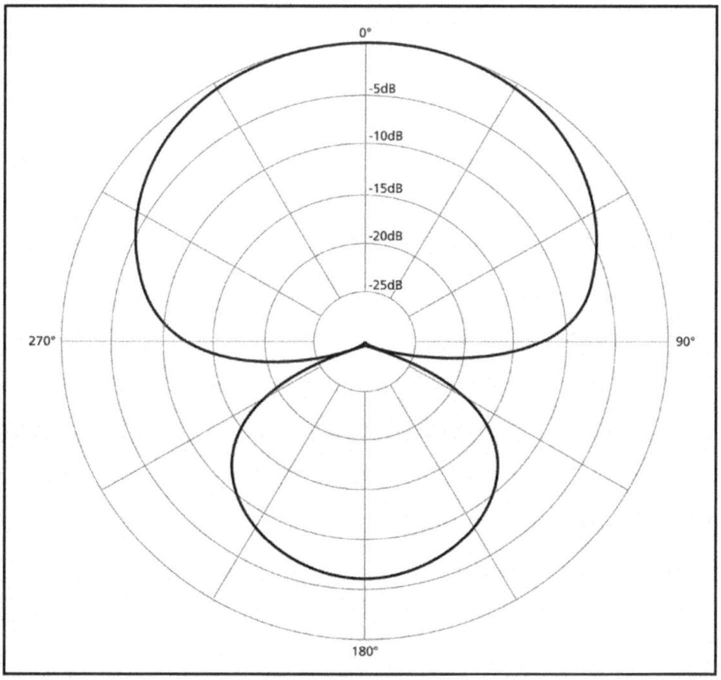

B

Figure 18–8. ***A.*** *Represents a supercardioid pattern.* ***B.*** *Represents a hypercardioid pattern. Reproduced under Creative Commons, © Galak76. https://en.wikipedia.org/wiki/Microphone#/media/File:Polar_pattern_supercardioid.png and https://upload.wikimedia.org/wikipedia/commons/\8/80/Polar_pattern_hypercardioid.png*

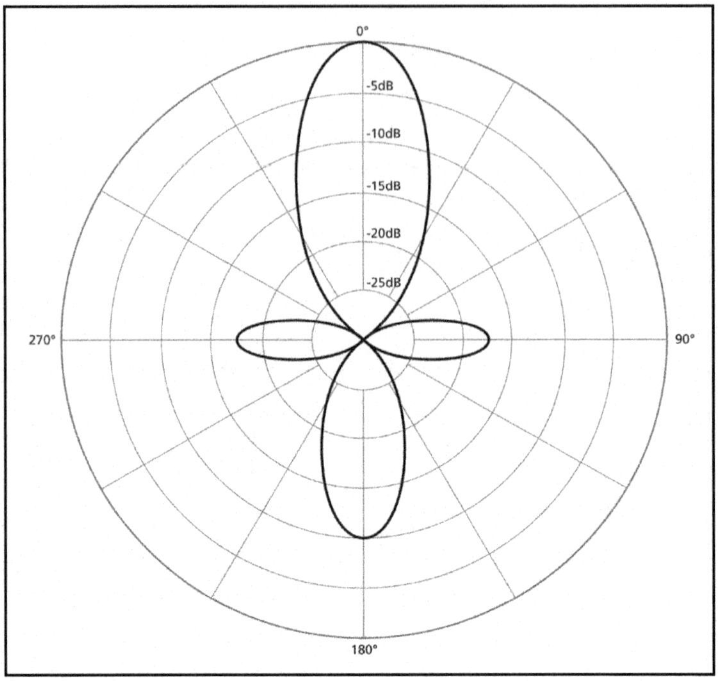

A

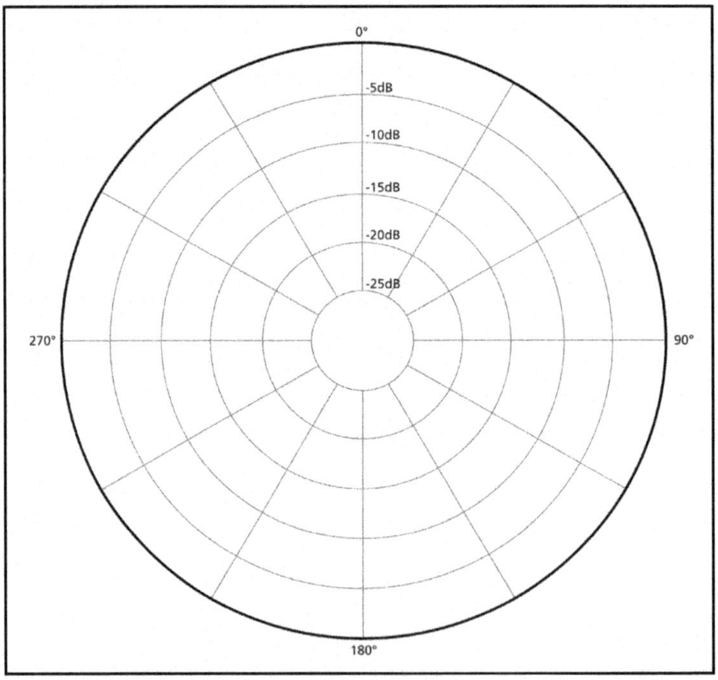

B

Figure 18–9.* A. *Represents a shotgun pattern.* B. *Represents an omnidirectional pattern. Reproduced under Creative Commons, © Galak76. https://en.wikipedia.org/wiki/Microphone#/media/File:Polar_pattern_directional.png and https://upload.wikimedia.org/wikipedia/commons/8/8d/Polar_pattern_omnidirectional.png

Implications for the Singer

Picking the right polar pattern can help alleviate problems with feedback and excess room noise. If you are performing with a floor monitor, a cardioid microphone is the best option. Since cardioid microphones have virtually no amplitude response from the posterior of the diaphragm, they will have only minimal response to the monitor. In some situations, such as recording a classical singer in a recital hall, you may want the microphone to respond to acoustic energy from more than one direction in order to capture the natural reverberation of the room. In that situation, a bidirectional or omnidirectional microphone is the better choice.

Frequency Response

Frequency response is a term used to define how accurately a microphone captures the audio spectrum of the acoustic signal. A "flat response" microphone captures the acoustic output with little to no alteration of the audio spectrum. Microphones that are not designated as "flat" have some type of attenuation or boost across one or more bands of frequencies within the audio spectrum.

When using a microphone with a polar pattern other than omnidirectional (a pattern that responds to sound equally from all directions), the user may encounter frequency response fluctuations in addition to amplitude fluctuations. Cardioid microphones in particular are known for their tendency to boost lower frequencies at close proximity to the sound source while attenuating those same frequencies as the distance between the sound source and the microphone increases. This is known as the "proximity effect."

Let us compare the frequency response curves of two microphones, the Shure SM-58 and the Oktava 319. The Shure SM-58 microphone attenuates or "cuts" the frequencies below 300 Hz and amplifies or "boosts" the frequencies in the 3-kHz range by 6 dB, the 5-kHz range by nearly 8 dB, and the 10-kHz range by approximately 6 dB (Figure 18–10). The Oktava 319 microphone cuts the frequencies below 200 Hz while boosting everything above 300 Hz with nearly 5 dB between 7 kHz and 10 kHz (see Figure 18–10). In practical terms, recording a bass singer with the Shure SM-58 would drastically reduce the amplitude of the fundamental frequency with a strong amplitude peak in the singer's formant zone. In contrast, the Oktava 319 would produce a slightly more consistent boost in the range of the singer's formant without reducing the amplitude of the lower frequencies. Either of these options could be acceptable depending on your needs, but the frequency response must be considered before making the recording.

Implications for the Singer

The frequency response of a microphone can significantly alter the balance of forward placement and fundamental of a singer's voice (called the singing power ratio). If a microphone significantly boosts the amplitude of the forward placement zone, it will alter the singing power ratio, thus altering our perception of the singer's voice. If a singer is struggling to find a reliable technical approach for boosting the upper frequencies of his or her voice, a microphone that boosts those frequencies could be beneficial. However, if a singer has an abundance of acoustic power in the upper frequencies of his or her voice, a microphone that boosts those frequencies

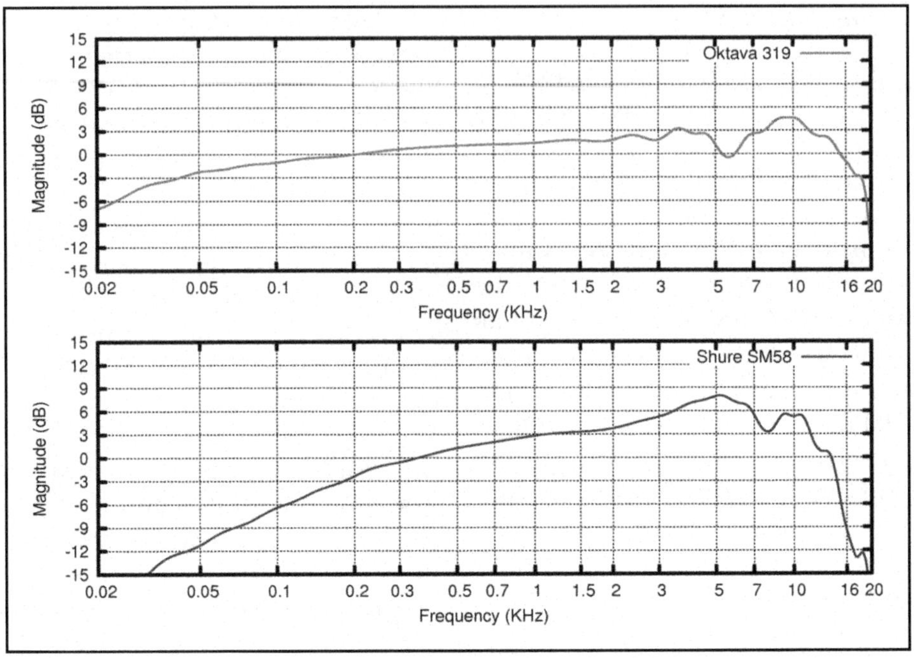

Figure 18–10. *Example frequency response graphs for the Oktava 319 and the Shure SM58. Reproduced under Creative Commons. https://commons.wikimedia .org/wiki/File:Oktava319vsshuresm58.png*

could artificially alter the singing power ratio in a manner that would cause the voice to be perceived as overly bright and perhaps harsh (Omori, Kacker, Carroll, Riley, & Blaugrund, 1996).

Singers should take the time to audition numerous microphones to see which one best complements their voice. Set several microphones in a row with the same settings at the soundboard and sing the same excerpt on each microphone. If possible, make a recording and listen for changes in the timbre from microphone to microphone.

MICROPHONE TECHNIQUE

Just as there are techniques that improve singing, there are also techniques that will improve microphone use. Understanding what a microphone does is only the first step to using it successfully.

Practicing With a Microphone

The best way to learn microphone technique is to practice with a microphone. Using a dynamic microphone, try the following:

- Position the microphone directly in front of your mouth, no further than 1 cm away. Sustain a comfortable pitch and slowly move the microphone away from your lips. Listen to how the sound quality changes. When the microphone is close to your lips, you should notice that the sound is louder and has more bass response. As you move away from the mic, there will be a noticeable loss in volume and the tone will become brighter.

- Next, try sustaining a pitch while rotating the handle down. You should notice that the sound quality changes in a similar fashion as when you moved the microphone away from your lips.
- Now try singing breathy with the microphone close to your lips. How little effort can you get away with and still sound good?
- Try singing bright, at a medium volume level, with a closed mouth and spread lips with the microphone placed approximately 1 to 3 cm from your mouth. In this position, you should be able to create aggressive sounds without over-singing.
- Next, cup both of your hands around the microphone and then sing into your hands. Try using a vocal fry in this position and experiment with death metal–style sounds. You should notice that the cupping of your hands increases the bass response and helps boost your vocal power without excess effort.
- Also, experiment with variations in your diction. Because the microphone amplifies everything, you may need to under-pronounce some consonants when singing on a microphone.

SIGNAL PROCESSING

Once the acoustic energy of the voice has been converted to an electrical signal by the microphone, the audio engineer can enhance the voice using various types of processing equipment. The components most commonly used by singers are equalization, reverb, delay, compression, and auto-tune.

Equalization (EQ)

Equalizers enable the audio engineer to alter the audio spectrum of the source in order to change the timbre of the instrument or singer. Equalizers come in three main types: shelf, parametric, and graphic.

Shelf

Shelf equalizers cut or boost the uppermost and lowermost frequencies of an audio signal (Figure 18–11). Although this type of equalization is not very useful for fine-tuning a singer's vocal quality, it can be very effective in removing room noise. For example, if an air conditioner creates a 60-Hz hum in the recording studio, the shelf can be set at 65 Hz. This setting eliminates frequencies below 65 Hz and effectively removes the hum from the vocal signal.

Parametric

Parametric units adjust a band of frequencies of the audio spectrum that fall within a defined width. The engineer selects a center frequency and adjusts the width of the bell curve surrounding that frequency by adjusting the "Q" (Figure 18–12). The engineer then boosts or cuts the frequencies within the bell curve to alter the audio spectrum.

Graphic

Graphic equalizers allow engineers to identify a specific frequency for boost or

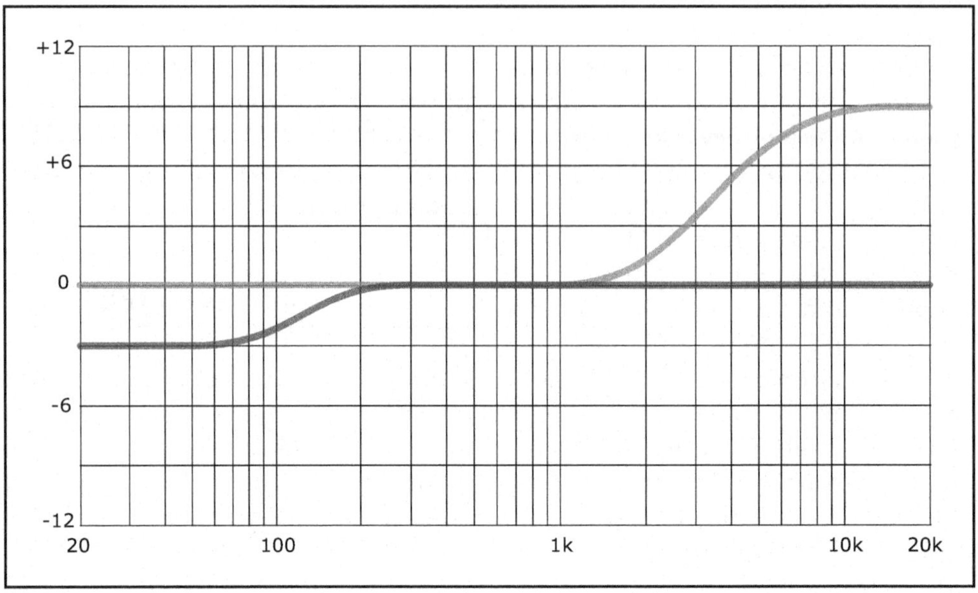

Figure 18–11. *The frequency amplitude curves above show the affect of applying a shelf EQ to an audio signal. Reproduced under Public Domain. https://en.wikipedia.org/wiki/Equalization_(audio)#/media/File:Shelving-eq.svg*

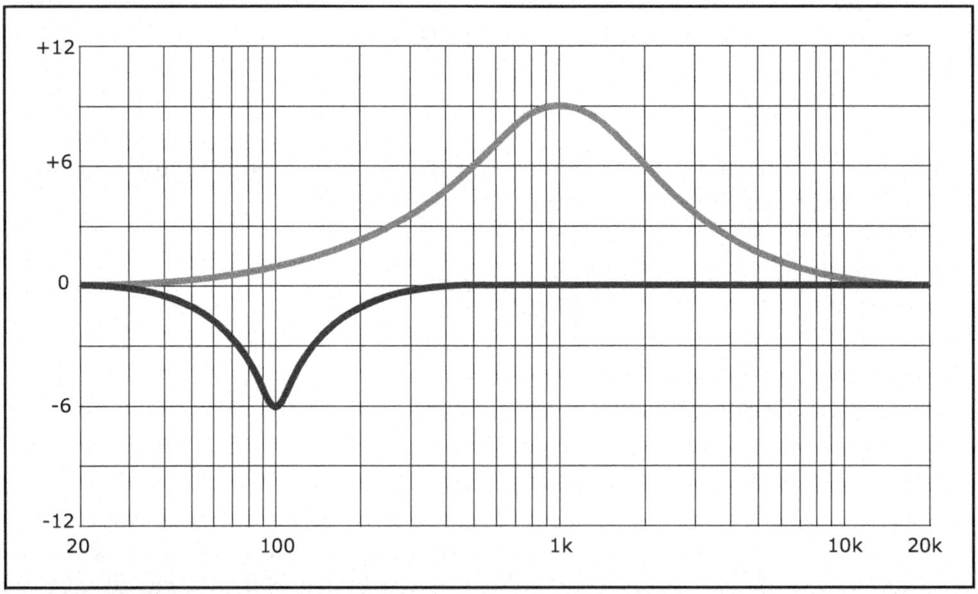

Figure 18–12. *The frequency amplitude curves above display two parametric EQ settings. The top curve represents a boost of +8 dB set at 1 kHz with a relatively large bell curve—a low Q. The lower curve represents a high Q set at 100 Hz with an attenuation of -6 dB. Reproduced under Public Domain. https://upload.wikimedia.org/wikipedia/commons/c/c6/Peaking-eq.svg*

cut with a fixed frequency bandwidth. A 10-band equalizer enables the audio engineer to adjust 10 specific frequencies, which typically include (in Hz): 31, 63, 125, 250, 500, 1k, 2k, 4k, 8k, and 16k (Figure 18–13). Graphic equalizers are often one of the final elements of the signal chain preceding only the amplifier and speakers. In this position, they can be used to adjust the overall sound quality of the entire mix.

Implications for the Singer

Equalization can be used in many different ways. When striving to replicate the natural timbre of the voice, you should audition several microphones and try to find an option that requires minimal equalization. If you are unable to find a suitable microphone, equalization adjustments can be used to compensate for the microphone's frequency response curve. If you would like to purposely alter the timbre of the voice, equalization is the best place to start. For example, if a singer's voice lacks forward placement, you could add power to the forward placement zone by boosting those frequencies with the equalizer. If a singer is sick and the natural ring of his or her voice is missing, you can use equalization to compensate. In both of these situations, equalization can be used to help a singer achieve the results he or she desires without resorting to constriction.

Compression

CCM singers often perform songs that feature extremes in both frequency and amplitude. Extreme variations in amplitude can prove problematic for the audio engineer who is usually attempting to maintain a balance between multiple instruments and/or voices. If the dynamic range is too extreme, engineers will often use compression to reduce amplitude fluctuations. Compressors limit the output of a sound source by a specified ratio. The user sets the maximum acceptable amplitude level for the output before compression, called the "threshold." The user then sets a ratio to reduce the output once it surpasses the threshold. The typical ratio for a singer is usually between 3:1 and 5:1. A 3:1 ratio indicates that for every 3 dB beyond the threshold level, the output will only increase by 1 dB. For

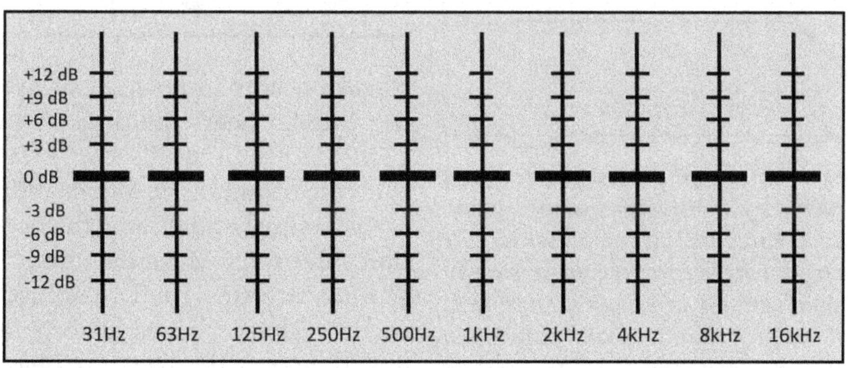

Figure 18–13. *The basic design of a 10-band graphic equalizer.*

example, if the singer went 21 dB beyond the threshold with a 3:1 ratio, the output would only be 7 dB beyond the threshold level (Figure 18–14).

Multiband Compression

If a standard compressor causes unacceptable alterations to the singer's timbre, engineers can use a multiband compressor. Rather than compressing the entire spectrum of sound, multiband compressors allow the engineer to isolate a specific frequency range within the audio signal and then set an individual compression setting for that frequency range. For example, if a singer creates a dramatic boost in the 4-kHz range every time that he or she sings above an A4, a multiband compressor can be used to limit the amplitude of the frequencies in only that part of the voice. By setting a 3:1 ratio in the 4-kHz range at a threshold that corresponds to the amplitude peaks that appear when the performer sings above A4, the engineer can eliminate vocal "ring" from the signal on only the offending notes while leaving the rest of the frequencies untouched. Multiband compressors are available for both live and studio use and can be a great alternative to compressing the entire signal.

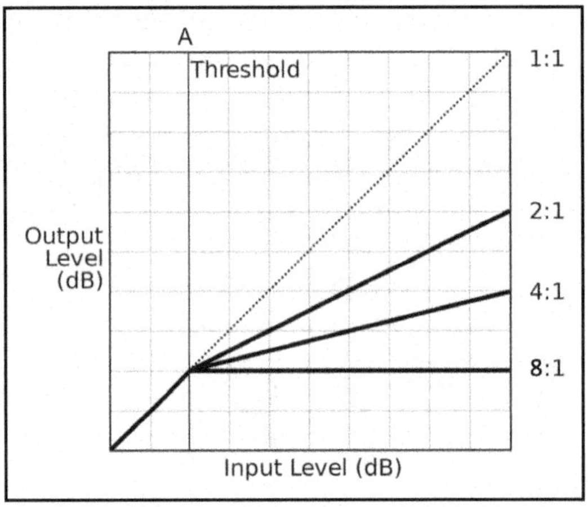

***Figure 18–14.** This graph represents the effects of various compression ratios applied to a signal. The 1:1 angle represents no compression. The other ratios represent the effect of compression on an input signal with the threshold set at line A. Reproduced under Public Domain. https://en.wikipedia.org/wiki/Dynamic_range_compression#/media/File:Compression_ratio.svg*

Implications for the Singer

Experienced artists will usually prefer microphone technique to compression. However, for inexperienced performers, those who sing aggressive styles such as rock, and those who move around a lot on stage, compression can be quite beneficial. Compression is also beneficial for those performers who sing in styles that exploit register breaks, flipping back and forth between chest and head voice. Without compression, there will be noticeable changes in dynamics as the singer flips over the break. However, with the right compression settings, the transition between chest and head will appear to be seamless.

Reverb

Reverb occurs in an acoustic space when the listener hears the direct signal of the voice and then, milliseconds later, hears the voice again as it reflects off the sidewalls, ceiling, and floor of the performance hall. Many CCM venues and recording studios are designed to inhibit natural reverb. These spaces absorb reflections and therefore the listeners hear only the direct signal of the voice. When performing in a venue that lacks natural reverb, even the best singer can sound harsh and amateurish. In such a space, reverb can significantly improve the quality of a performance.

Early reverb units transmitted the audio signal from the microphone through a metal spring or plate, which added supplementary vibrations to the sound. Although some engineers still use spring or plate reverb to obtain a specific effect, most now use digital units. Common settings on digital reverb units include wet/dry, bright/dark, and options for delay time. The wet/dry control adjusts the amount of direct signal (dry) and the amount of reverberated signal (wet). The bright/dark control helps simulate the effects of various surfaces within a natural space. For instance, harder surfaces such as stone reflect high frequencies and create a brighter tone quality while softer surfaces such as wood reflect lower frequencies and create a darker tone quality. The delay time, which is usually adjustable from milliseconds to seconds, adjusts the amount of time between when the dry signal and wet signal reach the ear. By adjusting these settings, engineers can transform almost any room into a chamber music hall or concert stadium.

Delay

Whereas reverb blends the wet and dry signals together to replicate a natural space, delay purposefully separates the two signals. With delay, you will hear the original signal first and then a digitally produced repeat of the signal several milliseconds to seconds later. The delayed signal may be heard one time or multiple times, and the timing of those repeats can be adjusted to match the tempo of the song.

Auto-Tune

Auto-tune was initially created by Antares Audio Technologies to clean up minor imperfections in otherwise perfect performances. It has now become an industry standard that many artists use, even if they are not willing to admit it (WENN.com, 2012). Although the name "auto-tune" seems to suggest that the process is completely automated, there are actually two ways that it can be applied, "auto" and "graphical." "Auto" auto-tune allows the engineer to set specific parameters for pitch correction that are then computer controlled. "Graphical" auto-tune tracks the pitch in the selected area of a recording and plots the fundamental frequency on a linear graph. The engineer can then select specific notes for pitch correction. The user can also drag selected pitches to a different frequency, add or reduce vibrato, and change formant frequencies above the fundamental. To simplify, the "auto" function makes general corrections while the "graphic" function makes specific corrections. The "auto" setting is usually used to achieve a specific effect (e.g., "I Believe" by Cher), while the "graphic" setting is used to correct small imperfections in a recorded performance.

Implications for the Singer

There are many factors that can cause a singer to struggle with pitch in the recording studio. Performers who are not accustomed to singing with headphones may experience difficulty singing accurately. Some singers find it helpful to remove one of the earphones while recording; others find it helpful to remove the vocal signal from their headphones. Another common factor that leads to unnecessary use of auto-tune is the signer's inability to stay in rhythm. Recording singers is like placing them under a microscope. Small rhythmic inaccuracies that are imperceptible in live performance can become quite obvious on a recording. Sometimes these rhythmic inaccuracies can lead singers to sustain notes beyond harmonic changes in the accompaniment. When this happens, they will often lose the center of the pitch. Another common problem is the use of vibrato. Although the pitch variations of vibrato are rarely noticed in live performance, on a recording, they can become quite obvious. Singers preparing to record in the studio should practice singing with straight tone. Learning to straight tone is especially helpful if the performer is planning on singing his or her own background harmonies.

Digital Voice Processors

Digital voice processors contain software that allows performers to duplicate the effects they used while recording their album during live performance. Although there are several brands of vocal effects processors available, the industry leader as of this printing is a company called TC-Helicon. TC-Helicon manufactures several different units that span from consumer to professional grade. TC-Helicon's premier performer controlled unit is called the VoiceLive 3. The VoiceLive 3 incorporates over 12 vocal effects, 11 guitar effects, and a multitrack looper with 250 factory presets and 250 memory slots for user presets. Onboard vocal effects include equalization, compression, reverb, and "auto" auto-tune. The unit also offers μMod (an adjustable voice modulator), a doubler (for thickening the lead vocal), echo, delay, reverb, and several other specialized effects (VoiceLive 3, 2014).

Monitors

Arguably the element most important to a singer in a live sound system, the monitor is simply a speaker that faces a performer. On-stage volume levels can vary considerably, with drummers often producing sound levels as high as 120 dB. Those volume levels make it nearly impossible for singers to receive acoustic auditory feedback while performing. Monitors improve aural feedback and help reduce the temptation to over-sing. Powered monitors have a built-in amplifier, which makes them convenient for use at home and when practicing with their band. Because powered monitors are lightweight and easy to transport, it can be beneficial for beginner and amateur artists to take a powered monitor with them to gigs in case the venue does not provide a monitor system. Professional and semiprofessional artists are likely to encounter in-ear monitors. In-ear monitor systems enable performers to receive their monitor feed through headphones, allowing them to move freely around the stage while maintaining their aural feedback.

THE IDEAL SETUP FOR THE SINGING VOICE SPECIALIST

If you are working with CCM singers on a regular basis, a small amplification system should be part of your studio. It is not necessary to purchase an elaborate setup; one that can amplify a single voice and guitar will be enough to instruct clients on the proper usage of audio equipment. For a microphone, I suggest the Shure SM-58. The SM-58 is a dynamic microphone with low sensitivity and is the most commonly used microphone in live performance venues. A powered monitor is a great option for providing amplification. Powered monitors can either be placed upright at ear level in the manner of a PA system, or they can be placed on the ground in monitor position. This enables you to give clients both experiences with one speaker. For low-cost options, I would suggest you research the products manufactured by Behringer, Peavey, and Yamaha.

In order to add digital effects, you will want to purchase a digital voice processor. I recommend the TC Helicon Voice Live Touch 2 or the TC Helicon Voice Live Play Acoustic. These are similar to the VoiceLive 3 but easier to use for those who are not planning on using the unit in live performances on a regular basis. Both units allow the user to connect a microphone and a guitar and both include presets that enable the user to easily add popular effects combinations to the vocals and are easy to operate.

TYPES OF CLIENTS

There are four types of clients you will encounter in your work with CCM singers: beginners, amateurs, semi-professionals, and professionals. Clients from each level will have unique needs and goals.

Beginners

Beginners are often still trying to find their own voice, are performing minimally, and lack formal voice training. Many of them do not own any audio equipment and may be rehearsing without amplification. When evaluating beginners, ask them how they rehearse to see if that is perhaps where troubles may be arising. If they do not understand how to use a microphone or a monitor, encourage them to purchase their own equipment and teach them how to use it.

Amateurs

Amateurs are slightly more advanced. They are beginning to perform more regularly and are often performing in venues that have minimal equipment or require the performers to bring their own. Depending on the stage of their career, they may or may not have begun recording.

If they work with you before recording, you have the opportunity to prevent future problems. Teach your client to sing with a metronome/click track and teach them to practice singing notes and rhythms accurately. This may help eliminate the need for auto-tune. Also encourage them to make informed decisions about what they lay down on record. Although a higher key may seem exciting in the heat of the moment, if they record a song in a key that is higher than they can comfortably sing on tour, they are setting themselves up for future trouble.

If they have already recorded, ask them about the recording process. How many days did they spend in the studio recording vocals? Did they do a lot of double tracking (recording a vocal multiple times and combining those tracks to make the voice appear larger than life)? Do they know what effects they used? Then try to determine if they are feeling pressure to produce the same results they captured in the studio during live performance. If it becomes apparent that they used extensive vocal effects in the studio, encourage them to purchase a digital effects processor and help them learn to use the system to their advantage.

Semi-Professionals

Semi-professionals are performing in venues with an experienced sound engineer or have their own engineer that works with them on a regular basis. They have usually already recorded and are accustomed to singing in venues with varying levels of audio feedback. Problems with this population are less likely due to improper use of audio technology. However, it is possible that they have recorded tracks with techniques that cannot be reproduced live without the proper equipment. If you suspect this may be the problem, talk with them about their recording process and how they are duplicating the recording studio effects during live performance. Be sure to have them sing both on and off microphone during their sessions.

Professionals

Professionals have achieved a level of success that allows them to tour with an expert engineer who has an in-depth knowledge of audio technology. Therefore, they are able to rely on that expert and focus solely on their performance. These performers usually require the least amount of coaching when it comes to using audio technology. However, as you are teaching them new techniques, you will want to work with them on a microphone, as well as acoustically, to make sure they like the results of the work you are doing with them. In some instances, hearing loss or poor auditory feedback may be causing the performer to over-sing. If you suspect that is the case, encourage them to talk with their sound engineer and ask for adjustments to the volume and equalization of their voice in the monitors. Boosting the frequencies in the forward placement zone can improve auditory feedback and reduce the urge to push.

EXAMPLE EXERCISES

Exercise 1

Problem: Singers often rely on raw vocal power instead of using the microphone as part of their instrument and allowing it to add the power they desire.

Objective: To teach performers the minimum effort level that they can successfully perform with and what that effort level will sound like off-microphone.

Method: Have the singers perform a song using a microphone and ask them to use as little effort as possible. Adjust the volume level of the amplifier to the performers' liking. This is an important step. You are trying to get them to reduce the volume level of their voice and to compensate for their reduction in power by boosting their volume with the sound system. Next, let them begin singing with amplification for 15 to 30 seconds. After they appear comfortable, turn the volume of the sound system all the way down or use the mute button if your system has one. Have them continue singing without amplification for 5 to 10 seconds and then turn the volume back up or unmute the system. Keep alternating between using amplification and muting the amplification for the duration of the song. Stop and ask them for feedback. Hopefully they will have noticed that they were able to sing with less effort and still attain a result that they were pleased with. Repeat this exercise several times until they begin to default toward singing at a lower volume level. It is not necessary for them to sing softly all of the time, but this can be a good exercise for those who tend to push. It can also be helpful for them to know how to back off and rely on the microphone when they are sick or fatigued.

Exercise 2

Problem: When singers struggle to hear themselves through the monitors, they will often over-sing.

Objective: To teach singers to adapt to various levels of auditory feedback while learning to resist the urge to push.

Method: Ask the singers to bring an instrumental track to their session. Play the instrumental track through the monitor and ask them to sing along with the track. While they sing, adjust the levels of the instrumental track and the voice until you find an acceptable balance between the two. Return to the beginning of the song and have them perform with the track. After 10 to 15 seconds, turn down their microphone and observe how they react. If needed, coach them to resist the urge to push. Bring the volume level of the vocals back to the level you began with, allow the singer to get comfortable, and then turn the vocals down again. Continue to alter the volume level of the vocals throughout the song. Next, go back to the beginning of the song and start with the optimal balance of the backing track and vocals. As the singers begin to perform, turn down the volume level of the backing track. Monitor their pitch accuracy and vocal effort. Coach them to listen for the instruments that provide the harmony and to focus on accuracy and ease of vocal production. Turn the backing track back up for a few seconds and then take the volume level down again. Repeat throughout the song. Discuss the experience of both variables and repeat the exercise(s) as needed.

Exercise 3

Problem: Rock singers often desire an "edgy" or "metallic" vocal quality that matches the timbre of an electric guitar. To produce those qualities, singers will often resort to vocal constriction. Although this will often produce the desired quality, it also puts singers at risk for vocal pathology.

Objective: To teach vowel modification coupled with microphone placement to reduce pushing in rock styles.

Method: Have the singers sustain a neutral /a/ vowel on a single pitch. Beginning with the microphone touching the lips, slowly pull the microphone away while listening to how the tone quality of the amplified signal changes. Using the SM-58, singers will notice that the microphone will make their voice sound fuller when up close and thinner the farther away the microphone is from the mouth. Next, place the microphone around 1 cm from the lips and sustain a neutral /a/ vowel. While sustaining the /a/ vowel, have the singers spread their lips into a smile position with their front teeth about 1 to 2 cm apart. Return to a neutral /a/ and bring the lips forward into a puckered position while allowing the jaw to drop. The singers should notice that in the smile position, the tone will get brighter and edgier and when the lips are brought forward the tone will get warmer. Next have them sing a section of a song or a vocal exercise in the smile position with the microphone 1 cm from their mouth. Coach them to adjust their mouth position as needed to help them take advantage of the boost in the upper harmonics produced by the SM-58's unique frequency response coupled with smile position resonance. If needed, slightly boost the treble using the equalizer. Discuss the results and see if there is a way to incorporate these ideas to reduce constriction in their songs.

Exercise 4

Problem: Many singers desire a breathy quality, but they often produce it through constriction. Because microphones are extremely sensitive to fluctuations in airflow, singers can take advantage of the microphone to produce a breathy quality without constriction.

Objective: To teach healthy breathy singing.

Method: Have the singers place a straw between their lips and blow air through the straw. Have them place one of their hands approximately 2 to 3 cm away from the end of the straw so that they can monitor their airflow. Next ask the singers to sustain an /o/ vowel through the straw. Coach them to produce the vowel with steady airflow and a breathy quality. You want to encourage transglottal airflow and head-mix/thin fold dominant vocal production. Repeat the sustained /o/ vowel and remove the straw after 3 to 4 seconds. Next try to produce the breathy /o/ without the straw. Finally, place the singers on a microphone so that they can hear the final product that is created when they increase transglottal airflow. When they feel comfortable on vowels, progress to songs.

CONCLUSION

It is normal for readers to be overwhelmed by all of the technical information associated with audio technology. Since this is primarily an overview, seek other resources to increase your understanding of these technical elements. Many great explanations are available online and can help clarify some of these difficult concepts. Check out your local library as well for books about audio recording or live sound. SoundOnSound.com and MixOnline.com both offer free articles detailing the recording process of famous artists as well as the live performance effects used by touring artists. Most important —experiment. The more you play around with equipment on your own, the better you will understand it.

REFERENCES

Benson, K. B. (1988). *Audio engineering handbook.* New York, NY: McGraw-Hill.

Campbell, M., & Greated, C. (1987). *The musician's guide to acoustics.* New York, NY: Schirmer Books.

McCoy, S. (2004). *Your voice: An inside view.* Princeton, NJ: Inside View.

Nair, G. (1999). *Voice-tradition and technology: A state-of-the-art studio.* San Diego, CA: Singular.

Omori, K., Kacker, A., Carroll, L. M., Riley, W. D., & Blaugrund, S. M. (1996). Singing power ratio: Quantitative evaluation of singing voice quality. *Journal of Voice, 10*(3), 228–235. Retrieved from http://www.ncbi.nlm.nih.gov/pubmed/8865093

Turner, R. P., & Gibilisco, S. (1985). *The illustrated dictionary of electronics* (3rd ed.). Blue Ridge Summit, PA: TAB Books.

VoiceLive3. (2014). Retrieved February 1, 2014, from http://www.tc-helicon.com/products/voicelive-3/

WENN.com. (July 4, 2012). Bieber admits studio vocal help. *Toronto Sun*. Toronto. Retrieved July 6, 2012, from http://www.torontosun.com/2012/07/04/bieber-admits-studio-vocal-help

CHAPTER 19

Using Apps in Voice Rehabilitation

Caroline Warren Banka

This discussion of apps for voice rehabilitation will cover general uses for apps in voice rehabilitation along with examples of several currently available apps. Although this information should be utilized in accordance with scope of practice (e.g., speaking voice therapy should be undertaken by professionals with the appropriate qualifications), much of what is included here will be useful for singing voice rehabilitation in any setting. Since this is a rapidly changing market, some of the apps discussed in this text may no longer be available after this is published, and there may be other new apps cherished by every clinician. At present, there are very few apps specifically designed for voice therapy, and few designed by speech-language pathologists (SLPs), so SLPs and singing voice rehabilitation specialists need to "think outside the box" and use apps designed for other purposes. When you are evaluating apps on your own, it may be helpful to review the voice literature, search app clearinghouses such as Happtique (http://www.happtique.com), search app stores, and review the app descriptions, user ratings, and reviews. In addition, conduct a social media query in your professional group. As you pilot the app, solicit feedback from your patients. Because there are currently no comprehensive clearinghouses for apps, it is impossible to canvas all current apps on all platforms. Therefore, this review focuses on the Apple operating system (iOS) but includes a few apps for the Android operating system where no comparable app was found for iOS.

There are many questions about the efficacy of using mobile apps to promote health. Research on these issues is in the early stages and is hampered by the constant proliferation of new apps and platforms. Here are just a few areas in question: Does having health information actually lead to behavior change? Do apps increase self-efficacy, thereby supporting behavior change? How accurate is self-monitoring of behavior, and how can this be improved? How do older people respond to apps, and how can apps be adapted to better meet their needs? What is the optimal way to deliver feedback and reminders to enhance learning and retention of the desired behavior? Can gamification make current voice apps more fun and motivating? Are there drawbacks to becoming dependent on apps to provide us information about ourselves when we might be better served by cultivating mindful awareness instead? In addition, questions about security of data will have to be addressed if protected health information from apps is transferred between the SLP or singing voice rehabilitation specialist and the patient or client (Boudreaux et al., 2014; Boulos, Brewer, Karimkhani, Buller, & Dellavalle, 2014; Dennison, Morrison, Conway, & Yardley, 2013; Payne, Lister, West, & Bernhardt, 2015; Van Stan, 2014; Zapata, Fernandez-Aleman, Idri, & Toval, 2015).

Despite the many questions yet to be fully addressed, the use of apps is widespread. SLPs and singing voice rehabilitation specialists should be familiar with ways in which apps can support voice rehabilitation and specific apps that provide the most benefit. Adherence to voice rehabilitation is challenging, and apps can encourage singers to practice outside the clinic if they have voice exercises on their phones. In the clinical setting, patients frequently report two obstacles to success in voice therapy: difficulty replicating the desired behavior without the SLP model present, and trouble remembering to practice (Van Leer, 2013). SLPs and singing voice rehabilitation specialists can use apps to address both of these obstacles, using apps for voice education, voice analysis, monitoring volume and pitch, recording voice samples for exercises, and using text to speech for voice rest, practice reminders, vocal hygiene trackers, and more.

VOICE EDUCATION (ANATOMY)

There are a number of apps with graphics and animations that can supplement text-based voice education. Although these apps do not contain the detailed information about diagnoses, surgical procedures, or voice therapy approaches that we typically include in our printed patient education handouts in the clinical setting, these graphics and animations help patients or clients understand complex laryngeal anatomy. Larynx ID (iOS $4.99, Blue Tree Publishing) has simple schematic drawings of the larynx from various views. It can display muscles and nerves, and it has animations and a drawing function. Vocal Folds ID (iOS $2.99, Blue Tree Publishing) focuses on the vocal folds alone, with animations and a drawing function. Respiratory Anatomy Atlas (iOS $0.99, Visible Body) has good illustrations of the respiratory support for the voice, but drawings of the larynx and vocal folds lack detail. It has some animations of rest breathing, but none for vocal fold vibration. drawMD ENT (available on iPad only; free) is an excellent tool with ability to draw on the illustrations. Draw! (Android, free) is a simple drawing tool without pictures.

iVoiceTherapy has an extensive voice education section, including laryngovideostroboscopic exams, ear training for perceptual evaluation, and detailed text explanations covering vocal hygiene and postoperative voice recommendations (see full discussion under iVoiceTherapy). However, it does not have the ability to draw on the images. Even without downloading an app, patients can use the video function on their smartphones to record their videostroboscopy exam. With their exam on their phone, they can review it and, if desired, play it to explain their diagnosis to family and friends.

VOICE ANALYSIS

SLPs may be skeptical of many apps on the market that claim to do voice analysis. As Van Leer (2013) points out, the problem with voice analysis apps is based on the fact that voice science has been slow to develop reliable acoustic measures of voice quality, even for desktop software programs. Voices that are too dysphonic can't be measured accurately because of problems with pitch tracking, and accurate acoustic measures of natural, connected speech (as opposed to sustained vowels) is also challenging. So the clinical utility of many standard desktop tools is lacking.

Another problem particular to voice analysis apps on mobile devices is the quality of the microphone combined with inconsistent placement of the speaker's mouth from the microphone. The average person may be less aware of the need for consistent microphone to mouth distance and consistent volume of voice for accurate measures over time. In the hands of untrained users, these apps may be less accurate than if used in the clinic by the SLP. With those caveats in mind, there are many mobile apps advertised as voice analyzers, and a few of them have some value. We should think of these as being useful for a client to take a baseline measurement for later comparison.

Among the many voice analysis apps, OperaVOX (iOS) leads the pack in studies showing reliability, but it is expensive. OperaVOX was developed by Oxford Research Wave Ltd., working with voice clinicians at University College London. The name stands for "On Person Rapid Voice eXaminer." It is available in three levels. OperaVOX Lite (free) records jitter and shimmer for sustained vowel. In addition to those capabilities, OperaVOX ($42.99) has additional features—recording maximum phonation time, analyzing reading and singing pitch ranges, and formant frequencies (F1, F2, F3, F4). To manage ambient noise and increase accuracy of measures, there is a volume-level sensor that prevents the user from completing an analysis if there is too much ambient noise. There is also a built-in color indicator that ensures the user will project the voice to the appropriate loudness. The internal mobile Apple device's microphone is deemed adequate. Results can be e-mailed to the SLP, and further analyses on audio files can be completed using MDVP (Multidimensional Voice Program), PRAAT, and so on.

OperaVOX has been validated, and in a study comparing OperaVOX to MDVP, OperaVOX was found to be comparable to MDVP and has high consistency for measuring F0 (fundamental frequency), jitter, and shimmer but not NHR (noise-to-harmonics ratio). Patients with type III voices (severe hoarseness) were excluded from this study (Baki et al., 2015). OperaVOXMulti is designed for professionals (ENTs and SLPs) and costs $399.99. It is intended for use in a clinic setting, and can analyze voice samples from multiple patients.

VOICE REHABILITATION

Monitoring Vocal Volume

There are several apps aimed at increasing loudness, such as Ah Up (iOS, Android, $0.99). This app requires the user to produce enough volume to keep an animated rocket in the air. Voice-O-Meter (iOS, $0.99) has data tracking and visual indication when the voice is in the "just right zone," providing reinforcement for increasing or decreasing volume, depending on the patient's goals.

Measuring Background Noise

Apps that measure noise can increase awareness of environmental noise levels that often lead to phonotrauma. These apps can be useful for singers with excessive loud voice use, whether due to personality or work environment. For these singers, knowing the level of ambient SPL (sound pressure level) at a party, concert, bar, or sports event may alert them to situations that put their voices at risk. This kind of information can also be used in vocal pacing, so that a singer might be given a guideline of 10 minutes of talking in an 80-dB environment, for example.

The National Institute for Occupational Safety and Health (NIOSH) has evaluated apps that measure SPL and published their results in the *Journal of the Acoustical Society of America* (Kardous & Shaw, 2014). They report that overall, iOS apps were found to be more accurate than Android apps because Android phones have many different manufacturers and use a variety of microphones and audio components. With iOS 6 in 2012, the iPhone added the ability to connect an external microphone through the headset input jack, allowing for more accurate recording. The ASA recommend these apps: SPLnFFT (iOS, $3.99) with a simple, color-coded sound meter; NoiseSee (no longer available); and SoundMeter (iOS, $29.99, Faber Acoustical).

Feedback on Pitch

These are plentiful, inexpensive, and provide support for Vocal Function Exercises, helping speakers habituate an optimal pitch zone and tracking pitch range. Pitch Perfect (iOS, free) has multiple ways to view a chromatic scale and play individual pitches. xPiano (iOS, Android, free) provides pitches from C1 to C7. Cleartune Chromatic Tuner (iOS, free) has a pitch wheel similar to a pitch pipe, for all octaves.

Breathing

There are many apps that teach lower abdominal breathing in isolation, but none that address the coordination of breathing with speaking. One of the best breathing apps is Breathe2Relax (iOS, free), with a detailed schematic animation of lower abdominal rest breathing and guided exercises accompanied by a pleasant voiceover narration. The voiceover can be turned off if desired, and there are text explanations as well. Inhale and exhale times are adjustable, allowing customization. Overall, this is an excellent introduction to lower abdominal breathing.

Voice Recorders to Record Voice Exercises

Most smartphones come with a voice memo function, and this can be used to record voice exercises. Van Leer (2013) notes that one of the main barriers to practice is the lack of an accurate model for practice. Recording the patient's voice exercises on his or her smartphone is an easy way for the patient to have an accurate model for home practice, available any time and any place. Van Leer suggests that it is even better to have the patients record themselves doing the exercises for home practice, since this increases self-efficacy and supports change. The patients can also record their home practice to share with the SLP at the next therapy session. Voice memos usually have a time and date stamp, so adherence to home practice can be documented. Although Van Leer's discussion focuses on voice therapy in the clinical setting, these features and strategies have obvious application and benefit for singing voice rehabilitation in any setting.

In addition to the voice memo function, there are many apps for audio recording. iTalk (iOS, Griffin Technologies, free) offers three quality levels for recording and records in AIFF (audio interchange file format), which is uncompressed and lossless, an advantage for recording voice quality. However, file size is large, so e-mailing is more problematic than with the compressed format, MP3. iTalk links with Dropbox for file transfer. Overall, this offers good quality recording, but the files are not easy to share.

DropVox (iOS, $1.99) records in MP3 and interfaces with Dropbox. Recordings of voice exercises can be e-mailed easily as long as the patient or client has a Dropbox account. Recorder & Editor (iSaid What?!) (iOS, $3.99) has a visual display similar to a waveform that shows peak clipping. The input level for the microphone can be adjusted accordingly. Recordings can be saved as WAV files and e-mailed or saved to a USB drive via iTunes. Clear Voice Premium (iOS, $0.99) also saves recordings as WAV files that can be e-mailed or linked to Dropbox.

Videos to Record Exercises

The singing voice rehabilitation specialist or the singer can use the smartphone's video function to record breathing, posture, stretches for the articulators—any exercise that needs more than audio for the singer to replicate the model at home. There are also many apps for creating videos, including Videolicious (iOS, free).

Practice Reminders

The alarms built into the iPhone can be programmed to provide repeatable reminders at the appropriate time. A different alarm can be programmed for each goal, whether that is a voice exercise, hydration, or a period of voice rest.

There are many calendar/reminder apps. Remember the Milk (iOS and Android, free) lets you enter a reminder, link to a time and location, and set an auditory or visual alert. Remember the Milk can be used to remind the singer to do voice exercises or to observe a "vocal nap" in support of vocal pacing. It syncs with many other platforms.

VoCal Voice Reminders (iOS, free) may provide an even more powerful reminder, in that it allows users to record a practice reminder in their own voice, which increases self-efficacy (Van Leer, 2013). For example, a singer can record her practice reminder using a resonant voice. VoCal combines a dictaphone, calendar, and alarm into one app—perfect for reminders to practice voice exercises or to observe a brief period of voice rest.

There are many apps for stopwatches and timers that can be used to record maximum phonation time. "Stopwatch%" (iOS, $0.99) is simple, with no sound.

iVOICETHERAPY

iVoiceTherapy (Infonet) was developed by Endo Education at University of California at Davis. Available on iOS for $12.99, it is one of the few voice therapy apps designed by SLPs. Unlike the vast majority of apps, it is not designed to be used without professional guidance. It is designed to complement the care of patients undergoing voice therapy in the clinical setting. The SLP programs the device for each patient, enabling the appropriate exercises for home practice. It contains a wealth of salient information for patients with voice disorders and some functions not found on other apps (e.g., cough and throat clear tracking, and a simple hydration tracker that takes into account caffeine and alcohol intake). Its weakness is that it has no graphic displays, aside from examples of videostroboscopic exams. Everything else is text, so that even descriptions of posture or descriptions of breathing exercises are without an image or movie. There is extensive audio material to serve as models for patient exercises. Although iVoiceTherapy provides well-structured audio exercises for patients, it lacks an easy way for the individual clinician to customize exercises in the app. Most voice clinicians have developed their own exercises for use with various patient populations. One can record a customized exercise in the Voice Sample function in iVoiceTherapy or use the Voice Memo already on the smartphone, but these can't be included in iVoiceTherapy's Play and Run function, where all the exercises are accessed as a unit and linked to programmed reminders.

iVoiceTherapy voice exercises include Vocal Yoga, Tone Flow, Breathing, Inflection and Emphasis, and Vowel Onsets. The exercises allow the patient to complete them simultaneously with clinician model or repeat after the model. All log-ons and task completions are time and date stamped, allowing the clinician to monitor compliance. Vocal Yoga (10 minutes) uses semi-occluded vocal tract sounds, such as humming, sustained /z/, trilled /r/ in sustained modal pitches, and then pitch glides, to enhance vocal fold pliability and pitch range. Tone Flow (6 minutes) teaches resonance and easy onset, using chanting and transitioning to conversational speech. Breathing (5 minutes) teaches breathing at rest (not coordinated with speaking) and is aimed toward patients with irritable larynx syndrome (ILS), cough, and vocal cord dysfunction (VCD). Inflection and Emphasis (3 minutes) is aimed at patients with Parkinson disease, MS (multiple sclerosis), and presbylarynges (vocal fold atrophy related to age). Vowel Onsets (2 minutes) teaches easy onset of phonation and includes negative practice. This is the only exercise on the iVoiceTherapy app that includes negative practice, and this feature can be helpful in other exercises as well.

The Play and Run feature allows the clinician to program in any of the above five exercises for the patient. There are additional features under the Exercise tab but not on the Play and Run list, including Sing, Cough & Throat Clearing, Volume, Voice Sample, Voice Conservation, Pitch, and Post-Operative. Using Sing, the clinician can create a playlist in iTunes, name it "iVoice," with songs appropriate for the particular patient to practice. Cough & Throat Clearing has features not currently found on other apps, including a cough timer that enables the patient to use a finger swipe for each cough/throat clear during the designated time (the time can be changed under Settings). The cough timer can be programmed for the patients to complete at a time when they are most symptomatic. The Volume exercise provides color visual feedback on volume, and it can be used with patients with Parkinson disease targeting the red range or, for patients who need to reduce their typical loudness, targeting the green range. For accurate measures, the microphone in the iPhone should be 12 inches from the mouth, or one can use the microphone on the iPhone earbuds. The Voice Sample allows the patient to record exercises or allows the clinician to record a tailored exercise for the patient. However, this customized exercise is not linked to the chosen exercises for Play and Run. Voice

Conservation includes a clever 20-point Voice Diet, for use with acute voice problems. Points are assigned for quiet, moderate, or loud talking; coughing; poor hydration; and missed reflux or allergy medications. The Pitch exercise provides real-time feedback on pitch. However, the print is small and not easy to read from any distance, and there is no graphic or color display.

The Post-Operative section allows the clinician to program in the dates for beginning and ending voice rest. Under Settings, the SLP can program in voice rest dates, along with the date to begin exercises, light talking, moderate talking, and so on. The dates programmed in drop into the reminder function.

iVoiceTherapy includes self-ratings, such as the Voice Handicap Index-10 (VHI-10), the Singing Voice Handicap-10 (SVHI-10), the Cough Severity Index (CSI), Dyspnea Index, and Reflux Symptoms Index. The Hydration rating is color-coded and accommodates intake not only of water but also of coffee and alcohol. Daily hydration entries are time and date stamped, keeping patients on track. There is also a journal section, allowing the patients to note patterns related to voice quality, coughing, reflux, or any subject they choose.

The Education tab in iVoiceTherapy includes Vocal IQ: Ear Training, Vocal IQ, Pathology Lab, Body Alignment, Irritable Larynx, Vocal Hygiene, and Post-Operative (with rationale for voice rest and postoperative recovery). Educational materials are included under each of these topics. In particular, the 12 videostroboscopic exams under Pathology Lab are a convenient and excellent teaching tool.

One might think the cost of the iVoiceTherapy app is prohibitive at $12.99. However, this app includes so many pertinent features that it is actually a great value for the price. Overall, this app is very well thought out but hampered by lack of ability for other SLPs to customize to their own approaches. As it stands currently, this app may be best used in conjunction with each SLP's prerecorded exercises, which would be downloaded for his or her patients. Aside from this, the app contains many of the features needed to support voice therapy, so the patient could avoid buying multiple apps to fill those needs.

VOICE HYGIENE

Hydration

There are many apps that are aimed at tracking hydration, but most only include daily water intake. Almost none account for overall hydration (water, other beverages, caffeine, alcohol), so there is room for improvement in this category. The only hydration app that includes other drinks besides water is Hydration Check (iOS, $0.99). Hydration Check covers many types of beverages, including caffeinated drinks, noncaffeinated beverages, and alcohol. It does not count caffeine or alcohol at the same value as water but does not subtract them from water intake either. Although many SLPs might disagree with how the app accounts for these beverages, it is the only app I found that allows you to keep track of everything you drink in a day. It does not provide reminders.

There are many other apps that track daily water intake, showing graphs over time and providing reminders. Waterminder (iOS, $1.99) has a tips section with facts about hydration, with customizable reminders and a history function to track water intake over time. To keep track of daily water intake, a simple line drawing of a person shows the water level rising from bottom up. Waterminder does not track caffeine. Waterlogged (iOS, free) uses a drawing of a water bottle, showing the level of water intake by day. Water Your Body (iOS, free) has a tips section with appealing photos of nature and motivating information about water.

Managing Medical Conditions Affecting Voice

The WebMD Allergy App (iOS, free) provides information tailored to your location. It provides allergy forecasts and allergy alerts and allows you to track exposure to allergens. Allergy Alert (iOS, Pollen.com, free) includes information on common pollens and allergens for people with allergies, asthma, cold, and cough. There are also apps that help track reflux, including GERD (Heartburn, GERD, and Acid Reflux Diary) (iOS, $4.99). There are many apps that help people manage asthma, including AsthmaMD (iOS, free), which tracks asthma symptoms, triggers and peak flows, has a diary function, and can show asthma symptoms over time in a graphical display.

Decreasing Throat Clearing, Cough, and Smoking

There are a vast number of apps supporting smoking cessation. One of the best is Smoke Free—Quit Smoking Now and Stop For Good (iOS, free), including over 20 techniques for smoking cessation. The only app that specifically targets coughing and throat clearing is part of iVoiceTherapy (see full discussion). However, there are many apps supporting habit change, and they can be customized to address a range of habits. HabitSeed (iOS, $0.99) can be customized for cough or throat clear.

VOICE REST AND VOCAL PACING

Although postoperative voice rest is essential for optimal recovery for singers who have had vocal fold surgery, voice rest is challenging, and the degree of compliance likely would increase with other options for communication. Rousseau et al. (2015) investigated the use of a text-to-speech (TTS) augmentative and alternative communication (AAC) device for voice rest. He found that patients on postoperative voice rest using the Lightwriter speech-generating device increased patient-perceived communication effectiveness. In addition, his study found that patients using TTS showed an increase in relative compliance with voice rest compared to those on voice rest without the benefit of TTS.

The array of text-to-speech apps enhances communication for patients on postoperative voice rest, likely leading to greater compliance. The most useful apps support preprogrammed speech, such as an explanation of why the person is unable to speak, so that this can easily be communicated to new acquaintances, avoiding a constant repetition of the same information. One can also prerecord any high-frequency phrases to save time.

Some of the best TTS apps include Speak It!, Verbally, Speech Assistant AAC, and iSpeech Text to Speech. Speak It! (iOS,

$1.99) has good quality voices, with a range of male and female voices, and British and American accents. It allows you to save high-use phrases. A copy/paste function allows the user to type a long text on the computer if desired, then e-mail it to the phone to be pasted into Speak It! for later use. Verbally (iOS, iPad only, free) has even more functionality, with its core words grid, core phrases grid, and text prediction, requiring less keystrokes. The premium version enables more personalization of these features. Speech Assistant AAC (Android, $4.39) allows the user to create topic categories with frequent words and phrases, which can be saved. It uses the voice loaded on the phone, or other voices can be purchased. iSpeech Text to Speech (iOS, free) is capable of saving and reusing frequent phrases. It comes with a male voice; other voices can be purchased for $0.99.

One other category of apps can help singers comply with voice rest or vocal pacing, where preplanning is essential. Calendar and scheduling apps are on most phones, and the user can program them to alert them to rest their voices at designated times.

REAL-TIME BIOFEEDBACK ON VOICE USE

The only mobile phone platform that accurately measures the amount of phonation is the Voice Health Monitor, which is under development and not yet commercially available. Other current ambulatory devices, such as the Ambulatory Phonation Monitor, VoxLog, and VocaLog, are not available on a smartphone platform (Van Stan, 2014). It has been demonstrated that our estimates of how much we use the voice are wildly inaccurate. It is well known that there are problems generally with self-reporting of behavior, and this may be especially true in the area of voice use. The Voice Health Monitor aims to provide more reliable and objective measures of voice use, with a user-friendly interface for voice use monitoring, daily sensor calibration, and periodic alert capabilities that can be audible, visual, or vibrotactile (Mehta, Zanartu, Feng, Cheyne, & Hillman, 2012). It uses a Nexus S smartphone with an Android operating system (OS) for data acquisition. Data are collected through a miniature accelerometer (ACC) worn on the neck. The advantage of the ACC versus a microphone is that the ACC is relatively immune from background noise, so the voice signal is not degraded (Mehta et al., 2012). The Voice Health Monitor uses three vocal dose measures: phonation time, cycle dose (number of vibrations per time frame), and distance dose (this combines cycle dose and amplitude based on SPL). At present, the Voice Health Monitor is not available commercially; it is intended to be used in clinics for research to help understand patterns of normal and hyperfunctional voice (Mehta et al., 2012).

For voice therapists, the potential of the Voice Health Monitor is great. Vocal pacing has become essential to the management of voice problems, especially for occupational and professional voice users, and patients with acute voice problems. This device will provide accurate data about how much the wearer actually uses the voice. This will allow individuals to better understand their own patterns of voice use, including what "dose" of phonation is optimal for them as individuals and how much recovery time they need.

In the area of clinical research, it may lead to clearer understanding of the relationship between voice use patterns and vocal pathology.

CONCLUSION

Singing voice rehabilitation specialists are likely to find their practice evolving to meet patients' interest in apps and will be rewarded by branching out into new technologies that can improve self-efficacy and overall progress in voice rehabilitation. Even without downloading an app, anyone with a smartphone has the ability to make an audio or video recording of their exercises, guided by the singing voice rehabilitation specialist. This meets an obvious need by providing a portable "substitute" for the provider model outside of the clinic. The singer and singing voice rehabilitation specialist can collaborate to decide upon most realistic times for voice practice, and practice alerts can be programmed onto singers' smartphones using their calendar function and alerts of their choice. Singers can use the video function on their phones to record their videostroboscopic exams and use other apps that explain laryngeal anatomy. Singers on postoperative voice rest will have a better experience if they use TTS apps. The iVoiceTherapy app, though expensive, is full of helpful features for voice patients in the clinical setting, and the Voice Health Monitor is likely to become the "Fitbit" for voice. There are many exciting developments in apps for voice rehabilitation, and voice professionals should work toward creating clearinghouses of best apps, complete research on efficacy in voice rehabilitation, and become active in developing apps specifically for voice. A summary of the apps discussed in this chapter is provided in Table 19–1, which may be used as an educational handout.

Table 19–1. Apps for Voice Rehabilitaiton

App Name	Platform	Cost	Description
Voice education (anatomy)			
Larynx ID	iOS	$4.99	Drawings of larynx from various views with animations and drawing function
Vocal Folds ID	iOS	$2.99	Simpler version showing vocal folds from various views, with animation and drawing function
Respiratory Anatomy Atlas	iOS	$0.99	Good for breathing mechanics, with animations, but not detailed for larynx
drawMD ENT	iPad only	Free	Detailed illustrations of larynx, with drawing function
Draw!	Android	Free	Simple drawing tool. Can use to write and erase during voice rest.
Voice analysis			
OperaVOX Lite	iOS	Free	Records jitter, shimmer, and F0
OperaVOX	iOS	$42.99	Records jitter, shimmer, F0, formant frequencies, MPT, reading and singing pitch ranges for individual user. Studies show comparable to PRAAT and MDVP for jitter, shimmer, and f0.
OperaVOX Multi	iOS	$399.00	Designed for use in clinics by professionals. Same functions as OperaVOX but can record multiple patients.
Monitoring vocal volume			
Voice-O-Meter	iOS	$0.99	Visual feedback for voice in "just right zone"
Monitoring ambient noise			
SPLnFFT	iOS	$3.99	Simple color-coded sound meter
SoundMeter	iOS	$29.99	Faber Acoustical
Pitch feedback			
xPiano	iOS	Free	Piano keys displayed C1 and up. Only Cs are labeled but has all octaves.
Pitch Perfect	iOS	Free	Pitch letters/notes displayed several ways
Cleartune chromatic tuner	iOS	Free	Pitches displayed on pitch wheel (like pitch pipe), with all octaves
Breathing			
Breathe2Relax	iOS	Free	Detailed animation of lower abdominal breathing. Pleasant voice over (on/off) and text. Inhale, exhale adjustable.

continues

Table 19–1. *continued*

App Name	*Platform*	*Cost*	*Description*
		Voice recorders to record exercises or reminders	
Voice memo function	iOS, Android	Free, on phone	Record voice exercises, reminders to practice
DropVox	iOS	Free	Saves in MP3, links to Dropbox, can be e-mailed
Recorder & Editor (iSaid What?!)	iOS	$3.99	Visual display like a waveform, shows peak clipping. Input level can be adjusted. Saves in WAV form; can be e-mailed.
Clear Voice Premium	iOS	$0.99	Saves as WAV file. Can be e-mailed or linked to Dropbox.
iTalk Recorder	iOS	$1.99	Griffin Technologies. Records in AIFF, which is uncompressed and high quality, but harder to share.
		Text to speech devices for voice rest	
Speak It!	iOS	$1.99	Male and female voices included
Speech Assistant AAC	Android	$4.39	Create categories with words/phrases. Uses voice on phone or can buy other voices. Saves phrases.
Verbally	iPad only	Free	Core words and phrases grids and text prediction.
iSpeech Text to Speech	iOS	Free	Save/reuse frequent phrases. Male voice and other voices $0.99 each.
		Practice reminders	
Voice memo function, comes with phone	iOS, Android	Free	Record reminders for practice, hydration, voice rest
Remember the Milk (RTM)	iOS, Android	Free	Enter reminders for practice, hydration, voice rest. Syncs with many platforms.
VoCal Voice Reminders	iOS	$0.99	GZero. Best when patient records practice reminder in the "target voice."
Alerts on phone	iOS, Android	Free	Program separate alert sounds for different exercises, hydration, voice rest.
		Stopwatches/timers	
Stopwatch%	iOS	$0.99	Simple, no sound. For MPT, VFE.
		Voice therapy—comprehensive	
iVoice Therapy	iOS	$12.99	SLP programs for patient. Voice exercises, biofeedback on pitch, volume, cough frequency. Tracks task completion. Self-ratings: VHI-10, SVHI-10, CSI. Education: strobes, irritable larynx, hygiene, postoperative care (and program in voice rest dates).

Table 19–1. *continued*

App Name	*Platform*	*Cost*	*Description*
		Vocal hygiene	
Hydration Check	iOS	$0.99	Includes many different beverages, including water, and subtracts for caffeinated drinks and alcohol. Does not provide reminders.
Waterlogged	iOS	Free	Simple. Does not track caffeine. Sends reminders.
Allergy	iOS Android	Free	Web MD. Sends allergy alerts based on user location, allergy forecast, allergy tracker.
Allergy Alert	iOS	Free	Pollen.com. Sends alerts pertinent to top allergens, has allergy diary.
Just Quit–Quit Smoking	iOS	Free	Has quit timer, quotes/suggestions, achievements, and notifications
		Real-time feedback—phonation monitor	
Voice Health Monitor	Android	Not for sale	Under development; currently used for clinical research. Accelerometer on neck measures F0, SPL, phonation time, cycle dose (number vibrations), and distance dose (combines cycle dose and amplitude based on SPL). Provides alerts when threshold is reached.

REFERENCES

Baki, M., Wood, G., Alston, M., Ratcliffe, P., Sandhu, G., & Rubin, J. S. (2015). Reliability of OperaVOX against Multidimensional Voice Program (MDVP). *Clinical Otolaryngology, 40*, 22–28.

Boudreaux, E., Waring, M. E., Hayes, R. B., Sadasivam, R. S., Muller, S., & Pagoto, S. (2014). Evaluating and selecting mobile health apps: strategies for healthcare providers and healthcare organizations. *Translational Behavioral Medicine, 4*, 363–371.

Boulos, M. N., Brewer, A. C., Karimkhani, C., Buller, D., & Dellavalle, R .P. (2014). Mobile medical and health apps: state of the art, concerns, regulatory control and certification. *Online Journal of Public Health Informatics, 5*(3), e229.

Dennison, L., Morrison, L., Conway, G., & Yardley, L. (2013). Opportunities and challenges for smartphone applications in supporting health behavior change: Qualitative study. *Journal of Medical Internet Research, 15*(4), e86.

Kardous, C. A., & Shaw, P. B. (2014). Evaluation of smartphone sound measurement applications. *The Journal of the Acoustical Society of America, 135*(4), EL186–EL192.

Mehta, D. D., Zanartu, M., Feng, S. W., Cheyne, H. A., & Hillman, R. E. (2012). Mobile voice health monitoring using a wearable accelerometer sensor and a smartphone platform. *IEEE Transactions on Biomedical Engineering, 59*(11), 3090–3096.

Payne, H. E., Lister, C., West, J. H., & Bernhardt, J. M. (2015). Behavioral functionality of mobile apps in health interventions: A systematic review of the literature. *Journal of Medical Internet Research Mhealth Uhealth, 3*(1), e20.

Rousseau, B., Gutmann, M., Mau, T., Francis, D., & Novaleski, C. (2015). Randomized controlled trial of supplemental augmentative and alternative communication versus voice rest alone after phonomicrosurgery. *Otolaryngology-Head and Neck Surgery, 152*(3), 494–500.

Van Leer, E. (2013). Using popular mobile devices in voice therapy. *ASHA Perspectives, 23*(3), 82–87.

Van Stan, J. (2014). Direct comparison of three commercially available devices for voice ambulatory monitoring and feedback. *ASHA Perspectives, 24*(2), 80–86.

Zapata, B. C., Fernandez-Aleman, J. L., Idri, A., & Toval, A. (2015) Empirical studies on usability of mHealth apps: A systematic literature review. *Journal of Medical Systems, 39*, 1–19.

APPENDIX 19–A

Vocal Health Apps

App Name	*Platform*	*Cost*	*Description*
Voice education (anatomy)			
Larynx ID	iOS	$4.99	Drawings of larynx from various views with animations and drawing function
Vocal Folds ID	iOS	$2.99	Simpler version showing vocal folds from various views, with animation and drawing function
Respiratory Anatomy Atlas	iOS	$0.99	Good for breathing mechanics, with animations, but not detailed for larynx
drawMD ENT	iPad only	Free	Detailed illustrations of larynx, with drawing function
Draw!	Android	Free	Simple drawing tool. Can use to write and erase during voice rest.
Voice analysis			
OperaVOX Lite	iOS	Free	Records jitter, shimmer, and F0
OperaVOX	iOS	$42.99	Records jitter, shimmer, F0, formant frequencies, MPT, reading and singing pitch ranges for individual user. Studies show comparable to PRAAT and MDVP for jitter, shimmer, and f0.
OperaVOX Multi	iOS	$399.00	Designed for use in clinics by professionals. Same functions as OperaVOX but can record multiple patients.
Monitoring vocal volume			
Voice-O-Meter	iOS	$0.99	Visual feedback for voice in "just right zone"
Monitoring ambient noise			
SPLnFFT	iOS	$3.99	Simple color-coded sound meter
SoundMeter	iOS	$29.99	Faber Acoustical
Pitch feedback			
xPiano	iOS	Free	Piano keys displayed C1 and up. Only Cs are labeled but has all octaves.
Pitch Perfect	iOS	Free	Pitch letters/notes displayed several ways
Cleartune chromatic tuner	iOS	Free	Pitches displayed on pitch wheel (like pitch pipe), with all octaves

continues

Appendix 19–A. *continued*

App Name	Platform	Cost	Description
		Breathing	
Breathe2Relax	iOS	Free	Detailed animation of lower abdominal breathing. Pleasant voice over (on/off) and text. Inhale, exhale adjustable.
		Voice recorders to record exercises or reminders	
Voice memo function	iOS, Android	Free, on phone	Record voice exercises, reminders to practice
DropVox	iOS	Free	Saves in MP3, links to Dropbox, can be e-mailed
Recorder & Editor (iSaid What?!)	iOS	$3.99	Visual display like a waveform, shows peak clipping. Input level can be adjusted. Saves in WAV form; can be e-mailed.
Clear Voice Premium	iOS	$0.99	Saves as WAV file. Can be e-mailed or linked to Dropbox.
iTalk Recorder	iOS	$1.99	Griffin Technologies. Records in AIFF, which is uncompressed and high quality, but harder to share.
		Text to speech devices for voice rest	
Speak It!	iOS	$1.99	Male and female voices included
Speech Assistant AAC	Android	$4.39	Create categories with words/phrases. Uses voice on phone or can buy other voices. Saves phrases.
Verbally	iPad only	Free	Core words and phrases grids and text prediction.
iSpeech Text to Speech	iOS	Free	Save/reuse frequent phrases. Male voice and other voices $0.99 each.
		Practice reminders	
Voice memo function, comes with phone	iOS, Android	Free	Record reminders for practice, hydration, voice rest
Remember the Milk (RTM)	iOS, Android	Free	Enter reminders for practice, hydration, voice rest. Syncs with many platforms.
VoCal Voice Reminders	iOS	$0.99	GZero. Best when patient records practice reminder in the "target voice."
Alerts on phone	iOS, Android	Free	Program separate alert sounds for different exercises, hydration, voice rest.
		Stopwatches/timers	
Stopwatch%	iOS	$0.99	Simple, no sound. For MPT, VFE.

App Name	*Platform*	*Cost*	*Description*
		Voice therapy—comprehensive	
iVoice Therapy	iOS	$12.99	SLP programs for patient. Voice exercises, biofeedback on pitch, volume, cough frequency. Tracks task completion. Self-ratings: VHI-10, SVHI-10, CSI. Education: strobes, irritable larynx, hygiene, postoperative care (and program in voice rest dates).
		Vocal hygiene	
Hydration Check	iOS	$0.99	Includes many different beverages, including water, and subtracts for caffeinated drinks and alcohol. Does not provide reminders.
Waterlogged	iOS	Free	Simple. Does not track caffeine. Sends reminders.
Allergy	iOS Android	Free	Web MD. Sends allergy alerts based on user location, allergy forecast, allergy tracker.
Allergy Alert	iOS	Free	Pollen.com. Sends alerts pertinent to top allergens, has allergy diary.
Just Quit–Quit Smoking	iOS	Free	Has quit timer, quotes/suggestions, achievements, and notifications
		Real-time feedback—phonation monitor	
Voice Health Monitor	Android	Not for sale	Under development; currently used for clinical research. Accelerometer on neck measures F0, SPL, phonation time, cycle dose (number vibrations), and distance dose (combines cycle dose and amplitude based on SPL). Provides alerts when threshold is reached.

CHAPTER 20

Singing Voice Rehabilitation Documentation: The Importance of Clinical Language

As you customize the rehabilitation plan for each singer you work with, you will need to develop an appropriate set of rehabilitation goals and document the progress of the singer throughout the rehabilitation process. The goals should encompass all the relevant elements of rehabilitation and should be designed to address the specific needs of the singer.

In a clinical setting, medical standards and insurance reimbursement practices require you to document rehabilitation goals in your initial evaluation report, and progress toward goals must be documented at each therapy session. These goals must be measurable, evidence based, and should indicate a rationale that draws a clear line between the goal and how achievement of the goal will contribute to the resolution of the underlying voice problem. The language you use should reflect your knowledge of voice disorders, voice science, and voice rehabilitation practices. It is best to avoid language that is vague, imagery based, or carries an instructional rather than a clinical connotation. Insurance companies (rightly) will not reimburse you if your rehabilitation plan looks like a series of voice lessons to them. Remember that the purpose of singing voice rehabilitation is to *restore function that has been lost*. Inevitably, principles of voice *habilitation* will inform rehabilitation activities, but all activities should be expressed in a way that focuses on the underlying anatomical, physiologic, acoustical, and behavioral principles that will yield the desired restoration of function.

Although the requirement for clinical documentation and language does not currently apply to the voice studio setting (where insurance billing considerations are not a factor), I would argue that the necessity for similar documentation habits pertains to the voice studio as well. If you are characterizing your work with a singer as rehabilitation—especially if medical providers are referring to you—you could be called upon to provide evidence of what went on in the sessions in case of liability or litigation. Even putting aside the liability issue, developing a treatment plan with clearly stated goals and regular documentation of progress demonstrates your professionalism and ensures that you remain focused on the underlying mechanical principles and how they interact with injury and dysfunction.

EXAMPLES OF CLINICAL LANGUAGE FOR SINGING VOICE REHABILITATION GOALS

A number of examples of scientific and evidence-based wording for singing voice rehabilitation goals are included in the following tables (Tables 20–1 through 20–8). Of course, your reporting of progress toward goals should use similarly scientific and clinical language, and examples of progress reporting are also provided herein.

Note that singing can be described as a "high-intensity/complex vocal task," as distinguished from speaking, which by comparison is less vocally athletic. Transitioning from vocalises to repertoire could be depicted as "short" versus "extended passages," as the progression of linguistic complexity is typically described for speaking voice tasks. "To rehabilitate voice to premorbid quality, stamina, and pitch and loudness range" can be used to express the goal of restoring lost vocal function.

These examples are not intended to be comprehensive or exhaustive, rather to provide a foundation for developing goals that are specific, customized, and that encompass the range of possible contributing factors.

CASE EXAMPLES

Case Example 1

The patient is a rock singer in a local cover band. She was a voice major in college and has many years of training in classical singing technique. She presents to you with a diagnosis of vocal fold nodules. When you have her demonstrate her typical warm-up routine, she exhibits mechanics and vocal quality consistent with classical singing; however, in a video of a performance, she is clearly belting. You note that in this performance, she demonstrates considerable vocal strain, and you conclude there is a disconnect between her technique in warm-ups and the requirements of her performance repertoire. You suspect that her inadequate technique relative to belting has contributed to her injury and must be remediated in order for her to recover. Among the areas you decide to target in rehabilitation is developing an exercise regimen that is better aligned with the vocal demands of her performance repertoire. In voice pedagogy terms, you need to teach her how to belt in a vocally healthy way. However, "belting" is clinically meaningless. A better formulation would be to use language that describes the scientific underpinnings of belting and what the singer must to do. She needs to:

Optimize resonance:

- The patient will utilize resonant voice to increase vocal tract inertance, facilitate vocal fold vibration, and lower phonation threshold pressure to decrease vocal hyperfunction, improve voice quality and projection, support resolution of underlying vocal injury and optimize vocal function.

Understand the difference between classical and belting technique:

- The patient will demonstrate understanding of different strategies for source-vocal tract interaction to enhance vocal sound, reduce forcefulness of vocal fold collision, and improve vocal fold vibration.

And achieve healthy belting:

- The patient will improve source-vocal tract interaction by utilizing megaphone mouth shape (with TA dominant adduction, high second harmonic energy, narrow epilarynx tube) in the range of F3–C5.

Now you have expressed your belting goals in language that is clinically meaningful and scientifically based.

Case Example 2

The patient is an adolescent male who has had a significant professional career as a boy soprano. Now entering puberty, he says "my voice has totally come unhinged." Perceptually, his voice is characterized by abnormally high pitch and nearly constant pitch breaks, during which modal phonation is sometimes briefly observed. Videostroboscopy reveals larynx structures that are within normal limits, but throughout the exam, he never achieves complete vocal fold adduction. The diagnosis is puberphonia. His speaking voice is dramatically affected, and his singing activities have come to a complete standstill: he can only sing in falsetto and cannot phonate at all below C4. You recognize that to achieve a normal voice, you must lead him to "discover" his "chest voice." He needs to:

Understand the mechanics of vocal registers and how his "chest voice" differs from "falsetto":

- The patient will demonstrate understanding of mechanical/physiologic/acoustical differences between TA dominant (moderately-fully contracted) and CT dominant (moderately-fully contracted) registration.

Phonate in chest register at age-appropriate pitch level rather than high-pitched falsetto register that is not age appropriate:

- The patient will utilize contraction of intrinsic laryngeal musculature (fully contracted TA) and lax vocal ligament to achieve developmentally appropriate fundamental frequency and to improve vocal stability, projection, and optimal coordination of respiratory/phonatory motor system in structured tasks and conversation.

And learn to transition from chest voice to falsetto to resume singing:

- The patient will improve vocal quality, pitch and dynamic range, and projection by maintaining appropriate balance of TA and CT muscle activation and degree of vocal ligament tension between 110 Hz and 440 Hz as measured by perceptual evaluation and absence of phonation/pitch breaks.

Table 20–1. ***Domain: Vocal Hygiene—Examples of Long- and Short-Term Singing Voice Rehabilitation Goals and Language for Reporting Progress***

Long-term goal: Patient/Client will improve vocal hygiene through improved hydration and decreased phonotraumatic behaviors.	
Short-term goals (criterion is 90% accuracy unless otherwise stated):	Sample progress reporting:
1. The Patient/Client will increase hydration for an eventual goal of eight glasses per day and limit caffeine intake (to maximum of 1–2, 8 oz. cups/day), as measured by Patient/Client report.	Reports approximately six glasses of water per day in the last week. Caffeine consumption is down to two servings/day of coffee.
2. The Patient/Client will eliminate phonotraumatic behaviors such as chronic throat clearing by substituting nontraumatic methods to clear mucus.	Independently used sip of water to avoid throat clearing five times during session. He reports that the urge to clear throat is strong and it takes effort to suppress.
3. The Patient/Client will avoid yelling/screaming/shouting by using alternative means of gaining attention (such as noise makers, bells, whistles, etc.), as measured by Patient/Client report.	Reports texting her kids to come to dinner rather than yelling for them across the house.
4. The Patient/Client will demonstrate understanding of phonotraumatic behaviors. Patient/Client will develop alternative behaviors to implement independently.	Discussed phonotraumatic nature of speaking in noisy environments. Brainstormed ideas. He came up with idea to go to a quieter location if he wants to have a conversation at a party so he is not standing near the audio speakers or other noisy area.

Table 20–2. *Domain: Vocal Pacing—Examples of Long- and Short-Term Singing Voice Rehabilitation Goals and Language for Reporting Progress*

Long-term goal: The Patient/Client will use vocal pacing and judicious voice use to facilitate resolution of vocal fold injury, reduce vocal fatigue, and optimize vocal stamina as measured by Patient/Client report.	
Short-term goals (criterion is 90% accuracy unless otherwise stated):	Sample progress reporting:
1. The Patient/Client will follow recommendations for perisurgical precautions, observing the surgeon's prescribed period of complete vocal rest for 7 days after surgery, and will follow guidelines for incremental return to normal voice use.	1 week after surgery: Reports adherence to recommendation with exception of a few (< 5) brief unintentional vocalizations (as when startled by loud noise) and one cough. Will now begin gradual resumption of speaking voice use starting with 10 minutes today, doubling duration each day as tolerated until next session (1 week).
2. The Patient/Client will follow guidelines for conservative voice use, including periods of complete voice rest (1 hour total daily), as measured by Patient/Client voice journal/diary.	Reviewed voice use journal together. She has established target of 10 minutes of voice rest for every one hour of talking at school, uses voice rest button to let students/staff know when she is on a voice break.
3. The Patient/Client will use amplification in speaking activities as needed to decrease voice overuse, as measured by Patient/Client report.	Purchased personal voice amplifier and is currently using it throughout the teaching day. She reports decreased vocal fatigue, which she associates with not having to speak as loudly as usual. "I can just turn up the volume to get them to listen."
4. The Patient/Client will complete high-intensity/complex vocal tasks for a minimum of 30 minutes without evidence of vocal fatigue, demonstrating appropriate coordination of respiratory/phonatory motor system.	Reports approximately 20 minutes of high-intensity/complex exercises 4/7 days since last week's session. She notes fatigue usually set in after about 15 minutes. During today's session, she reported fatigue after 20 minutes of high-intensity/complex exercises. Increased duration may reflect improved coordination resulting from immediate feedback/cueing from clinician.

Table 20–3. ***Domain: Vocal Coordination and Conditioning—Examples of Long- and Short-Term Singing Voice Rehabilitation Goals for Breath Support and Language for Reporting Progress***

Long-term goal: To optimize respiration mechanics during phonation to improve vocal fold vibration and decrease glottal pressing to support resolution of underlying vocal injury and optimize vocal function.	
Short-term goals (criterion is 90% accuracy unless otherwise stated):	Sample progress reporting:
1. The Patient/Client will demonstrate abdominal/diaphragmatic breathing patterns with adequate replenishing breaths during phonation to decrease hyperfunction and to optimize efficiency of breath flow on phonation, progressing through linguistic hierarchy: sound/syllable/word/phrase/sentence/paragraph reading/conversation.	Education regarding respiratory mechanics for phonation was provided, including video demonstration. He achieved low abdominal breathing pattern in isolation and at the sound level with moderate cues and full model: 70% accuracy. Postphonation exhalation was facilitating for maintaining breath flow through end of utterance.
2. The Patient/Client will use various feedback methods (visual, auditory, tactile, kinesthetic, proprioceptive) to achieve accurate low-abdominal breathing pattern.	Standing bent from the waist with arms stabilized by holding onto chair arms facilitated increasing her awareness of abdominal release during inhalation. Standing with the exercise ball suspended between abdomen and wall provided kinesthetic and tactile feedback, resulting in improved LAB pattern. Exhaling on /s/ and /z/ provided proprioceptive and auditory feedback for maintaining abdominal muscle activation and steady breath flow. Visual feedback from the mirror facilitated improved accuracy of self-assessment of abdominal vs. clavicular breathing pattern: achieved 90% accuracy in self-assessment at sound level.
3. The Patient/Client will achieve and maintain appropriate balance of thoracic expansion and abdominal compression during phonation to optimize vocal projection and minimize laryngeal strain in high-intensity/complex vocal tasks.	Tendency toward abdominal clenching noted in today's session. Worked on achieving adequate abdominal compression without clenching using model from clinician, tactile and visual feedback (mirror). He independently noted neck tension associated with abdominal clenching and used this awareness to successfully monitor abdominal clenching.

Table 20–4. ***Domain: Vocal Coordination and Conditioning—Examples of Long- and Short-Term Singing Voice Rehabilitation Goals for Resonant Voice and Language for Reporting Progress***

Long-term goal: The Patient/Client will utilize resonant voice to increase vocal tract inertance, facilitate vocal fold vibration, and lower phonation threshold pressure to decrease vocal hyperfunction, improve voice quality and projection, support resolution of underlying vocal injury, and optimize vocal function.	
Short term goals (criterion is 90% accuracy unless otherwise stated):	Sample progress reporting:
1. The Patient/Client will use semi-occluded vocal tract sounds to facilitate resonant voice, promoting favorable source-filter interaction and optimizing vocal tract inertance.	Education regarding benefits of semi-occluded vocal tract sounds was provided, including visual illustration with anatomical diagrams. Attempted small-straw phonation, lip trill, tongue trill. Tendency to use excessive subglottic pressure with small straw initially, resulting in cheek puffing and nasal air emission. Improved with cues to allow some air to escape around straw and "think lighter." Best coordination achieved with lip trill: 90% for sustained phonation at A3.
2. The Patient/Client will achieve resonant voice in speaking tasks following linguistic hierarchy of sound, syllable, word, phrase, sentence, paragraph reading, conversation.	Worked at sentence level today, continuing with /n/ initial words at the beginning of sentence. Periodically "recalibrated" reference sensation for resonant voice by briefly phonating through small straw. Achieved 90% accuracy. Excellent self-assessment demonstrated today.
3. The Patient/Client will demonstrate more anterior tongue carriage for improved oral resonance.	Achieved 100% accuracy on sustained phonation when humming with tongue protruded. Alternated protruding tongue and then allowing tongue to rest inside mouth with cue to keep tongue tip in contact with front teeth. She was ultimately able to maintain oral resonance without protruding tongue. Proceeded to /m/ initial syllables: 80% accurate.
4. The Patient/Client will release jaw tension and increase opening of oral cavity for improved resonance.	Worked on releasing jaw tension by humming with exaggerated chewing motion and /wau/ repetitions, 90% accurate at modal pitch. Visual feedback from the mirror was facilitating and promoted accurate self-assessment.

continues

Table 20–4. continued

5. The Patient/Client will demonstrate understanding of different strategies for source-vocal tract interaction to enhance vocal quality, reduce forcefulness of vocal fold collision, and improve vocal fold vibration to support resolution of underlying vocal injury and optimize vocal function.	Provided education regarding difference between megaphone mouth shape (with TA-dominant adduction, high second harmonic energy, narrow epilarynx tube) and inverted megaphone mouth shape (with lip rounding, elevated velum, narrow epilarynx tube, and clustering of third, fourth, and fifth vocal tract formants). She has historically received training in the latter, but proficiency in the former will be necessary to meet current vocal demands and professional voice activities. Visual and auditory illustrations were provided. She indicated understanding through asking insightful questions and correctly responding to clinician's questions.
6. The Patient/Client will improve source-vocal tract interaction by utilizing megaphone mouth shape (with TA-dominant adduction, high second harmonic energy, narrow epilarynx tube) in the range of F3–C5.	Inadequate lip widening persists, resulting in excessive reliance on vocal fold adduction to achieve desired sound output. Holding drinking straw horizontally under the tongue provided scaffolding for appropriate mouth shape. This mouth posture, combined with phonating on /æ/, helped raise first formant to reinforce second harmonic energy, and she was able to phonate to A4 successfully with greater ease of phonation, consistent with reduced forcefulness of vocal fold collision.
7. The Patient/Client will improve source-vocal tract interaction by utilizing inverted megaphone mouth shape (with lip rounding, elevated velum, narrow epilarynx tube, and clustering of third, fourth, and fifth vocal tract formants) in the range of C3–G4.	"Pushed" vocal quality, excessive laryngeal elevation, and evidence of excessive TA activation observed in range from C4–G4 today. Worked on lengthening resonator through increased lip rounding (phonation on /o/) and moderate cues to maintain "yawn" posture. This resulted in greater projection and "ringing" quality to voice with reduced effort, as demonstrated by his report of greater ease of phonation and clinician's perceptual evaluation.

Table 20–5. ***Domain: Vocal Coordination and Conditioning—Examples of Long- and Short-Term Singing Voice Rehabilitation Goals for Posture and Language for Reporting Progress***

Long-term goal: The Patient/Client will implement postural adjustments independently to optimize body alignment for respiration and phonation, and to decrease laryngeal hyperfunction to promote resolution of underlying injury.	
Short-term goals (criterion is 90% accuracy unless otherwise stated):	Sample progress reporting:
1. The Patient/Client will improve postural alignment to reduce laryngeal/neck/shoulder/articulatory tension and optimize breath support, oral resonance, and vocal projection.	Lordotic stance noted during exercises today. Provided model and kinesthetic cueing to rotate pelvis forward, resulting in improved alignment of head and spine. Visual feedback from the mirror was helpful for achieving target alignment. Tendency to elevate chin excessively, resulting in neck tension and excessive laryngeal elevation. Moderate verbal cues to "keep the floor of the mouth parallel with the floor of the room." Also, "imagine a thread going from the crown of the head to the ceiling." 80% correct by end of session. Decreased laryngeal strain noted with this posture adjustment. General propensity to drop rib cage by end of breath group is noted. Initially required maximal cues and manual positioning by clinician to maintain rib cage elevation. By the end of the session, she was able to achieve correct alignment independently with visual feedback from the mirror 80% of the time.
2. The Patient/Client will reduce laryngeal/neck/shoulder/articulatory tension by engaging core strength and reallocating stabilization strategy/effort to lower body.	Attempted a number of strategies to engage core strength for torso stability and to reduce laryngeal tension. This included sitting in chair and pulling up on the chair seat while also pushing her heels gently into the floor, sitting on fitness ball and bouncing during phonation tasks, and sitting in the chair while gently pushing back with heels to engage lower body for torso stability. The latter two were most facilitating today. Using these strategies, she was able to release muscle tension in the neck and achieve appropriate alignment of torso, neck, and head.
3. The Patient/Client will reduce laryngeal/neck/shoulder/articulatory tension by maintaining position of torso over pelvic floor.	Moderate cues to avoid leaning forward from the waist. Best alignment achieved by sitting on fitness ball.

Table 20–6. ***Domain: Vocal Coordination and Conditioning—Examples of Long- and Short-Term Singing Voice Rehabilitation Goals for Tension Reduction and Language for Reporting Progress***

Long-term goal: Patient/Client will eliminate maladaptive compensatory muscle tension to optimize coordination of respiratory/phonatory motor system and promote resolution of underlying injury.	
Short-term goals (criterion is 90% accuracy unless otherwise stated):	Sample progress reporting:
1. The Patient/Client will reduce maladaptive muscle tension by completing high-intensity/complex vocal tasks in short and extended passages demonstrating minimal base of tongue/jaw tension.	A number of strategies were attempted for reduction of base of tongue tension. These included (a) phonation while holding drinking straw horizontally under the tongue, (b) /ajal/ repetitions emphasizing excursion of base of tongue movement with jaw stabilized, (c) /m/ with tongue protruded, (d) phonating while holding protruded tongue tip with gauze, and (e) anchoring tongue tip behind bottom front teeth and protruding tongue dorsum over the bottom teeth during phonation. BOT tension was so severe that the only effective strategy was (d). Using this strategy, he was able to increase range by four semi-tones today, with audible improvement in resonance and projection.
2. The Patient/Client will decrease laryngeal and articulatory muscle tension by independently completing relaxation/stretching exercises.	Sequence of exercises was demonstrated. He executed exercises accurately following demonstration.

Table 20–7. Domain: Vocal Coordination and Conditioning—Examples of Long- and Short-Term Singing Voice Rehabilitation Goals for Vocal Exercise Regimen and Language for Reporting Progress

Long-term goal: Patient/Client will complete high-intensity/complex vocal tasks in short and extended passages demonstrating resonant voice quality, minimal maladaptive muscle tension, and adequate breath support.	
Short-term goals (criterion is 90% accuracy unless otherwise stated):	Sample progress reporting:
1. The Patient/Client will independently complete practice routine of ≥7 exercises without evidence of vocal fatigue and with adequate oral resonance and breath support to decrease phonotrauma, improve coordination of respiratory/phonatory motor system, and rehabilitate voice to premorbid quality, stamina, and pitch and loudness range. OR: 2. The Patient/Client will complete vocal fold stretching and contracting exercises spanning a range of ≥2 octaves without voice breaks or evidence of maladaptive muscle tension to improve vocal fold flexibility and coordination and proprioception of respiratory/laryngeal motor system and vocal tract.	In today's session: (1) Adductory power on small-straw phonation from 110 to 220 Hz, added crescendo-decrescendo today with good dynamic range; (2) 1-5-1 glide on lip trill from 98 to 349 Hz, strain noted on last two frequencies; (3) "swelling test" on 5-3-1 /hu/ staccato with ceiling at ~587 Hz, delayed onset of phonation noted ~494 Hz and above, but ceiling is increased by three semi-tones from last session, consistent with reduced vocal fold swelling; (4) 54321 scale on /i/ from 110 to 220 Hz, switched to /a/ and continued to 494 Hz, moderate cues to increase opening of oral cavity and maintain forward tongue position; (5) 13531 arpeggio on /jaɪ/ from 98 to 440 Hz with moderate cues to maximize excursion of base of tongue movement while stabilizing jaw position. Regular home practice is evident in progress today. Range has increased to >2 octaves, excluding falsetto.
3. The Patient/Client will execute high-intensity vocal tasks in short and extended passages between 220 Hz and 440 Hz without audible voice breaks.	Improved balance of thyroarytenoid (TA) and cricothyroid (CT) activation noted in this range today. Specifically, increased TA resulted in improved projection and decreased pitch breaks (twice in nine trials, decreased from 4/9 last session). Tendency to use excessive CT in this range is decreasing.
4. The Patient/Client will demonstrate awareness of healthy voice production through education, negative practice, and discrimination of voice samples of self and others.	Used playback from sections of today's session for self-assessment. Although she expressed concern that tone was "shrill" prior to listening to recording, afterward she agreed with clinician that tone is characterized by adequate oral resonance and improved breath support.

Note. *Example 1 emphasizes duration of routine, while Example 2 emphasizes using exercises to reach pitch range goal.*

Table 20–8. ***Domain: Vocal Coordination and Conditioning—Examples of Long- and Short-Term Singing Voice Rehabilitation Goals for Vocal Registers and Language for Reporting Progress***

Long-term goal: The Patient/Client will achieve appropriate balance of activation of intrinsic laryngeal musculature and vocal ligament to improve vocal stability and projection and to optimize coordination of respiratory/phonatory motor system.	
Short-term goals (criterion is 90% accuracy unless otherwise stated):	Sample progress reporting:
1. The Patient/Client will demonstrate understanding of mechanical/physiologic/acoustical differences between TA-dominant (moderately to fully contracted) and CT-dominant (moderately to fully contracted) registration.	Discussed mechanical/physiologic/acoustical differences between TA-dominant registration and CT-dominant registration and reference sensations for each. Visual illustrations provided via pictures and anatomical model. She demonstrated understanding through asking insightful clarifying questions and correctly answering clinician's questions.
2. The Patient/Client will achieve balance of activation of intrinsic laryngeal musculature through appropriate allocation of TA/CT activation.	She has a tendency to use inadequate TA activation in range C4–G4, resulting in poor projection, limited dynamic range, slightly breathy vocal quality. Explored sensations associated with TA-dominant register in range from G3–B3. She described feeling sensation of vibration in anterior throat and in the front part of the mouth. By using this reference sensation, she was able to increase TA activation, resulting in greater vocal fold adduction through F4 today, demonstrating improved projection, dynamic range, and decreased laryngeal strain.
3. The Patient/Client will complete high-intensity/complex vocal tasks in short and extended passages between A4 and A5 demonstrating predominantly CT muscle activation given minimal cues as measured by perceptual evaluation.	TA-dominant registration persists to D5, resulting in extreme laryngeal strain, poor dynamic range (loud only), and abrupt pitch ceiling. She was not able to phonate above D5. Worked on eliciting CT-dominant register via 5–1 glide on lip trill, progressing to /hu/. Ultimately achieved CT-dominant registration from A4–E5, although tone was quite breathy. This likely reflects underlying traumatic injury impairing closure in this pitch range. Will continue to work on strengthening CT-dominant registration with SOVT sounds, using positive oral pressure to decrease subglottal pressure and to promote improved closure and lowest phonation threshold pressure to support resolution of underlying injury.

CHAPTER 21

An Ounce of Prevention: The Singing Voice Rehabilitation Specialist as Vocal Health Educator

One of the most interesting and fulfilling aspects of a career in singing voice rehabilitation is that its hybrid nature affords opportunities to be involved in many different facets of the world of singing. The multiplicity of skills the profession requires of you—voice pedagogy, vocal performance, voice science, and clinical knowledge—provides a diverse and stimulating realm of vocational existence. If you've prepared thoroughly for the job, you will likely be engaged in your own performance activities and in *habilitation* —teaching students who do not have injuries—in addition to the work you do in the sphere of rehabilitation. I encourage you to take as many of those opportunities as you can. As we have explored at length in this text, the domains are intertwined and overlapping. Your activities in each area will inform the others, deepening your understanding, enriching your skills, and enlarging your empathy. Furthermore, continuing to be active as a performer and voice pedagogue can enhance your credibility as a singing voice rehabilitation specialist, help generate a broad pool of referral sources, and increase your visibility in the community.

Which brings us to the final bit of advice I would like to give you as we approach the end of our shared exploration: I invite you to consider how you can use your training, skills, and knowledge—in which you have invested so much of your time, talent, and financial resources —for the good of the community in which you live, and beyond. We have devoted the entirety of our time together to the topic of helping singers recover. It seems highly appropriate to spend at least a little time and a few pages contemplating how we can help singers (and everyone else, for that matter) avoid the need for voice rehabilitation.

At least once a week a patient in our clinic will make a comment to me along these lines: "I had no idea there could be any help for my problem," or "I thought I just had to live with this." Comments like these are what first inspired me to reach out to my community to let people know that there is help, there is hope, and that they can get better. And along the way,

I realized the power of vocal health education as a preventative tool. I think you will find this to be true in your practice, too. Why not share your ample resources for the cause of prevention?

WORLD VOICE DAY

A great way to get started on this venture is to create your own World Voice Day Celebration. World Voice Day began toward the end of the 20th century as Brazilian Voice Day. From there, it spread to the rest of the world and is now celebrated on April 16 each year. The website world-voice-day.org has a wealth of information, materials, ideas, and resources to get you started. Your celebration could be as simple as a small gathering at your practice or studio during which you provide information on vocal health, or you could join forces with other professionals to put on an event that might include vocal health presentations, medical information, voice screenings, vocal performances, teaching demonstrations, panel discussions, and/or celebrity speakers. Consider collaborating with voice colleagues in otolaryngology, speech-language pathology, academic music programs, private voice studios, public schools, places of worship, community choirs, opera and theater companies, recording studios, and radio and television stations—the possibilities are myriad and limited only by your imagination. Because it is recognized internationally, World Voice Day is a great vehicle for reaching out to your local media to get them involved in spreading the message of vocal health. This effort can be especially fruitful if you point out the importance of vocal health for broadcasters, and if you can illustrate the human interest impact of voice with a patient/client testimonial.

OTHER IDEAS FOR COMMUNITY ENGAGEMENT EVENTS AND ACTIVITIES

Your grassroots efforts in vocal health education aren't limited to World Voice Day. You can easily develop a vocal health presentation 30 to 60 minutes in length that is thorough, interesting, and engaging. Once you've put it together, it's simple to customize for specific audiences and take your show on the road. Here are a few suggestions for organizations to target:

- College and university music and theater programs: Target choirs, voice students, theater students, and faculty.
- Churches and synagogues: The choirs in most places of worship rehearse at a regular time, which makes it relatively easy to assemble forces. If you have a group that is interested, encourage them to collaborate with choirs from other churches or make the presentation open to the wider community to increase your audience and make your time investment more productive.
- Music educators: Many school districts already have a mechanism and resources for continuing education or teacher in-service training. Your presentation or workshop could be the perfect fit.

- There are state and regional chapters of national voice organizations such as National Association of Teachers of Singing (NATS), Voice and Speech Trainers Association (VASTA), and the National Association for Music Education (NAfME). Contact your state chapter and propose a session on vocal health.
- Find out what other voice-related organizations will be holding conferences or conventions in your area and submit a proposal for a vocal health presentation. In addition to those already mentioned, consider the American Choral Directors Association, Opera America, Kindermusik, Music Teachers National Association, and the Contemporary A Capella Society of America, to name just a few. Think outside the box as you cast your net wide to include organizations like the American Music Therapy Association or Barbershop Harmony Society.
- Science and art museums, libraries, and health organizations often have educational series that are open to the community. They usually have regular audiences and good advertising of events. The science of singing and vocal health would be interesting and relevant topics for a lecture series in any of these settings.

And don't forget:

- Music festivals
- Community choirs
- Community theater programs

Before you know it, these organizations will be reaching out to *you* to request your educational services and expertise.

BUILDING PERFORMING VOICE PARTNERSHIPS

You can promote vocal health by engaging with relevant institutions in your area. Reach out to local performing arts organizations (symphony orchestras, professional theater companies, opera companies, chamber music organizations, etc.) and performance venues to let them know about your professional services. Offer to provide vocal health information/brochures as a benefit for their visiting vocal artists. Depending on the setting in which you work, you might discuss expediting access to clinical services for performers with vocal emergencies. In addition, these organizations often host pre-performance lectures on a variety of topics and may be interested in singing science as a potential tie-in to a particular performance, or may wish to collaborate with you on community vocal health presentations or workshops. A bonus of staying active as a performer and teacher is that the contacts you will make and maintain can facilitate development of performing voice partnerships.

FOSTERING A VOCAL HEALTH EDUCATION PROGRAM

Your vocal health education efforts don't have to be limited to singing voice. Depending on your training and expertise, consider outreach to other voice populations. Occupational voice professionals, such as teachers, clergy, attorneys, call center operators, and customer service professionals, will also benefit from preventative vocal health education. If your background hasn't prepared you to work with these populations, recruit medical and speech-language pathology colleagues for collaboration.

Here are a few more ideas for developing your program:

- Depending on your resources, consider augmenting your grassroots community education events with vocal training programs. This could include singing classes or workshops that you teach or that feature local or national master teachers.
- Consider the role that you can provide in educating medical professionals on the special needs of singers. This could be part of medical grand rounds or continuing education for physicians, speech-language pathologists, and other allied health providers.
- Develop and maintain materials and resources for your vocal health education program such as printed brochures or handouts, vocal health resources on your website, or a vocal health blog. Your educational materials could include tips for vocal hygiene, vocal pacing, and voice training. Use social media to help spread the word about vocal health and to announce your upcoming events.

VOCAL HEALTH EDUCATION AS A MARKETING TOOL

Although vocal health education is a service that truly illustrates the concept of "paying it forward," keep in mind that your vocal health endeavors will yield a business benefit, too. Every time you engage with your community, you make the people around you aware that you are a valuable resource and that you care. In all likelihood, they will remember your expertise and generosity if they have a voice problem or know someone who does. It can be advantageous to document the number of referrals you get that can be attributed to your community engagement and vocal health education efforts. These data could help garner financial or time resources to continue to expand your vocal health program.

VOCAL HEALTH EDUCATION AS COMMUNITY SERVICE

This might seem like a lot of time and effort to expend, especially if you already have a busy caseload and are engaged in teaching and performance activities as well. Keep in mind that the ideas provided here are merely suggestions to spark your creativity—you can do as much or as little as your particular situation and interest will allow. Think of your vocal health education endeavors as the service aspect of your professional work. I think you will find it a worthwhile expense.

Index

Note: Page numbers in **bold** reference non-text material.

F

N

S

T

U

V

W

X

Y